Interventional Musculoskeletal Radiology

Guest Editors

Peter L. Munk, MD, CM, FRCPC

Wilfred C.G. Peh, MBBS, MHSM, MD, FRCPE, FRCPG, FRCR

RADIOLOGIC CLINICS OF NORTH AMERICA

www.radiologic.theclinics.com

May 2008 • Volume 46 • Number 3

SAUNDERS an imprint of ELSEVIER, Inc.

W.B. SAUNDERS COMPANY
A Division of Elsevier Inc.

1600 John F. Kennedy Boulevard • Suite 1800 • Philadelphia, Pennsylvania 19103-2899

http://www.theclinics.com

RADIOLOGIC CLINICS OF NORTH AMERICA Volume 46, Number 3
May 2008 ISSN 0033-8389, ISBN 13: 978-1-4160-6073-4, ISBN 10: 1-4160-6073-1

Editor: Barton Dudlick

Radiologic Clinics of North America (ISSN 0033-8389) is published bimonthly in January, March, May, July, September, and November by Elsevier Inc., 360 Park Avenue South, New York, NY 10010-1710. Business and Editorial Offices: 1600 John F. Kennedy Boulevard., Suite 1800, Philadelphia, PA 19103-2899. Customer Service Office: 6277 Sea Harbor Drive, Orlando, FL 32887-4800. Periodicals postage paid at New York, NY and additional mailing offices. Subscription prices are USD 290 per year for US individuals, USD 431 per year for US institutions, USD 142 per year for US students and residents, USD 339 per year for Canadian individuals, USD 530 per year for Canadian institutions, USD 394 per year for international individuals, USD 530 per year for international institutions, and USD 192 per year for Canadian and foreign students/residents. To receive student and resident rate, orders must be accompanied by name of affiliated institution, date of term and the signature of program/residency coordinatior on institution letterhead. Orders will be billed at individual rate until proof of status is received. Foreign air speed delivery is included in all *Clinics* subscription prices. All prices are subject to change without notice. **POSTMASTER:** Send address changes to *Radiologic Clinics of North America*, Elsevier Journals Customer Service, 6277 Sea Harbor Drive, Orlando, FL 32887-4800. **Customer Service: 1-800-654-2452 (US). From outside of the United States, call (+1) 407-563-6020. Fax: 407-363-9661. E-mail: JournalsCustomerService-usa@elsevier.com.**

Reprints. For copies of 100 or more of articles in this publication, please contact the Commercial Reprints Department, Elsevier Inc., 360 Park Avenue South, New York, New York 10010-1710. Tel.: (+1) 212-633-3812; Fax: (+1) 212-462-1935; E-mail: reprints@elsevier.com.

Radiologic Clinics of North America also published in Greek Paschalidis Medical Publications, Athens, Greece.

Radiologic Clinics of North America is covered in *MEDLINE/PubMed (Index Medicus), EMBASE/Excerpta Medica, Current Contents/Life Sciences, Current Contents/Clinical Medicine, RSNA Index to Imaging Literature, BIOSIS, Science Citation Index,* and *ISI/BIOMED.*

Printed in the United States of America.

Contributors

GUEST EDITORS

PETER L. MUNK, MD, CM, FRCPC
Professor of Radiology and Orthopedic Surgery; and Director, Musculoskeletal Radiology, Department of Radiology, Vancouver General Hospital, University of British Columbia, Vancouver, British Columbia, Canada

WILFRED C.G. PEH, MBBS, MHSM, MD, FRCPE, FRCPG, FRCR
Senior Consultant, Department of Diagnostic Radiology, Alexandra Hospital; and Clinical Professor, National University of Singapore, Republic of Singapore

AUTHORS

LOUIS A. GILULA, MD, FACR
Professor of Radiology, Orthopaedic Surgery, and Plastic and Reconstructive Surgery, Mallinckrodt Institute of Radiology, Washington University Medical Center, St. Louis, Missouri

APOORVA GOGNA, MBBS
Medical Officer, Department of Diagnostic Radiology, Changi General Hospital, Republic of Singapore

MANRAJ K.S. HERAN, MD, FRCPC
Clinical Assistant Professor of Radiology, Division of Neuroradiology, Vancouver General Hospital, University of British Columbia; and Clinical Assistant Professor of Radiology, Department of Radiology, British Columbia's Children's Hospital, University of British Columbia, Vancouver, British Columbia, Canada

GERALD M. LEGIEHN, MD, FRCPC
Clinical Assistant Professor of Radiology, Division of Interventional Radiology, Department of Radiology, Vancouver General Hospital, University of British Columbia, Vancouver, British Columbia, Canada

LUCK J. LOUIS, MD, FRCPC
Clinical Assistant Professor of Radiology, Sections of Musculoskeletal and Emergency Trauma Radiology, Department of Radiology, Vancouver General Hospital, University of British Columbia, Vancouver, British Columbia, Canada

JOHN E. MADEWELL, MD, BS
Professor and Chief, Musculoskeletal Section, Diagnostic Imaging, University of Texas MD Anderson Cancer Center, Houston, Texas

DAVID MALFAIR, MD, FRCPC
Assistant Clinical Professor, Department of Radiology, Vancouver General Hospital, University of British Columbia, Vancouver, British Columbia, Canada

PETER L. MUNK, MD, CM, FRCPC
Professor of Radiology and Orthopedic Surgery; and Director, Musculoskeletal Radiology, Department of Radiology, Vancouver General Hospital, University of British Columbia, Vancouver, British Columbia, Canada

PAUL J. O'SULLIVAN, FFRRCSI, MRCPI
Assistant Professor, Diagnostic Imaging, University of Texas MD Anderson Cancer Center, Houston, Texas

RICHARD J.T. OWEN, MB BCh, MRCP, FRCR
Assistant Professor, Radiology and Diagnostic Imaging, University of Alberta, Edmonton, Alberta, Canada

WILFRED C.G. PEH, MBBS, MHSM, MD, FRCPE, FRCPG, FRCR
Senior Consultant, Department of Diagnostic Radiology, Alexandra Hospital; and Clinical Professor, National University of Singapore, Republic of Singapore

FAISAL RASHID, MBBS, FRANZCR
Fellow, Department of Radiology, Musculoskeletal Division, Vancouver General Hospital, Vancouver, British Columbia, Canada

ERIC M. ROHREN, MD, PhD
Section Chief, Positron Emission Tomography; and Associate Professor, University of Texas MD Anderson Cancer Center, Houston, Texas

ANDREW D. SMITH, MBChB, FRANZCR
Diagnostic Neuroradiology Fellow, Division of Neuroradiology, Vancouver General Hospital, University of British Columbia, Vancouver, British Columbia, Canada

WILLIAM C. TORREGGIANI, MBBCh, MRCPI, FRCR, FFRRCSI
Department of Radiology, Adelaide and Meath Hospitals (incorporating the National Children's Hospital), Tallaght, Dublin, Ireland

EMILY WARD, MBBChBAO, MRCPI
Department of Radiology, Adelaide and Meath Hospitals (incorporating the National Children's Hospital), Tallaght, Dublin, Ireland

Contents

> Joint injections remain a valuable modality in the detection and treatment of intra-articular pathology. Over the past several decades, various diagnostic and therapeutic indications for joint injections have been developed. Imaging guidance for joint injection generally increases accuracy in joint aspirations and diagnostic blocks. Confirming intra-articular placement with steroid injections improves efficacy and reduces local complications. Administering intra-articular contrast can improve the diagnostic performance of CT and MR imaging in many circumstances. This article focuses on the rationale for injections at different sites and describes different fluoroscopic approaches for common joints.

> Image guidance allows safe passage of needles, often into small and otherwise inaccessible lesions, and into the portions of the lesion most likely to yield useful samples, while avoiding damage to important structures. This article hopes to provide a useful guide to image-guided musculoskeletal biopsy for radiologists in practice and in training.

> Positron emission tomography (PET)–computed tomography (CT) is a useful device in identifying musculoskeletal lesions that require biopsy. It can be used to localize the primary lesion, identify a site to biopsy, and evaluate metastatic lesions that require follow-up biopsies. Not all malignant tumors have hypermetabolic activity, and there are many benign lesions and physiologic processes that do have increased F-18 fluorodeoxyglucose uptake. Knowledge of these issues is important when reviewing PET-CT and directing subsequent musculoskeletal biopsies.

> The field of spinal injection procedures is growing at a tremendous rate. Many disciplines are involved, including radiology, anesthesiology, orthopedics, physiatry and rehabilitation medicine, as well as other specialties. However, there remains tremendous variability in the assessment of patients receiving these therapies, methods for evaluation of outcome, and in the understanding of where these

procedures belong in the triaging of those who require surgery. In this article, we attempt to highlight the biologic concepts on which these therapies are based, controversies that have arisen with their increasing use, and a description of complications that have been reported.

Ultrasound scan is an invaluable tool in the diagnosis and treatment of disorders of the musculoskeletal system. Core concepts that are common to most ultrasound-guided procedures are reviewed, including an in-depth discussion regarding the use of injectable corticosteroids. Various aspects of intra-articular, intratendinous, bursal, and ganglion cyst intervention are discussed and promising advances in the treatment of chronic tendon disorders are presented.

Transarterial embolization should be considered in the treatment algorithm of primary or secondary bone tumors. Specific benefit is present where there is a high risk of bleeding at surgery, where there is spinal involvement and neural encroachment, where active bleeding is present, or in awkward surgical locations where prolonged surgery is anticipated.

Venous malformations are categorized as low-flow vascular malformations within the domain of vascular anomalies and are the most common vascular malformation encountered clinically. Venous malformations are by definition present at birth, undergo pari passu growth, and present clinically because of symptoms related to mass effect or stasis. Although diagnosis can usually be made by clinical history and examination, differentiation from other vascular and nonvascular entities often requires an imaging work-up that includes ultrasound, CT, MR imaging, and diagnostic phlebography. All decisions regarding imaging work-up and decision to treat must be coordinated though referral and discussions with a multidisciplinary team and be based on clearly defined clinical indications. Percutaneous image-guided sclerotherapy has become the mainstay of treatment for venous malformations and involves the introduction of any one of a number of endothelial-cidal sclerosants into the vascular spaces of the lesion, with each sclerosant possessing its own unique spectrum of advantages and disadvantages.

Radiofrequency Ablation is the use of low-voltage high-frequency electrical energy to heat and destroy abnormal tissues within the human body. It has gained increasing acceptance as both a primary and secondary form of treatment in the musculoskeletal system because of its excellent safety profile, ease of use, and technical success. In the musculoskeletal system, radiofrequency ablation may be used to treat a wide range of lesions that include primary lesions such as osteoid osteomas and a variety of metastases both within the osseous skeleton as well as those lying within the muscles and soft tissues. In this chapter, a background to the principles, physics, and indications of radiofrequency is presented as well as an in-depth description of radiofrequency ablation techniques that may be utilized in the musculoskeletal system.

Wilfred C.G. Peh, Peter L. Munk, Faisal Rashid, and Louis A. Gilula

Percutaneous vertebroplasty is a safe, inexpensive, and effective interventional vertebral augmentation technique that provides pain relief and stabilization in carefully selected patients with severe back pain due to vertebral compression. Complications from percutaneous vertebroplasty can be devastating, but are rare and avoidable with application of a meticulous technique. Percutaneous vertebroplasty has a role in the management pathway of patients presenting with painful vertebral compression fractures. Kyphoplasty uses a balloon tamp with the aim of restoring vertebral body height, improving kyphotic deformity, and creating a cavity into which bone cement is injected. Kyphoplasty is as effective and safe as vertebroplasty in treatment of painful vertebral compression fractures. Skyphoplasty, a modification of kyphoplasty, is a promising new technique.

Radiologic Clinics of North America

THE CLINICS ARE NOW AVAILABLE ONLINE!

Access your subscription at:
www.theclinics.com

GOAL STATEMENT

The goal of the *Radiologic Clinics of North America* is to keep practicing radiologists and radiology residents up to date with current clinical practice in radiology by providing timely articles reviewing the state of the art in patient care.

ACCREDITATION

The *Radiologic Clinics of North America* is planned and implemented in accordance with the Essential Areas and Policies of the Accreditation Council for Continuing Medical Education (ACCME) through the joint sponsorship of the University of Virginia School of Medicine and Elsevier. The University of Virginia School of Medicine is accredited by the ACCME to provide continuing medical education for physicians.

The University of Virginia School of Medicine designates this educational activity for a maximum of 15 *AMA PRA Category 1 Credits*™. Physicians should only claim credit commensurate with the extent of their participation in the activity.

The American Medical Association has determined that physicians not licensed in the US who participate in this CME activity are eligible for 15 *AMA PRA Category 1 Credits*™.

Credit can be earned by reading the text material, taking the CME examination online at http://www.theclinics.com/home/cme, and completing the evaluation. After taking the test, you will be required to review any and all incorrect answers. Following completion of the test and evaluation, your credit will be awarded and you may print your certificate.

FACULTY DISCLOSURE/CONFLICT OF INTEREST

The University of Virginia School of Medicine, as an ACCME accredited provider, endorses and strives to comply with the Accreditation Council for Continuing Medical Education (ACCME) Standards of Commercial Support, Commonwealth of Virginia statutes, University of Virginia policies and procedures, and associated federal and private regulations and guidelines on the need for disclosure and monitoring of proprietary and financial interests that may affect the scientific integrity and balance of content delivered in continuing medical education activities under our auspices.

The University of Virginia School of Medicine requires that all CME activities accredited through this institution be developed independently and be scientifically rigorous, balanced and objective in the presentation/discussion of its content, theories and practices.

All authors/editors participating in an accredited CME activity are expected to disclose to the readers relevant financial relationships with commercial entities occurring within the past 12 months (such as grants or research support, employee, consultant, stock holder, member of speakers bureau, etc.). The University of Virginia School of Medicine will employ appropriate mechanisms to resolve potential conflicts of interest to maintain the standards of fair and balanced education to the reader. Questions about specific strategies can be directed to the Office of Continuing Medical Education, University of Virginia School of Medicine, Charlottesville, Virginia.

The authors/editors listed below have identified no financial or professional relationships for themselves or their spouse/partner:
Barton Dudlick (Acquisitions Editor); Louis A. Gilula, MD, FACR; Apoorva Gogna, MBBS; Manraj Kanwal Singh Heran, MD, FRCPC; Theodore E. Keats, MD (Test Author); Gerald M. Legiehn, MD; FRCPC; Luck J. Louis, BSc, MD, FRCPC; John E. Madewell, MD, BS; David M. Malfair, MD, FRCPC; Paul J. O'Sullivan, FFRRCSI, MRCPI; Richard J.T. Owen, MBBCh, MRCP, FRCR; Wilfred C.G. Peh, MBBS, MHSM, MD, FRCPE, FRCPG, FRCR (Guest Editor); Faisal Rashid, MBBS, FRANZCR; Eric T. Rohren, MD, PhD; Andrew D. Smith, MBChB, FRANZCR; William C. Torreggiani, MBBCh, MRCPI, FRCR, FFRRCSI; and Emily Ward, MBBChBAO, MRCPI.

The authors/editors listed below have identified the following financial or professional relationships for themselves or their spouse/partner:
Peter L. Munk, MD, FRCPC (Guest Editor) serves on the Speaker's bureau for Cook Canada, Inc. and Boston Scientific.

Disclosure of Discussion of Non-FDA Approved Uses for Pharmaceutical and/or Medical Devices
The University of Virginia School of Medicine, as an ACCME provider, requires that all authors identify and disclose any "off label" uses for pharmaceutical and medical device products. The University of Virginia School of Medicine recommends that each physician fully review all the available data on new products or procedures prior to clinical use.

TO ENROLL

To enroll in the Radiologic Clinics of North America Continuing Medical Education program, call customer service at 1-800-654-2452 or sign up online at http://www.theclinics.com/home/cme. The CME program is available to subscribers for an additional annual fee USD 205.

Preface

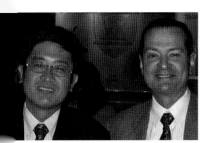

Wilfred C.G. Peh, MBBS, MHSM, MD,
FRCPE, FRCPG, FRCR
Peter L. Munk, MD, CM, FRCPC
Guest Editors

If an issue of the *Radiologic Clinics of North America* had been published on the subject of interventional musculoskeletal radiology 30 years ago, it would have looked quite different from the one you see before you today. Although in the past interventional radiologists and musculoskeletal radiologists used needles only for occasional joint injections or biopsies and little else, their use has now become an important component of both disciplines.

Although joint injections in the appendicular skeleton and the spine have been performed for many years, their role in the management of joint pain has expanded dramatically, particularly in an aging population. The number of possible interventions in the spine has grown, often resulting in marked variations in the types of procedures performed and indications for their use. These topics are explored in this issue of *Radiologic Clinics of North America*.

The article on vertebral augmentation reflects the explosive expansion of the use of these techniques in the management of compression fractures in the spine. With a greater awareness of the clinical sequela of osteoporosis in an ageing population in the Western world, the use of spinal augmentation has found an important role in improving quality of life in an increasingly large cohort of patients. As interventional musculoskeletal radiologists, we have found this to be an extraordinarily rewarding aspect of our practice, providing dramatic, rapid improvement in patients' symptoms. The strong positive feedback from patients is gratifying, especially to radiologists who do not always find themselves in the position of receiving this.

Although musculoskeletal imaging-guided biopsy has been performed for many years, many centers still rely on open biopsy. Our centers, like many others, have switched over almost exclusively to imaging-guided biopsy as a rapid, safe, effective, and inexpensive way of making a diagnosis in patients who have tumors. The use of positron emission tomography CT has helped refine the selection of patients and facilitated the planning of procedures.

Additional articles on musculoskeletal ultrasonography have also been included in this issue, because sonographic units are widely available throughout the world and allow many procedures to be performed even in centers that do not have very extensive and sophisticated facilities available to them. Two articles on vascular interventions have also been included. Embolization of tumors has been an important adjunct in the management of many musculoskeletal lesions for the past 40 years. More recently, a better appreciation of sclerotherapy and transarterial and transvenous embolization in the management of venous malformations has developed. These latter lesions are particularly difficult and challenging to manage by surgical techniques, and this procedure has revolutionized the treatment of this group of patients.

All of the authors are highly experienced in their areas of musculoskeletal intervention and are up-to-date practitioners whom we trust provide a useful and contemporary review of their subject. It has been rewarding to be involved in the development and popularization of these techniques, and musculoskeletal intervention has an

Radiol Clin N Am 46 (2008) xi–xii
doi:10.1016/j.rcl.2008.07.001

radiologic.theclinics.com

increasingly bright and important role to play in the future.

Peter L. Munk, MD, CM, FRCPC
Musculoskeletal Division
Department of Radiology
Vancouver General Hospital
University of British Columbia
899 West 12th Avenue
Vancouver, BC V5Z 1M9
Canada

Wilfred C.G. Peh, MBBS, MHSM, MD, FRCPE, FRCPG, FRCR
Department of Diagnostic Radiology
Alexandra Hospital
378 Alexandra Road
Singapore 159964
Republic of Singapore

E-mail addresses:
Peter.Munk@vch.ca (P.L. Munk)
Wilfred@pehfamily.per.sg (W.C.G. Peh)

Therapeutic and Diagnostic Joint Injections

David Malfair, MD, FRCPC

KEYWORDS

- Joints • Arthrography • Injection • Shoulder • Wrist
- Knee • Hip

Over the past several decades, various diagnostic and therapeutic indications for joint injections have been developed. Conventional arthrography often provides useful diagnostic information and may be coupled with CT or MR imaging to enhance the performance of these modalities. Relief after injection of local anesthetic strengthens diagnostic confidence that symptoms arise secondary to internal derangement. Intra-articular steroids have been shown to provide weeks of therapeutic relief in various circumstances. Imaging-guided needle placement may also be required for aspiration to rule out infection or crystal arthropathy. Ultrasound and fluoroscopy are commonly used in imaging-guided joint injection. This article focuses on the rationale for injections at different sites and describes different fluoroscopic approaches for common joints.

Temporary relief from intra-articular injection of local anesthetic confirms internal derangement as the source of pain. In many cases, symptomatic improvement after diagnostic block is associated with improved outcome after surgical intervention.[1,2] The presence of an anatomic lesion may be incidental to the clinical presentation. For example, labral tears of the hip are often found in asymptomatic patients. At the author's institution, bupivicaine, a medium-acting local anesthetic, is added as a diagnostic block to MR arthrograms. Relief of pain with activity in the hours following the examination increases clinical confidence that a visualized articular abnormality is the source of symptoms. Intra-articular lidocaine is less useful in this respect because its effects are attenuated by the time the MR imaging examination is completed. The medium-acting local anesthetic also ameliorates the delayed discomfort that patients report due to capsular distention, especially after shoulder and hip arthrograms. Recent literature suggest deleterious effects of the bupivicaine on cartilage.[3,4] Though this has not been found to occur in diagnostic or therapeutic injections, this evolving literature should be known.

Injected steroid is commonly used as a therapeutic strategy for treatment of articular disorders. These steroids are powerful anti-inflammatories that provide short- and medium-term relief and are used by most orthopedic surgeons and rheumatologists.[5–7] The most common local complication is a sterile synovitis causing discomfort within the first days of injection. It is hypothesized that this synovitis occurs secondary to the particulate nature of the injectate.[8] The effect of steroids on articular cartilage is debated. Several investigators have reported deleterious effects, including thinning and chondromalacia of the articular cartilage.[9,10] Other investigators presume that cartilage changes are subclinical because no changes in radiographic appearance or joint replacement rates were found after the use of steroids, compared with controls.[11,12] Local complications include tendon tears and soft tissue atrophy in the setting of extra-articular extravasation, including skin atrophy and depigmentation,[13] important possible complications in superficial injections of the hands and feet. Cases of avascular necrosis and Charcot arthropathies after intra-articular steroid administration have been

Department of Radiology, Vancouver General Hospital, University of British Columbia, 899 West 12th Avenue, Vancouver, BC V5Z 1M9, Canada

E-mail address: dmalfair@gmail.com

Radiol Clin N Am 46 (2008) 439–453

doi:10.1016/j.rcl.2008.02.007

reported.[14,15] Systemic complications may occur but are rare.

Conventional arthrography often offers diagnostic information but is more commonly combined with advanced modalities such as MR imaging or CT. Direct injection of gadolinium into joints improves diagnostic performance in several ways. Distension of the capsule assists in the delineation of small, complex, intra-articular structures. Extension of gadolinium into small defects in cartilage, tendons, and ligaments increases the conspicuity of these lesions. MR arthrography allows the use of primarily T1-weighted sequences, which boast a high signal-to-noise ratio. Finally, extravasation of gadolinium into the adjacent soft tissues, or abnormal communications between adjacent joints, provides critical diagnostic information.

GENERAL TECHNIQUE

Relevant imaging should be reviewed before the procedure to confirm the clinical diagnosis, recognize coexistent pathology, and assist planning. Informed consent includes a brief description of the procedure and discussion of the benefits and risks. The risks of arthrography can be divided into local or systemic complications. Local complications include infection, bleeding, and damage to intra-articular structures. Sterile synovitis was more common in the past when ionic contrast agents were used. Systemic complications include allergic and vasovagal reactions. Overall, the risks of arthrography are low. In a survey of 57 radiologists who had performed 126,000 arthrographic studies, no deaths, 3 cases of infection, and 56 cases of hives were reported.[16] In another series, of 25,000 arthrograms, one infection and 20 mild allergic reactions occurred.[17]

Imaging guidance is used to localize the injection site with the patient in an appropriate position. Proper positioning permits patient comfort and optimal anatomic access for performing the procedure. After the patient is prepped and draped, local anesthetic is infiltrated at the needle entry site. For larger joints such as the shoulder, hip, and knee, a 22-gauge spinal needle is most commonly used. If infection is suspected, an 18-gauge needle is better suited to the aspiration of tenacious secretions. Most peripheral joints are easily accessed with a 25-gauge 3.5-cm needle. Once in the appropriate position, an attempt at aspiration is performed, to rule out infection. Gross infection presents a risk for septicaemia if subsequent arthrography pressurizes the joint capsule.[18] An effusion should be aspirated as much as possible when found. The presence of an effusion decreases the concentration of gadolinium or steroid and may decrease the diagnostic performance o therapeutic outcome. The optimal gadolinium concentration for T1 contrast on a 1.5T scanne has been reported to be 2 mmol/liter.[19]

Measurement of pain relief is an important par of a diagnostic block with intra-articular loca anesthetic. The level of pain preceding the procedure is compared with the level immediately following the procedure. One method of rating discomfort is on a simple verbal scale of 0 to 10, with 10 being the worst pain ever experienced. Visual analog scores are effective and commonly used in the research setting.[20] If the pain only occurs during certain movements or exercises, the patient is encouraged to attempt these provocative maneuvers in the hours following the injection. Because steroids generally have more delayed effects, the patient is encouraged to keep a pain diary for the referring clinician, to improve the therapeutic response measurement over the following weeks.

SHOULDER
Rationale

Administration of intra-articular gadolinium for direct MR arthrography is the most common indication for glenohumeral joint injection in the radiology department. Direct MR arthrography boasts several advantages over routine MR imaging evaluation of the shoulder. Improved accuracy in diagnosing full-thickness and partial-thickness articular surface tears has been reported.[20–23] Extension of contrast into the subacromial bursa is nearly diagnostic of a full-thickness tear of the rotator cuff. The evaluation of labral pathology is a key advantage of MR arthrography, compared with conventional MR imaging.[24,25] Coexistent, unsuspected labral pathology is often present in young patients, leading some investigators to recommend arthrography in patients younger than 40 years of age.[26] In the postoperative patient, diagnostic difficulty in distinguishing a tear from postsurgical granulation tissue is a common problem in routine MR imaging. Gadolinium extending into the lesion distinguishes a tear from postsurgical changes.[27,28] The rotator interval and biceps pulley are also best assessed with MR arthrography.[29]

Adhesive capsulitis is effectively diagnosed on arthrography. It is generally difficult to inject more than 5 mL of contrast material, and joint recesses are usually absent in patients who have this condition. Symptomatic improvement of adhesive capsulitis has been reported with intra-articular steroids and distention arthrography. In a randomized control trial, steroids and physiotherapy resulted in the greatest clinical improvement, compared with placebo.[30] However, steroids alone also resulted in a statistically significant improvement, compared with physiotherapy alone. Weeks of symptomatic and functional improvement after distention arthrography compared with placebo has been reported in other randomized controlled trials.[31] A posterior approach is preferred to the anterior approach, which can be challenging because of fibrosis in the axillary pouch. After intra-articular placement of the needle is confirmed with contrast, a mixture of steroids and bupivicaine is injected. Twenty to 50 mL of sterile normal saline is infused after the medication until the pain threshold is reached or capsular rupture occurs. The patient should be aware that this procedure may be painful and that discomfort is common the following day.

The significance of acromioclavicular (AC) arthropathy has been debated. AC degenerative changes are frequently asymptomatic and are nearly universal in patients older than 50 years of age.[32–34] Despite this, many patients will have significant improvement of symptoms after a diagnostic block of this joint. Medium-term pain relief and improved function have been reported with the administration of intra-articular local anesthetic and steroid.[35,36] Imaging findings have been associated with the painful AC joint. Strobel and colleagues[36] described improved result of diagnostic block in patients who had capsular hypertrophy measuring more than 3 mm. Other investigators suggest that the presence of clavicular edema is an insensitive but specific sign for symptomatic degenerative changes.[37] Although these associations reach a statistical significance, no single imaging finding or group of imaging findings can accurately distinguish the symptomatic AC joint from the large prevalence of asymptomatic degenerative AC joint changes. For this reason, a diagnostic injection of lidocaine is usually performed to confirm that symptoms arise from the AC joint, before surgical treatment. Fluoroscopic-guided injection reduces the chance of inadvertent injection of the subacromial-subdeltoid bursa.

The accuracy of anterior blind injection of the shoulder is poor. Anterior glenohumeral injections have demonstrated an accuracy of 27% to 42%.[38,39] Accurate needle placement was associated with improved clinical outcome after injection with steroids. Improved accuracy has been described using a modified posterior approach without imaging guidance. In one study by Catalano and colleagues,[40] 125 of 147 (85%) patients were successfully injected on the first attempt. The posterior approach is also a common method

for sonographic injection of the glenohumeral joint.[41,42] In one study, only 16 of 24 blind AC joint injections were purely intra-articular.[35]

Technique

Numerous techniques have been described in the fluoroscopic injection of the shoulder. Those used most often are the anterior, posterior, and rotator interval approaches. The anterior (Schneider) technique is the most commonly used and involves an anterior approach with the patient supine and with the arm partially externally rotated.[43] External rotation makes more articular surface available for the anterior approach. However, extreme external rotation should be avoided because it increases tension on the anterior capsule and increases the risk for extra-articular extravasation of injected contents. In the anteroposterior (AP) supine view, the anterior glenoid rim lies medial to the humeral head. A wedge may be used to achieve close to a Grashey view of the glenohumeral articulation. In either patient position, it is critical that the needle be placed at least a few millimeters lateral to the medial cortex of the humerus, to avoid inadvertent contact with the labrum (**Fig. 1**). The anterior method does have some disadvantages. It traverses the expected needle path of the glenohumeral ligaments and subscapular tendon, and the anterior labrum, and may penetrate these

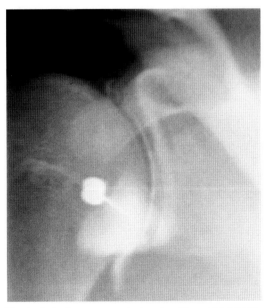

Fig. 1. Anterior approach to shoulder arthrogram. Patient is in supine position. Ideal needle position is a few millimeters lateral to the humeral cortex to avoid inadvertent contact with the glenoid labrum.

structures.[44] More often, inadvertent extravasation during injection makes diagnostic evaluation of these critical anterior structures more challenging.

A modified anterior approach is the rotator interval approach, performed with the patient supine.[45] A short (3.5-cm) needle is advanced to the medial upper quadrant of the humeral head (**Fig. 2**). It is important to avoid internal rotation of the arm, to avoid inadvertent puncture of the long head of the biceps. This technique is easily learned and avoids the glenohumeral ligaments and the labrum. However, it can also lead to diagnostic difficulties, especially with increasing interest in the imaging of the coracohumeral ligament and the rotator interval.

The posterior approach is performed with the patient prone, with the arm in external rotation. The palm should be facing down, and a bolster is placed under the symptomatic shoulder to obtain a Grashey view.[46] The needle is advanced to the medial aspect of the humeral head, approximately 5 mm lateral and 10 mm superior to the inferomedial cortex (**Fig. 3**). External rotation of the arm results in laxity of the posterior capsule, which enhances the ease of intra-articular placement. Most important, continuous downward pressure while the needle tip abuts the bone is gradually released during the test injection, which allows the injectate to find the potential space between the

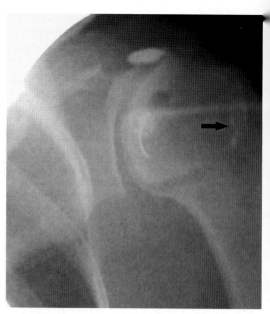

Fig. 3. Posterior approach to shoulder arthrogram. Patient is in prone position with arm in external rotation and bolster used to achieve Grashey view of glenohumeral joint. Needle target is the medial aspect of the humeral head, one centimeter above the inferior aspect of the joint. Intra-articular contrast commonly extends into the biceps sheath (*arrow*).

humerus and the posterior joint capsule. If injection is made without downward pressure on the needle initially, injection into the posterior rotator cuff is a frequent result. Although slightly more technically challenging, the posterior approach is preferred at the author's institution. The posterior shoulder anatomy is less variable and less commonly affected by pathology, and it has fewer stabilizing structures than the anterior aspect of the shoulder. A rotator interval or conventional anterior approach is performed if posterior labral pathology is clinically suspected.

The AC joint is injected under fluoroscopic guidance, with the patient in a supine position. A 25-gauge needle is placed from either an anterior or superior approach. A small amount of contrast can be injected to confirm position before injection of local anesthetic.

ELBOW
Rationale

Although MR imaging examination of the elbow is most often performed without contrast, MR arthrography may provide additional information in some circumstances. Arthrography is most often used to distend the joint and aid in the diagnosis of osteochondral bodies. Ossific bodies

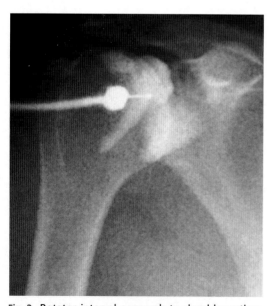

Fig. 2. Rotator interval approach to shoulder arthrogram. Patient is in supine position with arm externally rotated to move the biceps tendon out of the needle path. Needle target is the superomedial aspect of the humeral head.

near the joint may represent intra-articular bodies or periarticular ossification. MR or CT arthrography is also helpful in distinguishing them. Routine MR imaging demonstrates excellent accuracy for full-thickness, ligamentous tears but limited sensitivity for detecting partial tears. Partial tears of the anterior band of the ulnar collateral ligament at its insertion on the sublime tubercle of the coronoid process may be difficult to detect on routine MR imaging.[47] MR arthrography demonstrates high sensitivity and specificity in detecting partial tears and small avulsion fractures at this attachment.[48]

Technique

In elbow arthrography, the lateral approach is used most often. The patient is placed in a prone position, with the elbow placed above the head in 90° flexion. A lateral view of the elbow is obtained and the needle is placed within the radiocapitellar joint (**Fig. 4**). The primary disadvantage of this technique is the diagnostic dilemma that can occur with gadolinium extravasation around the radial collateral ligaments. A posteromedial approach avoids this drawback. The patient is positioned supine, with the elbow above the head, pronated and flexed to 30°. The medial epicondyle is palpated and the needle is placed between the medial epicondyle and the olecranon. The needle entry site is approximately 1 cm lateral to the

medial epicondyle to reduce the chance of inadvertent contact with the ulnar nerve. The needle pathway has an anterolateral orientation, with the target being the olecranon fossa (**Fig. 5**).

WRIST
Rationale

Wrist arthrography is performed most often to assess the triangular fibrocartilage complex (TFC) or the intrinsic ligaments. Knowledge of the anatomy of these structures is critical to accurate interpretation of wrist arthrography. The intrinsic interosseous ligaments, the scapholunate (SL) and lunotriquetral (LT) ligaments, consist of strong volar and dorsal components composed primarily of type I collagen. A central component is composed of fibrocartilage. The TFC includes volar and dorsal components composed of type 1 collagen. An additional central portion is avascular and composed of weaker, obliquely oriented sheets of collagen fibers. The radial aspect of the TFC attaches directly to the cartilage of the ulnar aspect of the radius. The peripheral attachments include the proximal foveal attachment and a distal attachment near the meniscal homolog and adjacent lunate and triquetrum.

The key challenge in detecting clinically significant intrinsic ligament and TFC lesions is the high prevalence of degenerative attritional tears of these structures, which are often symptomatic. These attritional tears of the intrinsic ligaments and TFC are

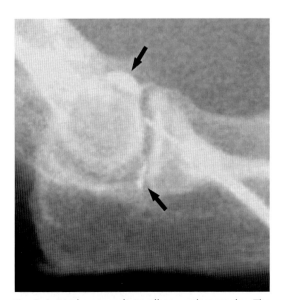

Fig. 4. Lateral approach to elbow arthrography. The patient is prone with the arm above head and elbow flexed at 90°. The lateral side of elbow faces upward. Needle enters the radiocapitellar joint and contrast (*arrows*) is placed to confirm intra-articular position.

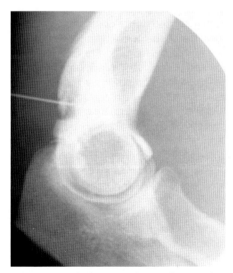

Fig. 5. Posteromedial approach to elbow arthrography. The patient is supine with arm above head and elbow flexed at 90°. Skin entry site is one centimeter lateral to the medial epicondyle to avoid contact with the ulnar nerve.

seldom present in teenagers but are found with a near 50% prevalence in older patients.[49] Differentiation of traumatic from attritional tears is best achieved with a careful history. A young patient who has recent trauma and a deficiency of an intrinsic ligament or TFC tear is more likely to suffer a symptomatic lesion. Imaging appearances may also help differentiate a traumatic from an attritional tear. Central perforations of the TFC tend to occur in asymptomatic patients, whereas radial or ulnar avulsions are usually traumatic.[50] Adjacent degenerative changes in the triscaphe or radioscaphoid joints suggest an attritional SL tear. Similarly, a chronic LT tear is often found in the setting of ulnar impaction and is associated with perforations of the TFC and lunate chondromalacia. Attritional tears most often involve the entire intrinsic ligament or only the central component. Isolated dorsal tears or joint space widening are more common with traumatic, symptomatic lesions.[51]

Wrist arthrography demonstrates moderate-to-strong sensitivity and excellent specificity in detecting TFC tears and tears of the intrinsic ligaments, when compared with arthroscopy as a gold standard.[52,53] Full-thickness tears of the SL ligament can be missed on triple-compartment arthrography, possibly because of a redundant torn ligament preventing the flow of contrast.[54] These types of false-negative arthrograms are uncommon when evaluating the LT ligament or TFC. The ability to distinguish attritional tears from symptomatic traumatic lesions relies on the visualization of the dorsal, central, and volar components of the intrinsic ligaments. Special conventional arthrographic maneuvers may evaluate these volar and dorsal components. This topic is beyond the scope of this article but an excellent discussion can be found in the review article by Linkous and Gilula.[55] MR imaging or CT following conventional arthrography may further delineate the components of the intrinsic ligaments and the TFC. In a study comparing conventional CT arthrography with arthroscopy, both correlated with high sensitivity and specificity for tears seen on arthroscopy.[56] However, CT arthrography was better able to ascertain the precise location of the tear, a quality that helps distinguish acute tears from attritional lesions. The superior sensitivity and improved interobserver reliability of CT arthrography, compared with conventional MR imaging, in the detection of dorsal tears of the SL ligament have been demonstrated.[56] A direct comparison of CT arthrography and MR arthrography has not been performed because it would likely require two different injections at different times to avoid diffusion of contrast into adjacent structures in the interval between studies.

Technique

Wrist arthrography is a complex procedure that should be tailored to answer the clinical question. The three main types of arthrography are midcarpal injections, radiocarpal injections, and distal radioulnar joint (DRUJ) injections. These are ideally performed with a C-arm, which can be rotated to profile the SL and LT joints in turn. A midcarpal injection is used at the author's institution to assess the integrity of the intrinsic ligaments. A midcarpal injection provides improved intrinsic ligaments compared with radiocarpal arthrography.[57] Contrast in the dorsal recess of the radioscaphoid joint may obscure visualization of these structures. TFC tears are diagnosed on radiocarpal injection. If this is unremarkable, an additional DRUJ arthrogram may detect partial tears and tears of the foveal attachment.[58]

The midcarpal injection is performed with a 1-inch 25-gauge needle with placement at the triquetrolunohamate space from a dorsal approach (**Fig. 6**). Normal midcarpal injection may extend to involve the carpometacarpal joints of the second through fifth digits. Extension between the SL and LT articulations is also noted. Communication with the radiocarpal joint is limited by the SL and LT ligaments along the proximal aspects of these joints. Extension into the radiocarpal joint suggests deficiency in one or both of these ligaments. After removal of the needle, the wrist is examined in radial and ulnar deviation with first, the SL, and then, the LT joint in profile. CT or MR imaging is performed after arthrography to characterize more fully the ligamentous defects and to

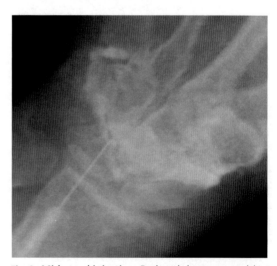

Fig. 6. Midcarpal injection. Patient is in prone position with arm above head, elbow flexed, and wrist pronated. Needle target is the joint space between the hamate, capitate, lunate, and triquetrum.

determine whether they involve the dorsal, volar, or central portions of the ligament.

The radiocarpal injection is performed most easily at the level of the radioscaphoid joint from a dorsal approach (**Fig. 7**). The dorsal lip of the radius overlaps the joint slightly, and a needle entry site a few millimeters distal to the joint is recommended to avoid this prominence. Care is also taken to avoid the region of the SL ligament. Communication with the DRUJ or midcarpal joint signals TFC and intrinsic ligament pathology, respectively. Injection of contrast is usually performed with cine fluoroscopy, which confirms the location of communication. In approximately 75% of cases, the radiocarpal joint communicates with the pisiform-triquetral joint.[59,60] In patients who do not have this communication, a diagnostic block may be required before surgery for treatment of pisiform-triquetral arthritis. In this setting, direct arthrography of this joint can be performed from an ulnar approach, with the hand pronated and in mild flexion.[60]

The key to successful DRUJ arthrography is needle placement. The needle should be placed adjacent to the ulnar, rather than at the center of the joint, a few millimeters proximal to the distal ulnar surface. Approximately 1 mL of contrast is injected (**Fig. 8**). The dorsal sensory branch of the ulnar nerve may be irritated by this approach[61] and the patient should be alerted to this possibility before the procedure.

HIP
Rationale

The hip is the most commonly injected joint under fluoroscopy at the author's institution. The spine, sacroiliac joints, and supporting soft tissues are common sources for hip pain and can present diagnostic uncertainty. A positive preoperative diagnostic block with local anesthetic is a reliable indicator of internal derangement and a good predictor of improvement after surgical intervention.[1,62,63] Intra-articular steroids may also provide weeks to months of relief in nonsurgical candidates or act as a temporizing measure before surgery.[5]

MR arthrography is commonly advocated for the evaluation of the hip. The key advantage of intra-articular gadolinium is the improved characterization of labral pathology. Czerny[64] reported a diagnostic accuracy of 91% using this modality, compared with conventional MR imaging, in the identification of labral tears. Improved visualization of chondral defects and loose bodies is also noted.[65] A diagnostic block with local anesthetic added to the MR arthrogram may suggest the presence of an intra-articular abnormality that is occult on imaging.[62]

Hip injection is also important in the postoperative hip. Aspiration identifies an infected prosthesis before revision, with sensitivity rates ranging from 83% to 98%.[66,67] Some investigators recommend aspiration before most hip revisions because unsuspected infection is not infrequently found.[66] Other investigators have found a 2% prevalence of unsuspected infection and a 13% incidence of false-positives on specimen cultures.[68] These investigators recommend aspiration only in selected patients. Bupivicaine injection into the pseudocapsule of the joint prosthesis also predicts a good outcome if the patient goes on to revision.[69]

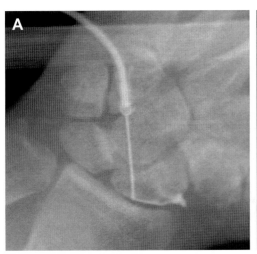 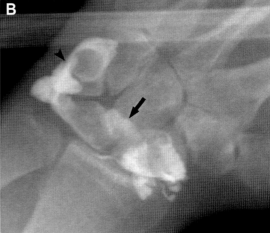

Fig. 7. Radiocarpal injection. (*A*) Skin entry site is a few millimeters distal to the joint space to avoid the dorsal rim of the radius. (*B*) Progressive injection of contrast fills the dorsal recess (*arrow*), which may obscure visualization of the intrinsic ligaments. Communication with the pisotriquetral joint (*arrowhead*) is commonly seen.

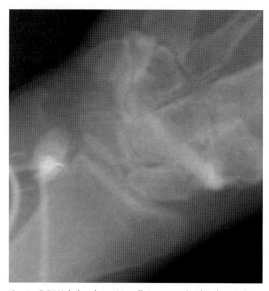

Fig. 8. DRUJ injection. Needle target is the lateral aspect of the ulnar cortex. Following contact, the needle is placed more radially, deeper into the joint. Note recent midcarpal injection.

If no frank infection is identified, conventional arthrography can demonstrate loosening, synovitis, and fistulae. Arthrographic studies of femoral cemented components are sensitive and specific tests in the evaluation of prosthetic loosening, especially when performed with digital subtraction arthrography.[70] Criteria to diagnose a loose femoral component include contrast extension past the intertrochanteric line in a standard component or halfway down the component of a long-stem prosthesis. Inconsistent literature is noted in regards to the acetabular component, with a specificity of only 58% in one study.[71] Maus and colleagues also found predicting acetabular loosening to be challenging. They recommended arthrographic criteria for acetabular loosening that included the presence of contrast extending underneath the middle third of the component, or the presence of 2-mm–thick contrast extending under the component.[70] A common cause of false-negatives in hip arthrography is the decompression of the hip capsule with extension into the greater trochanter or pseudobursae. In these cases, intra-articular pressure may be insufficient to force contrast underneath the loosened component. In the setting of recurrent infection, postarthrogram radiographs may demonstrate fistulae connecting to soft tissue abscesses.[72] These fistulae may become more conspicuous if the radiographs are obtained after the patient has ambulated for a brief period after the procedure.

Swan and colleagues[73] first identified the limitations of arthrography in detecting aseptic loosening in the noncemented prosthesis, and these limitations were corroborated in subsequent larger studies.[74,75] Arthrography has been shown to demonstrate only moderate accuracy in detecting loosening/infection of noncemented acetabular (68%) and femoral components (63%).[75] In one comparison study, plain radiography demonstrated better overall accuracy than conventional arthrography, nuclear arthrography, or scintigraphy in the detection of aseptic loosening in the noncemented prosthesis.[76] Diagnosis of aseptic loosening using conventional or nuclear arthrography is the absence of plain film findings should be made with care in the noncemented hip arthroplasty. Although the sensitivity will increase, the specificity of these modalities has been measured at 70%.[76]

Iliopsoas bursa injection may be requested in patients who have a clinical diagnosis of anterior snapping hip.[77] Opacification of the bursa with contrast shows the tendon in relief, and administering corticosteroids can help ameliorate symptoms at the same time. Ultrasound has become increasingly popular in the diagnosis and treatment of a snapping hip. Iliopsoas bursitis may be present in the absence of a snapping iliopsoas tendon. Aspiration may also be required to rule out septic bursitis. Relief with intra-articular local anesthetic within the iliopsoas bursa also confirms the clinical suspicion as a source for anterior hip pain.

Injection of the hip using only anatomic landmarks has been reported. Studies boast a high accuracy in blind placement, as confirmed by visualization of the needle over the femoral neck on postprocedure fluoroscopy.[78] When injection of arthrographic dye is used to confirm placement after surface anatomy technique, accuracy is found to be around 80%.[79]

Technique

Numerous injection techniques of the hip have been described in the literature. The most commonly used fluoroscopic technique is a straight AP approach that parallels the radiograph beam. Needle placement along the lateral aspect of the cortex at the femoral head–neck junction is often advocated because it avoids the potential damage to the femoral vessels and anesthesia to the femoral nerve (**Fig. 9**). Advocates of needle placement along the medial aspect of the femoral neck suggest that injection and aspiration are easier in this area because of the more redundant capsule in this portion of the joint. Needle placement in the middle of the femoral neck has been shown to present a three-times-greater risk for contrast extravasation, and it should be avoided.[80] A lateral

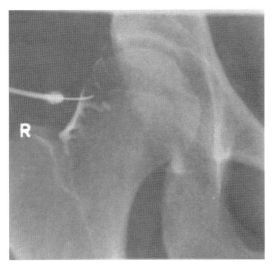

Fig. 9. Anterior approach to hip arthrogram. Patient is in supine position. Needle target is the lateral aspect of the femoral head–neck junction.

approach following standard arthroscopy portals can also be used.[81] This approach avoids the neurovascular structures but can be more challenging because the depth and position of the needle tip are more difficult to ascertain. Cranial angulation is used in obese patients to avoid pannus. AP positioning of the needle in this circumstance may inadvertently transgress the peritoneum in these patients (**Fig. 10**).

In patients who have already undergone hip arthroplasty, the AP technique can be modified. The skin entry site is placed just lateral to the neck of the prosthesis (**Fig. 11**), which allows

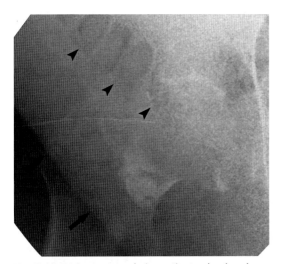

Fig. 10. Anterior approach in patient who has large body habitus. An oblique approach with long spinal needle is used to avoid pannus. A direct AP approach may transgress peritoneum and bowel (*arrowheads*).

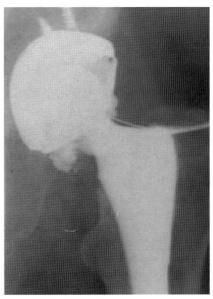

Fig. 11. Hip arthrography in patient who has hip arthroplasty. An anterior approach is performed with skin entry site slightly lateral to the prosthesis, allowing visualization of needle path.

visualization of the needle path as it is advanced to the lateral aspect of the prosthetic neck. Brandser and colleagues[82] describe a technique of spinning the bevel away from the neck to place the needle an extra 1 to 2 cm posterior to the lateral aspect of the femoral neck. The dry tap rate was only 2.4% using this method. Aspiration should be performed before the injection of additional material. If a strong concern exists regarding loosening or infection of a hip arthroplasty, dedicated postprocedure radiographs are performed after the patient has ambulated briefly, which allows the contrast to extend into areas of component loosening or soft tissue fistula (**Fig. 12**). Needle tip position at the midpoint of the intertrochanteric line will lead to the highest success rate when attempting to aspirate a hip with a Girdlestone arthroplasty (**Fig. 13**).[83]

Injection of the iliopsoas bursa is performed with the patient in a supine position. The ideal location for needle placement is along the anterior rim of the acetabulum, at a line drawn between the ipsilateral lesser trochanter and the inferior aspect of the ipsilateral sacroiliac joint (**Fig. 14**). The needle enters the iliopsoas bursa most easily while contrast is being injected because downward pressure of the needle on the bone is released.

KNEE
Rationale

Knee joint injections are often performed blindly with good success, especially in the presence of

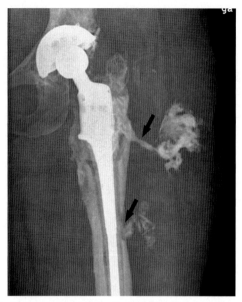

Fig. 12. Hip arthrography in patient who has recurrent infections of total hip arthroplasty. AP radiograph performed after hip arthrography followed by patient ambulation. Contrast extends into two fistula connecting to soft tissue abscesses (*arrows*).

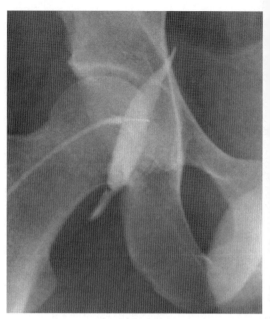

Fig. 14. Iliopsoas bursogram. Patient is in supine position. Needle target is the anterior rim of the acetabulum on a line drawn between the lesser trochanter and the inferior aspect of the sacroiliac joint.

a knee effusion. In patients who do not have an effusion, correct placement can be more difficult. Jackson and colleagues[84] found a 71% and 75% rate of accurate placement in those patients

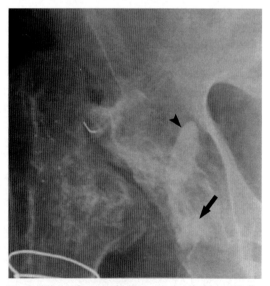

Fig. 13. Hip arthrography in patient who has Girdlestone arthroplasty. Patient is in supine position. Needle target is at a point bisecting the intertrochanteric line. Administration of contrast demonstrates contrast communication with the pseudocapsule at the level of the acetabulum (*arrow*) with extension into the iliopsoas bursa (*arrowhead*).

injected from the anterolateral and anteromedial approaches, respectively. A blind patellofemoral approach resulted in a higher accuracy (93%), a success rate that has been reproduced.[85] Patients who have inadvertent extra-articular injections have been shown to have decreased response, compared with those with proper placement. Although most procedures can be performed without imaging guidance, obese patients or patients who have patellofemoral arthritis may be sent for imaging-guided knee injection.

Knee joint injections may be diagnostic and therapeutic with the intra-articular placement of local anesthetic and steroid. In randomized trials, steroid has shown good short-term improvement in symptoms, compared with placebo.[6,86] Novel therapies, such as hyaluronic acid, are also used. Small amounts of these novel therapies are expensive, and imaging is often used to ensure correct intra-articular delivery.

Another use for knee injections is for MR or CT arthrography, most commonly used in the postoperative knee in an attempt to improve detection of meniscal tears after previous meniscectomy.[87] In patients who had prior resection of more than one fourth of their meniscus, MR arthrography increased accuracy by 10% to 20%, when compared with conventional arthrography, in one study.[88] Characterizing osteochondritis dissecans is another strength of MR arthrography.[89]

Technique

Knee arthrography is usually performed at the patellofemoral joint, from either a medial or lateral approach. This approach is usually straightforward, especially in the presence of an effusion. The patellar is manually displaced away from the needle with one hand while the other guides the needle (**Fig. 15**). This technique can be challenging in those patients who have patellofemoral arthritis or large body habitus. An anterior method may also be used, which may be achieved from either a lateral or a medial approach. The needle is placed just medial to the patellar tendon near the inferior patellar pole. The needle is advanced slightly cephalad until it abuts the medial femoral condyle (**Fig. 16**).[90] An anterolateral approach has also been advocated.[91] Less discomfort was noted with a needle target site of lateral femoral condyle rather than with an approach closer to midline. The investigators postulated that this difference was secondary to the increased innervation of Hoffa's fat pad.

ANKLE
Rationale

Therapeutic hindfoot injections provide valuable diagnostic information to the clinician. It is often difficult to differentiate pain arising from the tibiotalar joint, subtalar joint, or talocalcaneonavicular joint from an extra-articular cause. In general, the degree of arthritis on imaging does correlate to relief from local anesthetic.[92] Relief from injection localizes the abnormal joint and distinguishes the joint as a source of pain rather than an extra-articular source such as tenosynovitis, heel pad injury,

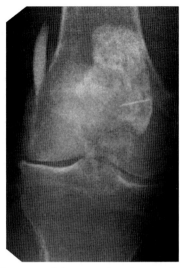

Fig. 16. Anteromedial approach to knee arthrogram.

or plantar fascial injury. It is important to mix contrast with the diagnostic block. Subtalar and ankle joints communicate in 10% of the population.[93] Similarly, following trauma, capsular disruption may result in abnormal communications between joints of the hindfoot and midfoot. This communication occurred in 4 out of 32 patients in one series.[92] The recognition of these communications may alter surgical planning. For example, without the administration of contrast, the communication between the subtalar and talocalcaneonavicular joint would not be identified. Pain arising from the talocalcaneonavicular joint in this setting may be falsely localized after relief with subtalar injection. Relief of symptoms after diagnostic block correlates with significant pain relief after surgical management.[2]

Administration of intra-articular gadolinium may also be useful in selected indications. Direct MR arthrography improves the detection and characterization of cartilage abnormalities.[94] Visualization of osteochondral bodies is also improved because of distention of the joint. MR arthrography may improve the assessment of ankle impingement syndromes.[95,96] MR arthrography also improves the accuracy of detecting lateral ligamentous injury.[97,98]

Technique

Generally, 25-gauge needles are sufficient to interrogate the ankle joints. The tibiotalar joint is straightforward to inject. With the patient lying in a decubitus position, the needle is advanced into the anterior aspect of the joint. Care is taken to avoid anterior tendons and the dorsalis pedis

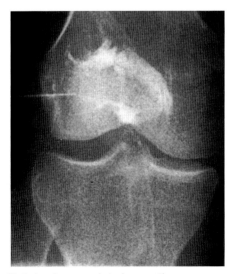

Fig. 15. Lateral approach to knee arthrogram.

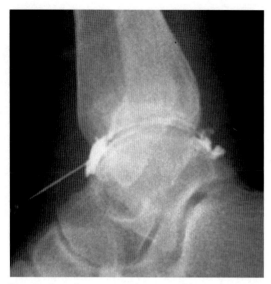

Fig. 17. Anterior approach to ankle arthrogram. Patient is in decubitus position with ankle bolstered to achieve true lateral position. Needle is inserted medial to anterior tibial tendon.

artery. Confirmation of correct placement with contrast is then obtained (**Fig. 17**).

The subtalar joint consists of an anterior and posterior portion. The posterior portion is injected from a lateral approach, just below the fibula. A slightly cephalad approach facilitates intra-articular placement (**Fig. 18**). Palpation of the peroneal tendons is performed before injection.

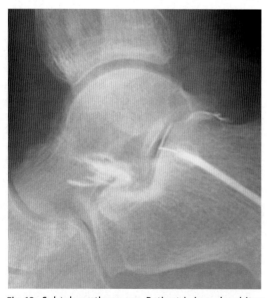

Fig. 18. Subtalar arthrogram. Patient is in a decubitus position with a slightly cephalad needle path.

SUMMARY

Joint injections remain a valuable modality in the detection and treatment of intra-articular pathology. Imaging guidance for joint injection generally increases accuracy in joint aspirations and diagnostic blocks. Confirming intra-articular placement with steroid injections improves efficacy and reduces local complications. Administering intra-articular contrast can improve the diagnostic performance of CT and MR imaging in many circumstances.

REFERENCES

1. Crawford RW, Gie GA, Ling RS, et al. Diagnostic value of intra-articular anaesthetic in primary osteoarthritis of the hip. J Bone Joint Surg Br 1998; 80(2):279–81.
2. Khoury NJ, el-Khoury GY, Saltzman CL, et al. Intraarticular foot and ankle injections to identify source of pain before arthrodesis. AJR Am J Roentgenol 1996; 167(3):669–73.
3. Gomoll AH, Kang RW, Williams JM, et al. Chondrolysis after continuous intra-articular bupivacaine infusion: an experimental model investigating chondrotoxicity in the rabbit shoulder. Arthroscopy 2006;22(8):813–9.
4. Piper SL, Kim HT. Comparison of ropivacaine and bupivicaine toxicity in human articular chondrocytes. J Bone Joint Surg Am 2008;90:986–91.
5. Robinson P, Keenan AM, Conaghan PG. Clinical effectiveness and dose response of image-guided intra-articular corticosteroid injection for hip osteoarthritis. Rheumatology (Oxford) 2007;46(2): 285–91.
6. Ravaud P, Moulinier L, Giraudeau B, et al. Effects of joint lavage and steroid injection in patients with osteoarthritis of the knee: results of a multicenter, randomized, controlled trial. Arthritis Rheum 1999; 42(3):475–82.
7. Hochberg MC, Perlmutter DL, Hudson JI, et al. Preferences in the management of osteoarthritis of the hip and knee: results of a survey of community-based rheumatologists in the United States. Arthritis Care Res 1996;9(3):170–6.
8. McCarty DJ, Hogan JM. Inflammatory reaction after intrasynovial injection of microcrystalline adernocorticosteroid esters. Arthritis Rheum 1964;7:359–67.
9. MacLean CH, Knight K, Paulus H, et al. Costs attributable to osteoarthritis. J Rheumatol 1998;25(11): 2213–8.
10. Mankin HJ, Conger KA. The acute effects of intra-articular hydrocortisone on articular cartilage in rabbits. J Bone Joint Surg Am 1966;48:1383–8.
11. Roberts WN, Babcock EA, Breitbach SA, et al. Corticosteroid injection in rheumatoid arthritis does not

increase rate of total joint arthroplasty. J Rheumatol 1996;23(6):1001–4.

12. Raynauld JP, Buckland-Wright C, Ward R, et al. Safety and efficacy of long-term intraarticular steroid injections in osteoarthritis of the knee: a randomized, double-blind, placebo-controlled trial. Arthritis Rheum 2003;48(2):370–7.

13. Konttinen YT, Friman C, Tolvanen E, et al. Local skin rash after intraarticular methyl prednisolone acetate injection in a patient with rheumatoid arthritis. Arthritis Rheum 1983;26(2):231–3.

14. Fitzgerald RH Jr. Symposium on arthritis in older persons. Section II. Drugs and intrasynovial steroid therapy. Intrasynovial steroid therapy: uses and abuses. J Am Geriatr Soc 1977;25(2):57–8.

15. McCarty DJ, McCarthy G, Carrera G. Intraarticular corticosteroids possibly leading to local osteonecrosis and marrow fat induced synovitis. J Rheumatol 1991;18(7):1091–4.

16. Newberg AH, Munn CS, Robbins AH. Complications of arthrography. Radiology 1985;155(3):605–6.

17. Frieberger RH, Kaye JJ, editors. Arthrography. New York: Appleton-Century-Crofts; 1979. p. 2–3.

18. Jarvik JG, Dalinka MK. Case report 743: urographic opacification following arthrography of the hip. Skeletal Radiol 1992;21(5):346–8.

19. Montgomery DD, Morrison WB, Schweitzer ME, et al. Effects of iodinated contrast and field strength on gadolinium enhancement: implications for direct MR arthrography. J Magn Reson Imaging 2002; 15(3):334–43.

20. Huskisson EC. Measurement of pain. Lancet 1974; 2(7889):1127–31.

21. Palmer WE, Brown JH, Rosenthal DI. Rotator cuff: evaluation with fat-suppressed MR arthrography. Radiology 1993;188(3):683–7.

22. Flannigan B, Kursunoglu-Brahme S, Snyder S, et al. MR arthrography of the shoulder: comparison with conventional MR imaging. AJR Am J Roentgenol 1990;155(4):829–32.

23. Meister K, Thesing J, Montgomery WJ, et al. MR arthrography of partial thickness tears of the undersurface of the rotator cuff: an arthroscopic correlation. Skeletal Radiol 2004;33(3):136–41.

24. Chandnani VP, Yeager TD, DeBerardino T, et al. Glenoid labral tears: prospective evaluation with MRI imaging, MR arthrography, and CT arthrography. AJR Am J Roentgenol 1993;161(6):1229–35.

25. Palmer WE, Brown JH, Rosenthal DI. Labral-ligamentous complex of the shoulder: evaluation with MR arthrography. Radiology 1994;190(3): 645–51.

26. Rowan KR, Andrews G, Spielmann A, et al. MR shoulder arthrography in patients younger than 40 years of age: frequency of rotator cuff tear versus labroligamentous pathology. Australas Radiol 2007; 51(3):257–9.

27. Rand T, Freilinger W, Breitenseher M, et al. Magnetic resonance arthrography (MRA) in the postoperative shoulder. Magn Reson Imaging 1999;17(6): 843–50.

28. Probyn LJ, White LM, Salonen DC, et al. Recurrent symptoms after shoulder instability repair: direct MR arthrographic assessment–correlation with second-look surgical evaluation. Radiology 2007; 245(3):814–23.

29. Morag Y, Jacobson JA, Shields G, et al. MR arthrography of rotator interval, long head of the biceps brachii, and biceps pulley of the shoulder. Radiology 2005;235(1):21–30.

30. Carette S, Moffet H, Tardif J, et al. Intraarticular corticosteroids, supervised physiotherapy, or a combination of the two in the treatment of adhesive capsulitis of the shoulder: a placebo-controlled trial. Arthritis Rheum 2003;48(3):829–38.

31. Buchbinder R, Green S, Forbes A, et al. Arthrographic joint distension with saline and steroid improves function and reduces pain in patients with painful stiff shoulder: results of a randomised, double blind, placebo controlled trial. Ann Rheum Dis 2004;63(3):302–9.

32. Zanca P. Shoulder pain: involvement of the acromioclavicular joint. (Analysis of 1,000 cases). Am J Roentgenol Radium Ther Nucl Med 1971;112(3): 493–506.

33. Bonsell S, Pearsall AW 4th, Heitman RJ, et al. The relationship of age, gender, and degenerative changes observed on radiographs of the shoulder in asymptomatic individuals. J Bone Joint Surg Br 2000;82(8):1135–9.

34. Needell SD, Zlatkin MB, Sher JS, et al. MR imaging of the rotator cuff: peritendinous and bone abnormalities in an asymptomatic population. AJR Am J Roentgenol 1996;166(4):863–7.

35. Partington PF, Broome GH. Diagnostic injection around the shoulder: hit and miss? A cadaveric study of injection accuracy. J Shoulder Elbow Surg 1998;7(2):147–50.

36. Strobel K, Pfirrmann CW, Zanetti M, et al. MRI features of the acromioclavicular joint that predict pain relief from intraarticular injection. AJR Am J Roentgenol 2003;181(3):755–60.

37. Shubin Stein BE, Ahmad CS, Pfaff CH, et al. A comparison of magnetic resonance imaging findings of the acromioclavicular joint in symptomatic versus asymptomatic patients. J Shoulder Elbow Surg 2006;15(1):56–9.

38. Sethi PM, Kingston S, Elattrache N. Accuracy of anterior intra-articular injection of the glenohumeral joint. Arthroscopy 2005;21(1):77–80.

39. Eustace JA, Brophy DP, Gibney RP, et al. Comparison of the accuracy of steroid placement with clinical outcome in patients with shoulder symptoms. Ann Rheum Dis 1997;56(1):59–63.

40. Catalano OA, Manfredi R, Vanzulli A, et al. MR arthrography of the glenohumeral joint: modified posterior approach without imaging guidance. Radiology 2007;242(2):550–4.

41. Zwar RB, Read JW, Noakes JB. Sonographically guided glenohumeral joint injection. AJR Am J Roentgenol 2004;183(1):48–50.

42. Cicak N, Matasović T, Bajraktarević T. Ultrasonographic guidance of needle placement for shoulder arthrography. J Ultrasound Med 1992;11(4):135–7.

43. Schneider R, Ghelman B, Kaye JJ. A simplified injection technique for shoulder arthrography. Radiology 1975;114(3):738–9.

44. Chung CB, Dwek JR, Feng S, et al. MR arthrography of the glenohumeral joint: a tailored approach. AJR Am J Roentgenol 2001;177(1):217–9.

45. Dépelteau H, Bureau NJ, Cardinal E, et al. Arthrography of the shoulder: a simple fluoroscopically guided approach for targeting the rotator cuff interval. AJR Am J Roentgenol 2004;182(2):329–32.

46. Farmer KD, Hughes PM. MR arthrography of the shoulder: fluoroscopically guided technique using a posterior approach. AJR Am J Roentgenol 2002;178(2):433–44.

47. Schwartz ML, Andrews JR. Preoperative evaluation of the ulnar collateral ligament by magnetic resonance imaging and computed tomography arthrography. Evaluation in 25 baseball players with surgical confirmation. Am J Sports Med 1994;22(1):26–31.

48. Nakanishi K, Masatomi T, Ochi T, et al. MR arthrography of elbow: evaluation of the ulnar collateral ligament of elbow. Skeletal Radiol 1996;25(7):629–34.

49. Wright TW, Del Charco M, Wheeler D. Incidence of ligament lesions and associated degenerative changes in the elderly wrist. J Hand Surg [Am] 1994;19(2):313–8.

50. Viegas SF, Patterson RM, Hokanson JA, et al. Wrist anatomy: incidence, distribution, and correlation of anatomic variations, tears, and arthrosis. J Hand Surg [Am] 1993;18(3):463–75.

51. Palmer AK. Triangular fibrocartilage complex lesions: a classification. J Hand Surg [Am] 1989;14(4):594–606.

52. Linkous MD, Pierce SD, Gilula LA. Scapholunate ligamentous communicating defects in symptomatic and asymptomatic wrists: characteristics. Radiology 2000;216(3):846–50.

53. Weiss AP, Akelman E, Lambiase R. Comparison of the findings of triple-injection cinearthrography of the wrist with those of arthroscopy. J Bone Joint Surg Am 1996;78(3):348–56.

54. Theumann N, Favarger N, Schnyder P, et al. Wrist ligament injuries: value of post-arthrography computed tomography. Skeletal Radiol 2001;30(2):88–93.

55. Linkous MD, Gilula LA. Wrist arthrography today. Radiol Clin North Am 1998;36(4):651–72.

56. Schmid MR, Schertler T, Pfirrmann CW, et al. Interosseous ligament tears of the wrist: comparison of multi-detector row CT arthrography and MR imaging. Radiology 2005;237(3):1008–13.

57. Wilson AJ, Gilula LA, Mann FA. Unidirectional joint communications in wrist arthrography: an evaluation of 250 cases. AJR Am J Roentgenol 1991;157(1):105–9.

58. Levinsohn EM, Rosen ID, Palmer AK. Wrist arthrography: value of the three-compartment injection method. Radiology 1991;179(1):231–9.

59. Theumann NH, Pfirrmann CW, Chung CB, et al. Pisotriquetral joint: assessment with MR imaging and MR arthrography. Radiology 2002;222(3):763–70.

60. Pessis E, Drapé JL, Bach F, et al. Direct arthrography of the pisotriquetral joint. AJR Am J Roentgenol 2006;186(3):800–4.

61. Gilula LA, Hardy DC, Totty WG. Distal radioulnar joint arthrography. AJR Am J Roentgenol 1988;150(4):864–6.

62. Byrd JW, Jones KS. Diagnostic accuracy of clinical assessment, magnetic resonance imaging, magnetic resonance arthrography, and intra-articular injection in hip arthroscopy patients. Am J Sports Med 2004;32(7):1668–74.

63. Illgen RL 2nd, Honkamp NJ, Weisman MH, et al. The diagnostic and predictive value of hip anesthetic arthrograms in selected patients before total hip arthroplasty. J Arthroplasty 2006;21(5):724–30.

64. Czerny C, Hofmann S, Urban M, et al. MR arthrography of the adult acetabular capsular-labral complex: correlation with surgery and anatomy. AJR Am J Roentgenol 1999;173(2):345–9.

65. Schmid MR, Nötzli HP, Zanetti M, et al. Cartilage lesions in the hip: diagnostic effectiveness of MR arthrography. Radiology 2003;226(2):382–6.

66. Somme D, Ziza JM, Desplaces N, et al. Contribution of routine joint aspiration to the diagnosis of infection before hip revision surgery. Joint Bone Spine 2003;70(6):489–95.

67. O'Neill DA, Harris WH. Failed total hip replacement: assessment by plain radiographs, arthrograms, and aspiration of the hip joint. J Bone Joint Surg Am 1984;66(4):540–6.

68. Barrack RL, Harris WH. The value of aspiration of the hip joint before revision total hip arthroplasty. J Bone Joint Surg Am 1993;75(1):66–76.

69. Crawford RW, Ellis AM, Gie GA, et al. Intra-articular local anaesthesia for pain after hip arthroplasty. J Bone Joint Surg Br 1997;79(5):796–800.

70. Maus TP, Berquist TH, Bender CE, et al. Arthrographic study of painful total hip arthroplasty: refined criteria. Radiology 1987;162(3):721–7.

71. Murray WR, Rodrigo JJ. Arthrography for the assessment of pain after total hip replacement. A

comparison of arthrographic findings in patients with and without pain. J Bone Joint Surg Am 1975;57(8): 1060–5.

72. Steinbach LS, Schneider R, Goldman AB, et al. Bursae and abscess cavities communicating with the hip. Diagnosis using arthrography and CT. Radiology 1985;156(2):303–7.

73. Swan JS, Braunstein EM, Wellman HN, et al. Contrast and nuclear arthrography in loosening of the uncemented hip prosthesis. Skeletal Radiol 1991; 20(1):15–9.

74. Barrack RL, Tanzer M, Kattapuram SV, et al. The value of contrast arthrography in assessing loosening of symptomatic uncemented total hip components. Skeletal Radiol 1994;23(1):37–41.

75. Cheung A, Lachiewicz PF, Renner JB. The role of aspiration and contrast-enhanced arthrography in evaluating the uncemented hip arthroplasty. AJR Am J Roentgenol 1997;168(5):1305–9.

76. Temmerman OP, Raijmakers PG, Deville WL, et al. The use of plain radiography, subtraction arthrography, nuclear arthrography, and bone scintigraphy in the diagnosis of a loose acetabular component of a total hip prosthesis: a systematic review. J Arthroplasty 2007;22(6):818–27.

77. Vaccaro JP, Sauser DD, Beals RK. Iliopsoas bursa imaging: efficacy in depicting abnormal iliopsoas tendon motion in patients with internal snapping hip syndrome. Radiology 1995;197(3):853–6.

78. Mauffrey C, Pobbathy. Hip joint injection technique using anatomic landmarks: are we accurate?: A prospective study. The Internet Journal of Orthopedic Surgery 2006;3(1).

79. Leopold SS, Battista V, Oliverio JA. Safety and efficacy of intraarticular hip injection using anatomic landmarks. Clin Orthop Relat Res 2001;391(10):192–7.

80. Duc SR, Hodler J, Schmid MR, et al. Prospective evaluation of two different injection techniques for MR arthrography of the hip. Eur Radiol 2006;16(2): 473–8.

81. Kilcoyne RF, Kaplan P. The lateral approach for hip arthrography. Skeletal Radiol 1992;21(4):239–40.

82. Brandser EA, El-Khoury GY, FitzRandolph RL. Modified technique for fluid aspiration from the hip in patients with prosthetic hips. Radiology 1997; 204(2):580–2.

83. Swan JS, Braunstein EM, Capello W. Aspiration of the hip in patients treated with Girdlestone arthroplasty. AJR Am J Roentgenol 1991;156(3):545–6.

84. Jackson DW, Evans NA, Thomas BM. Accuracy of needle placement into the intra-articular space of the knee. J Bone Joint Surg Am 2002;84(9):1522–7.

85. Bliddal H. Placement of intra-articular injections verified by mini air-arthrography. Ann Rheum Dis 1999;58(10):641–3.

86. Pendleton A, Arden N, Dougados M, et al. EULAR recommendations for the management of knee osteoarthritis: report of a task force of the Standing Committee for International Clinical Studies Including Therapeutic Trials (ESCISIT). Ann Rheum Dis 2000;59(12):936–44.

87. Chung CB, Isaza IL, Angulo M, et al. MR arthrography of the knee: how, why, when. Radiol Clin North Am 2005;43(4):733–46.

88. Applegate GR, Flannigan BD, Tolin BS, et al. MR diagnosis of recurrent tears in the knee: value of intraarticular contrast material. AJR Am J Roentgenol 1993;161(4):821–5.

89. Kramer J, Recht MP, Imhof H, et al. Postcontrast MR arthrography in assessment of cartilage lesions. J Comput Assist Tomogr 1994;18(2):218–24.

90. Zurlo JV, Towers JD, Golla S. Anterior approach for knee arthrography. Skeletal Radiol 2001;30(6): 354–6.

91. Moser T, Moussaoui A, Dupuis M, et al. Anterior approach for knee arthrography: tolerance evaluation and comparison of two routes. Radiology 2008; 246(1):193–7.

92. Mitchell MJ, Bielecki D, Bergman AG, et al. Localization of specific joint causing hindfoot pain: value of injecting local anesthetics into individual joints during arthrography. AJR Am J Roentgenol 1995; 164(6):1473–6.

93. Resnick D. Radiology of the talocalcaneal articulations. Anatomic considerations and arthrography. Radiology 1974;111(3):581–6.

94. Cerezal L, Abascal F, García-Valtuille R, et al. Ankle MR arthrography: how, why, when. Radiol Clin North Am 2005;43(4):693–707.

95. Robinson P, White LM, Salonen DC, et al. Anterolateral ankle impingement: MR arthrographic assessment of the anterolateral recess. Radiology 2001; 221(1):186–90.

96. Jordan LK 3rd, Helms CA, Cooperman AE, et al. Magnetic resonance imaging findings in anterolateral impingement of the ankle. Skeletal Radiol 2000;29(1): 34–9.

97. Chandnani VP, Harper MT, Ficke JR, et al. Chronic ankle instability: evaluation with MR arthrography, MR imaging, and stress radiography. Radiology 1994;192(1):189–94.

98. Lee SH, Jacobson J, Trudell D, et al. Ligaments of the ankle: normal anatomy with MR arthrography. J Comput Assist Tomogr 1998;22(5):807–13.

Image-Guided Musculoskeletal Biopsy

Apoorva Gogna, MBBS[a],
Wilfred C.G. Peh, MBBS, MHSM, MD, FRCPE, FRCPG, FRCR[b],*,
Peter L. Munk, MD, CM, FRCPC[c]

KEYWORDS

- Bone biopsy • Musculoskeletal biopsy
- Musculoskeletal diseases • Musculoskeletal intervention
- Orthopedic imaging

Sampling of bone and marrow for analysis has been recognized for millennia;[1] however, image-guided bone biopsy is a relatively recent development. Since the description of percutaneous biopsy for diagnosis of skeletal lesions by Coley in 1931,[2,3] and fluoroscopic-guided procedures by Lalli in 1970,[3,4] image-guided bone biopsy has developed significantly, led by innovations in imaging and intervention. It has become an essential part of managing musculoskeletal lesions, including primary and secondary bone tumors[5,6] and infections.[7,8]

Although early reports dismissed minimally invasive bone biopsy only as a "simple, primary diagnostic procedure" with significant inconclusive or misleading results,[9,10] later reports increasingly recognized their low morbidity, lower cost (compared with open biopsy),[11] high accuracy, and repeatability in the event of an inconclusive result.[3,5,12–27] This has led to greater importance of image-guided bone biopsy, which has replaced open surgical biopsy in many instances. The advantages of the procedure even have translated to veterinary applications.[28,29] The accurate characterization based on the small tissue samples obtained is often challenging, however.[30–36]

Image guidance allows safe passage of needles, often into small and otherwise inaccessible lesions, and into the portions of the lesion most likely to yield useful samples, while avoiding damage to important structures. This article hopes to provide a useful guide to image-guided musculoskeletal biopsy for radiologists in practice and in training.

PREPARATION
Why Must One Perform This Biopsy?

The presence of a bony or soft tissue lesion does not automatically imply the need for histology. Clinical information, laboratory findings, and imaging features may be sufficient to provide high diagnostic confidence for certain lesions, allowing for a conservative management or therapeutic trial. In addition, a clearly benign lesion for which therapy is not indicated does not require biopsy. A range of benign bone lesions has been described in the literature and familiarity with these may help avoid an unnecessary biopsy.[37–41] The history, physical examination, and laboratory and imaging findings for each patient should be reviewed thoroughly and the case discussed with the referring clinicians. The indication and approach to image-guided biopsy must be tailored for each patient.

Indications and Contraindications

The recognized indications and contraindications for biopsies in general are outlined in **Box 1**.[42–44]

[a] Department of Diagnostic Radiology, Changi General Hospital, 2 Simei Street 3, Singapore 529889, Republic of Singapore
[b] Department of Diagnostic Radiology, Alexandra Hospital, 378 Alexandra Road, Singapore 159964, Republic of Singapore
[c] Department of Radiology, University of British Columbia, Vancouver General Hospital, 899 West 12th Avenue, Vancouver, BC V5Z 1M9, Canada
* Corresponding author. Department of Diagnostic Radiology, Alexandra Hospital, 378 Alexandra Road, Singapore 159964, Republic of Singapore.
E-mail address: wilfred@pehfamily.per.sg (W.C.G. Peh).

Radiol Clin N Am 46 (2008) 455–473
doi:10.1016/j.rcl.2008.04.014
0033-8389/08/$ – see front matter © 2008 Elsevier Inc. All rights reserved.

These should be considered carefully in reference to each patient. The most common indications for bone biopsies are tumor and infection. For known primary tumors, biopsy may be indicated for solitary bone lesions if identification of the bone lesion will influence therapy. For example, in a patient who has known colon carcinoma and extensive liver and lung metastases, finding multiple new vertebral osteolytic lesions clearly does not need biopsy of these vertebral lesions, as it will not alter the patient's management. In contrast, a patient who has a known colon carcinoma with no solid organ metastases and a single vertebral osteolytic lesion may be considered for vertebral biopsy, because the outcome will affect the stage of tumor and subsequent management.

Patients with tumors in remission after treatment who subsequently present with a new bone lesion may need biopsy. For known, radiographically stable, bone metastases, biopsy may be needed to determine tumor viability, especially if scintigraphic studies (eg, fluorodeoxyglucose [FDG] positron emission tomography [PET]) are equivocal. Often, biopsy may be the only method of exclusion of sinister solitary bone lesions in the absence of classic benign features, especially when the history is suggestive.[41] Primary musculoskeletal tumors require identification, grading, and often cytogenetic analysis, for prognosis and treatment. Even in definite bone metastases, biopsy may be useful for identifying a primary lesion when this is not apparent. Tumor markers are recognized to be unhelpful in identifying an unknown primary lesion, except for possibly prostate-specific antigen (PSA).[45]

Early stages of spondylodiskitis may be difficult to differentiate from degenerative Modic 1 changes, inflammatory lesions (eg, seronegative spondiloarthropathy), amyloidosis, or crystal deposition disease[8,46] on MR imaging, and scintigraphy.[47] Hence, biopsy may be required to help to make a distinction.

Perhaps the only absolute contraindication to performing a biopsy is a lesion that can be diagnosed on imaging with a high degree of certainty and where no additional information will be obtained from the biopsy to aid in patient management. Examples include the classic benign lesion (the "do not touch lesion") and definite metastases from a known primary (eg, multiple bone metastases of prostate cancer).

Biopsy in certain sites increases the hazard, and alternative biopsy routes may be more appropriate. For example, C1 and odontoid biopsy may be conducted by means of a transpharyngeal route by the otorhinolaryngologic surgeon with a lower risk of complications than computed tomography (CT)-guided percutaneous biopsy if no other less hazardous site is apparent. Uncooperative or pediatric cases may require referral for general anesthesia. The risk–benefit ratio of percutaneous versus open biopsy should be reconsidered, if the patient ultimately will require general anesthesia. Severe coagulopathy or thrombocytopenia should be corrected before the procedure. For certain cases, a hematological consultation may be required to deal with coagulopathies that the radiologist may not have experience in correcting.

Percutaneous or Open Biopsy?

Percutaneous biopsy has several advantages over open biopsy. It is minimally invasive, allowing access to different parts of the lesion rather than just the surgically exposed area. The imaging modality often can direct the biopsy needle to the areas most likely to yield suitable specimens. The minimally invasive approach reduces recovery time and patient morbidity. The procedure has a high reported accuracy, which ranges from 68% to 97%.[14,15,17–20] There is also lower cost incurred for the patient.[11,48–50] For example, Ward and Kilpatrick,[11] in a study of 66 consecutive fine-needle aspiration cytology (FNAC) biopsies of primary bone tumors, estimated total charges for FNAC to be $1968 compared with $4312 for open biopsy, based on an intent-to-diagnose approach. Of their 66 biopsies, 73% were diagnostic, 8% partially diagnostic, and 18% nondiagnostic.

Limitations of percutaneous biopsy include a small but real risk of having a negative sample (ie, no diagnostic information is derived). The most common cause is insufficient material obtained, which may be because of too few passes, and sampling of necrotic or sclerotic areas that do not yield adequate number of cells for confident analysis. Diagnosis of benign and metastatic tumors is easier than primary soft tissue and bone tumors on percutaneous biopsy, and many studies report high accuracy in classifying lesions as benign or malignant, but lower accuracy in specifying exact pathology and grade. For example, in a study of 155 patients who had sarcoma, Welker and colleagues[27] reported that needle biopsy was 92.4% accurate in differentiating benign from malignant lesions, 88.6% accurate in providing exact grade, and 72.7% accurate in determining exact pathology.

When is it Safe and Appropriate to Proceed?

What is expected from the biopsy? Biopsy of musculoskeletal tumors ideally is performed at the institution where definitive management is expected to occur, as part of a multidisciplinary team that includes an orthopedic oncologist, musculoskeletal radiologist, bone pathologist, and oncologist. The difficulty in diagnosis of a bone and soft tissue sarcoma is recognized. The institution also requires the services of an experienced cytopathologist to interpret fine-needle biopsy specimens. A hastily done, incorrectly sited biopsy may not yield desired results, and will affect further imaging, compromise further biopsy attempts, and worst of all, adversely impact the prognosis of the patient.

Primary musculoskeletal tumors may be eligible for curative resection; hence, each case requires close discussion and agreement among the operating surgeon, musculoskeletal radiologist, and bone pathologist to facilitate route and type of biopsy needed. Anatomic compartments not involved by tumor must not be breached by the biopsy device, as this may predispose to local recurrence and require limb amputation, where limb conservation otherwise may have been feasible. In many centers, palpable lesions and primary limb tumors usually are biopsied by the orthopedic oncologist, while relatively inaccessible lesions requiring image-guided biopsy (eg, CT-guided) are performed by the radiologist after discussion with the treating orthopedic surgeon (**Fig. 1**).

Appropriate imaging should be completed before the biopsy[44] for two main reasons. First, the findings influence the procedure itself, and second, lesion characteristics may be altered by postbiopsy changes. For example, scintigraphic studies for suspected bone metastasis should be scheduled first, as other (potentially more easily accessible) lesions may be demonstrated.[16] Accuracy of percutaneous disc biopsy has been reported to be as low as 47.5% for spondylodiskitis. When the diagnosis of osteomyelitis or diskitis is obvious, biopsy for the sole purpose of obtaining material for culture must be performed with caution because of high rates of negative cultures, reported to be up to 60%.[8,51–54] Paravertebral collections and intervertebral disc space fluid are often sterile.[8] In addition, there is the risk of seeding adjacent noninfected tissue with microbes. Furthermore, because the most commonly found organism is *Staphylococcal aureus* (in 50% to 60% of cases),[54–56] it is reasonable to consider a therapeutic trial in such cases, without first doing a biopsy.

Platelet count, hemoglobin, prothrombin time (PT), and activated partial thromboplastin time (APTT) should be performed before most procedures. Platelet levels above $100,000/mm^3$ are adequate for most procedures, while levels below $50,000/mm^3$ require prophylactic transfusion just before the procedure (because of short half-life of transfused platelets). Patients on anticoagulants should have them stopped before the biopsy, particularly for core biopsy. Aspirin causes permanent inhibition of platelet activity, and between 4 to 10 days may be required for return of normal function. Uremia in renal failure causes platelet

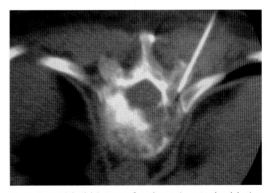

Fig. 1. CT-guided biopsy of a thoracic vertebral lesion performed with the patient lying prone and using a costovertebral approach.

dysfunction, which can be reversed by scheduling hemodialysis before the procedure.

Patients on antimicrobials may need to stop taking them for about 48 hours before the biopsy to facilitate microbiological assessment.[57] Diet adjustment usually involves fasting for 8 to 12 hours, with oral medications allowed up to the morning of the procedure, taking only sips of water. Patients who have insulin-dependent diabetes mellitus should be instructed to take only half their normal dose of insulin and a 5% dextrose- containing infusion started before the procedure, along with hypocount monitoring. In the authors' center, warfarin is stopped for 3 days before a biopsy. For selected cases where anticoagulation is critical (eg, prosthetic heart valves), heparin may be used up to 4 hours before the procedure, usually in consultation with the patient's cardiologist. Prophylactic antibiotics are usually not necessary.

Postprocedure monitoring in the hospital may be required if there is increased risk of developing a complication of biopsy. Planning for admission should be done early and the patient forewarned appropriately. Some practitioners schedule a pre-procedural visit, which provides a valuable opportunity to establish rapport, allay the patient's fears, engage in a risk–benefit discussion, discuss alternatives, and provide relevant details of the procedure.[58,59] Informed consent should be obtained during this visit, and pre-/postprocedure instructions conveyed, usually by means of printed information sheets.

TECHNIQUE AND EQUIPMENT
Preliminary Preparation

The patient's vital signs are monitored continually and recorded every 15 minutes by a trained person who is not involved in performing or assisting with the procedure, preferably a nurse. All patients should have an intravenous (IV) line in situ. The operator should don sterile gloves and eye-protective gear after scrubbing up. Premedications are given if necessary, including sedatives and antianxiety drugs. The authors usually titrate IV doses of midazolam and fentanyl or meperidine, with monitoring of vital signs and pulse oximetry. Platelet, fresh frozen plasma, or cryoprecipitate cover also is initiated if required. Prophylactic antibiotics are not indicated.

The skin is cleansed with povidone iodine and alcohol or chlorhexidine, and sterile drapes placed around the biopsy site. Local anesthetic is delivered from the planned site of entry up to the lesion. The adjacent muscles and the periosteum of bone also may be infiltrated to help minimize pain.

Positioning

Patient position should facilitate needle access and maximize comfort for the patient and operator. For prolonged procedures, the risk of inducing pressure sores over bony prominences should be borne in mind, especially for the debilitated patient. For biopsy of the thoracic and lumbar spine, the patient usually is positioned prone, but alternative positions include lateral decubitus and oblique positions to facilitate needle entry and patient comfort.

In the cervical spine, an anteriorly located lesion requires supine positioning (**Fig. 2**), while lesions in the pedicles or posterior elements may be approached posteriorly with the patient prone or prone oblique in position (**Fig. 3**).[57] Retroperitoneal lesions can be approached posteriorly or occasionally anteriorly (transperitoneal). The posterior approach usually is used, especially when larger core samples are needed. As the anterior approach entails transgressing bowel, only a 20G or smaller needle should be used, and only when absolutely necessary. A patient who has had recent abdominal surgery may not be able to lie prone for biopsy, and alternative positioning will become necessary. The patient's body habitus may preclude usage of certain modalities, and alternatives may be needed (eg, fluoroscopy or open biopsy).

Ideally, prior imaging using the modality to be used for biopsy guidance should be performed. A lesion demonstrated on one modality (eg, MR imaging) may not be visualized adequately on another modality (eg, CT fluoroscopy) or even on the same modality without IV contrast enhancement. The radiologist, with tactile skills and anatomic knowledge, is equipped to direct the biopsy needle into CT-occult lesions. The radiation dose to the patient should be considered, especially for anticipated difficult or long procedures, where repeated imaging can be anticipated.

Route

For primary long bone tumors, where limb-sparing surgery (LSS) is a possibility, strict adherence to anatomic compartments is important. Bone sarcomas may known to recur locally because of tumor seeding along core needle biopsy track,[60,61] requiring resection of the biopsy track with a core of adjacent tissue along with the tumor at definitive surgery.[62] Additional chemotherapy or radiation therapy may be required because of inappropriate initial image-guided and open biopsy.[63] Discussion with the operating team is hence vital, and preferably the biopsy should be performed in the same center as the planned

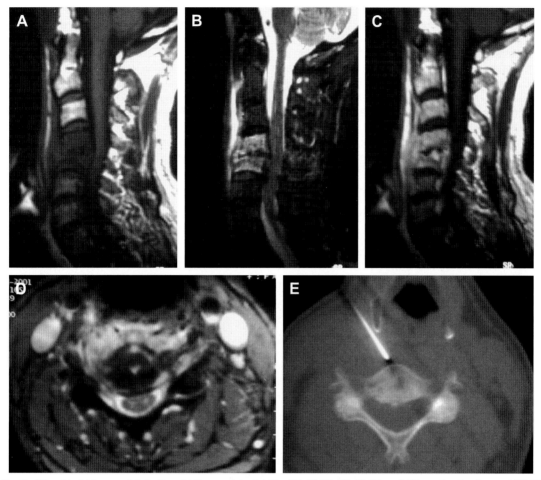

Fig. 2. CT-guided biopsy of infective C4/5 spondylodiskitis. (A) T1-W, (B) T2-W and (C) contrast-enhanced T1-W sagittal, and (D) T2-W axial MR images show involvement of C4 and C5 vertebral bodies with anterior soft tissues. (E) The needle is directed into the lesion with the patient lying supine, using the right anterolateral approach and avoiding the vital neck structures.

surgery. Nevertheless, actual risks of seeding of tumor by FNAC are remote, estimated at three to nine cases per 100,000 patients.

The biopsy track should be planned such that uninvolved anatomic compartments and neurovascular bundles are not crossed by the biopsy needle.[57] In certain cases, the most direct route to the lesion may be inappropriate. Readers are referred to reviews on anatomic compartments and guidelines for core-needle biopsy of primary and soft tissue tumors.[64–67]

Types of Lesion/Lesion Characteristics

For multiple lesions, biopsy of the largest and most superficial lesion is often the best. The integrity of the underlying bone, however, should be considered. Preferably, the biopsy should be placed in a nonweight-bearing portion of bone to prevent iatrogenic fracture. The identity and proximity of

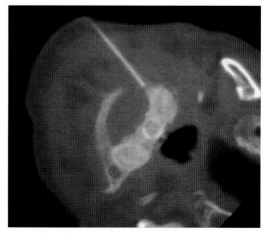

Fig. 3. CT-guided biopsy of the C2 vertebral neural arch in a patient who had both metastases and septicemia. The patient is in a prone oblique position, and the needle approach is posterolateral.

adjacent vital structures must be considered. An iliac biopsy thus may be safer than thoracic vertebral biopsy for multiple bone metastases in a patient with an unknown primary tumor.

If infection is suspected in the spine, the disc and adjacent subchondral bone should be included in the specimen. The soft tissue component of a bone lesion also should be sampled. Ideally, all samples should be sent for histology, cytopathology, and microbiology. CT-guided biopsy has been found to be accurate for active bacterial disc infections, but less reliable for fungal infections. Cytopathology improves sensitivity for fungal infections.

Mixed sclerotic–lytic lesions should be biopsied over their lytic portions. Clearly necrotic and cystic areas of the lesion have a lower yield compared with the solid margins. Ultrasound is particularly useful in identifying solid areas in a predominantly cystic tumor. The radiologist should identify the most appropriate areas to biopsy on the preliminary scan. Enhancing areas of the tumor are more likely to yield viable cells. By correlation with the contrast-enhanced diagnostic study, CT fluoroscopy still can be used to direct the needle into these areas (**Fig. 4**). Areas of the lesion showing color flow on power Doppler imaging should be targeted preferentially.

Needle Types

The needle type is determined by the nature of the lesion to be biopsied and the preference of the operator.[11,17,27,57,58,68–72] The chosen needle

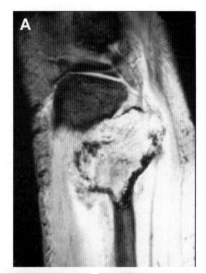

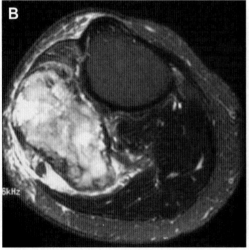

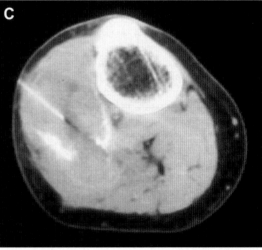

Fig. 4. CT-guided biopsy of a fibular osteosarcoma with avoidance of compartmental contamination. (*A*) Contrast-enhanced T1-W sagittal and (*B*) T2-W axial MR images show a large tumor arising from the fibular head, with soft tissue extension. (*C*) CT-guided biopsy of this lesion was performed.

should be long enough to reach the lesion and provide an adequate core of tissue. Smaller needles reduce patient discomfort, have a smaller risk of injury to adjacent structures, and are expected to cause less bleeding, especially from vascular lesions. They are best applied for aspiration of fluid, for cytology of soft tissue lesions, and for sampling disc contents for culture or cytology. Cutting needles can obtain greater cores of tissue from bone and soft tissue. Biopsy needles can be divided into three categories: fine aspiration needles (eg, Chiba, Cook, Bloomington, Indiana); cutting needles (eg, Tru-cut, Baxter Healthcare, Deerfield, Illinois; Quick-core, Cook, Bloomington, Indiana; Temmo, Bauer Medical, Clearwater, Florida), and trephine (Ostycut, Angiomed/Bard, Karlsruhe, Germany; Craig, George Tiemann, Hauppage, New York; Ackerman, Cook, Bloomington, Indiana). Sizes range from 22G for fine-needle aspiration sets to 11G for trephine biopsy.

Fine needles (20 to 22G) are ideal for cytology and aspiration of fluid; they have a lower risk of hemorrhage (eg, in suspected hemangiomas or vascular metastases such as renal cell carcinoma) and a lower risk of tract seeding (**Fig. 5**). They tend to bend while targeting deep lesions, however, and they are difficult to redirect without reinsertion. Additionally, they are unable to penetrate intact bone and provide small specimens, which may be under-representative of the whole lesion. Larger bore needles are more likely to provide adequate material for subtyping, especially in suspected small cell lymphoma. They can be drilled into bone, allowing coaxial insertion of smaller needles. The coaxial technique also allows multiple passes through a single skin puncture (see **Fig. 5**B and C).

When the bony cortex has been breached by the lesion, and a soft tissue component exists, biopsy can be obtained using an aspiration or cutting needle (**Fig. 6**). Where there is a thick overlying cortex, this first must be breached using various techniques, including a trephine needle, which has a cutting tip to allow penetration of bone, or drill-based systems (**Fig. 7**). To avoid repeat punctures through bone, using a coaxial system allows multiple passes through a single bone window (**Fig. 8**).

Techniques

For deep lesions, the coaxial method allows multiple passes by means of a single track (see **Figs. 5 and 8**). For FNAC biopsy of lesions more than 10 cm deep, using a 20G rather than a 22G needle[58] is preferable, as it is more resistant to bending. For intact bone, the lesion may be accessed using a drill tip with a coaxial sheath. Sclerotic lesions are sampled best with a trephine needle, of at least 15G size, followed by a 22G or smaller FNAC needle inserted coaxially. Osteolytic lesions in bone should be sampled with a trephine needle. Spring-loaded cutting needles used for soft tissue biopsy usually are not advised for biopsy of bone lesions that have overlying intact cortex.

A cytotechnologist should be available on site, especially for lesions where there may be doubt about adequacy (eg, lesions with significant necrosis or sclerosis), and in small lesions where only limited number of passes can be attempted.

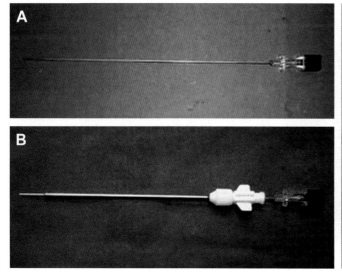
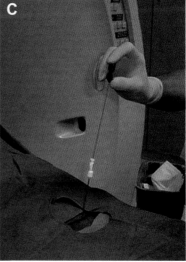

Fig. 5. Aspiration needle. (*A*) 22G Chiba needle (Cook, Bloomington, Indiana). (*B, C*) Chiba needle that has been placed coaxially within a shorter 14.5G trephine needle.

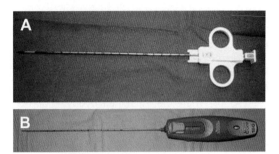

Fig. 6. Examples of cutting needles; all are 18G in size and have spring-loaded firing mechanisms (biopsy guns). (*A*) Quickcore needle (Cook, Bloomington, Indiana). (*B*) Easycore needle (Boston Scientific, Natick, Massachusetts).

At least three passes should be made, if the cytotechnologist is not available. For suspected infections, aspirated blood clots can be sent for microbiology in a sterile container.[57]

Does Size Matter?

Fine-needle biopsy provides cells that can be analyzed for ultrastructural abnormalities. Core biopsy yields histology for assessing intercellular relationship. For primary malignant tumors, the latter is crucial. Although there are several reports of

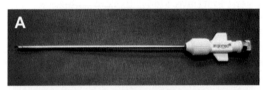

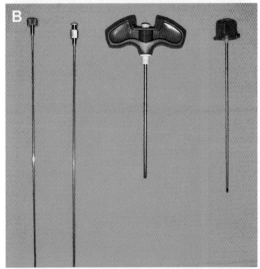

Fig. 7. Examples of trephine bone biopsy needles. (*A*) 14.5G Ostycut needle (Angiomed/Bard, Karlsruhe, Germany). (*B*) 11G Cook bone biopsy needle (Cook, Bloomington, Indiana).

fairly good accuracy with FNAC for primary tumors alone, the results are variable and often positively influenced by a large number of benign lesions in the study population. As these benign tumors are easier to diagnose, this increases the perceived accuracy of FNAC in some studies. Mesenchymal tumors are among the most difficult of pathologies to diagnose,[27] and while FNAC is the modality of choice for epithelial tumors, the reported results are variable for mesenchymal tumors. In contrast, multiple institutions report consistently good results for core-needle biopsy.[27] Hence, core biopsy is recommended for primary tumors.

For lymphoma, core specimens often are required for subtyping, especially for small cell lymphomas. For lesions with hemorrhagic potential (eg, in suspected hemangiomas or vascular metastases from primaries such as renal cell carcinoma), fine- needle sampling usually is recommended. For metastatic tumors and infections, fine- needle aspiration is often sufficient.[17] As a general principle, samples from all suspected infections also should be sent for cytopathology, and at least one sample from suspected tumors should be sent for microbiologic assessment.

The spindle cell tumors are difficult to diagnose by FNAC, but core biopsy often can provide adequate material for tissue pattern and histochemical analysis.[35,36] Welker and colleagues,[27] however, reported two cases of misdiagnosed spindle cell tumors on core biopsy. The first was a low-grade spindle cell sarcoma detected on open incisional frozen section biopsy, which was diagnosed as giant cell tumor on needle biopsy. Detailed analysis revealed a low-grade bone sarcoma, with giant cells and small foci of high-grade osteosarcoma variant. The second initially was diagnosed as pseudosarcomatous fascitis of the posterior thigh. The lesion was thought to be low to intermediate-grade fibrosarcoma on open biopsy, eventually revised to a high-grade malignant fibroid histiocytoma after sampling a second area that was involving the sciatic nerve. These highlight the difficulties created by sampling error in these difficult mixed mesenchymal tumors. The authors concluded that open biopsy offers minimal information beyond that revealed by needle biopsy.

For certain conditions, even the larger core biopsy specimen may prove to be inadequate, as pathologic differentiation from other similar disease conditions may be impossible, requiring radiological and clinical correlation. For example, osteofibrous dysplasia can be very difficult to distinguish from its main differentials of adamantinoma and monostotic fibrous dysplasia, especially on a small biopsy specimen.[18] Other lesions that have been reported to be misdiagnosed on percutaneous biopsy include

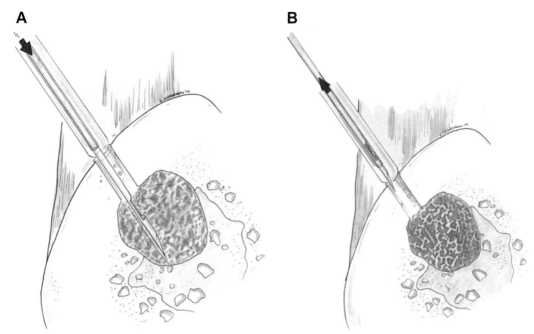

A   **B**

Fig. 8. (A, B) Diagrams show coaxial passage of a cutting needle through a trephine needle.

dedifferentiated chondrosarcoma,[11,34] hemangioendothelioma,[11] and chondroblastoma of bone.[32]

Image Guidance Modality and Biopsy Techniques

The lesion ideally should be well-visualized on the modality to be used to guide biopsy, and a formal assessment already should have been done with that same modality. Information from several modalities, however, may have to be combined in the mind of the radiologist to achieve optimum targeting (eg, the metabolically active, non-necrotic, and nonsclerotic portions of a large mixed tumor). The imaging modality should be safe and provide adequate visualization of relevant anatomy to allow a safe approach to the lesion.

Fluoroscopy

Fluoroscopy, ideally biplanar, is used most often to guide biopsy in long bones. Positioning is usually more comfortable for the patient. Patient movement does not degrade image quality as severely as for CT or MR imaging.[73] Fluoroscopy is also more widely available, is cheaper, and delivers a lower radiation dose compared with CT for the same imaging duration. Visualization of small intramedullary lesions and soft tissue component of bone tumors, however, is poor. Also, small lesions in complex-shaped bones (eg, pelvis and vertebrae) may be difficult or hazardous to access on fluoroscopic guidance.

Ultrasound

Ultrasound is used most frequently to guide biopsy of soft tissue lesions (**Fig. 9**). Ultrasound also can be used for lesions on or near a bone surface, especially if there is an associated soft tissue component.[73–77] Strengths of ultrasound include real-time imaging, multiplanar visualization, no ionizing radiation exposure, and more flexible positioning for the patient.[58] Color Doppler can be used to identify tumor neovascularity and the relationship of the tumor to the neurovascular bundle.[78] Clearly cystic or necrotic areas can be avoided,[73] and areas showing blood flow on Doppler imaging can be targeted preferentially. Nearby vascular structures can be identified on color imaging and thus avoided. Deep lesions, lesions encased by bone, and those with overlying air-containing structures (eg, bowel loops in the case of a pelvic bone mass), however, cannot be visualized well.

In ultrasound-guided biopsy,[78] the lesion to be targeted is visualized in two planes, and a solid area of tumor is identified, preferably with evidence of neovascularity seen on color Doppler. If the lesion is hypovascular, then sampling of the tumor margin is done. Using the biopsy function of the ultrasound machine, the distance and angle to lesion are calculated in a suitable plane that avoids important intervening structures. The probe

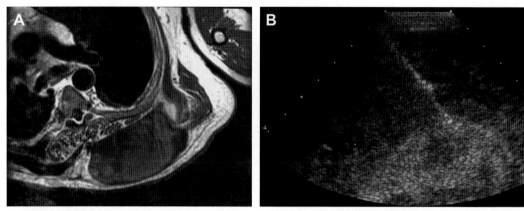

Fig. 9. Ultrasound-guided biopsy of a superficial soft tissue mass. (*A*) Axial T1-W MR image shows a large solid subcutaneous mass located in the posterior chest wall. (*B*) Ultrasound image shows direction of the echogenic needle tip into the lesion.

is placed in a sterile probe cover, and a sterile transparent drape is applied to the ultrasound console to facilitate adjustment of control dials. A sterilized biopsy transducer guide may be applied to the probe if required.

The echogenic needle tip should be visualized during approach to the lesion and documented within the lesion on two planes before obtaining the biopsy specimen. Color Doppler can be applied to guide the needle to perfused areas. A screw stylet can be used to increase visualization of the needle tip. Enhanced needle tips are also available (eg, Biosponder needle, Advanced Technology Laboratories, Bothel, Washington). Another tip is to trap a tiny bubble of air in the needle tip by withdrawing and reinserting the stylet before inserting the needle.

MR imaging

MR imaging guidance is attractive for its lack of radiation and superior delineation of pathology often not visible in other modalities. Equipment compatibility issues, patient positioning, cost, and availability of MR imaging scan room time, however, are all factors to consider and preclude MR imaging as a routine modality for guiding biopsy.

Computed tomography

Technical advances in high-speed array processors, partial reconstruction algorithms, slip ring technology, and higher heat capacitance of radiography tubes have allowed near real-time visualization of structures on CT.[79] Images can be reconstructed up to six frames per second. CT fluoroscopy has become the cornerstone of image-guided biopsy of the nonpalpable lesion, especially deep lesions and in patients who have significant respiratory movement.

Radiation dose is an important consideration. In contrast to fluoroscopy, where radiation doses are several centigrays per minute, in CT fluoroscopy, the dose delivered is in the order of several centigrays per second. CT fluoroscopy doses are small compared with conventional CT, however, and this can be minimized by using short bursts of imaging.

Paulson and colleagues[80] assessed CT fluoroscopy doses to radiologists performing various procedures using low millicurie (10 mA) settings and predominantly intermittent imaging. Most procedures used the quick check method, where only a few consecutive slices are imaged at a time, and the needle is advanced after studying these images. For spine biopsy, radiation doses to whole body, ocular lens, and skin (measured outside the lead gown) ranged from 0.66 to 2.8 mrem, 1.0 to 2.8 mrem, and 1.5 to 2.8 mrem, respectively, when the quick check method was used (occupational whole body limit = 5000 mrem ie, 50 mSv per year). The average fluoroscopy time was also considerably shorter, about one-fourth to one-seventh that reported by other authors, and average patient doses were 3.2 cGy per procedure. Hence, with appropriate settings, CT fluoroscopy doses for the operator can be negligible.

In CT fluoroscopy-guided biopsy in the authors' center, the monitor is set up to show three consecutive slices reconstructed in a 256 × 256 matrix and displayed on a 768 × 768 matrix. The slice number is noted, and the operator and staff stand behind a lead glass screen during imaging to reduce radiation exposure.[57] The couch top can be moved by the console or manually. For console operation, the authors use a transparent sterile cover to drape the console to allow the operator to adjust the table independently.

The lesion-to-skin distance and trajectory angle are estimated by assessing the preliminary images. The representative slice number is marked. A grid can be placed on the patient's skin, or alternatively, a skin surface marker is placed. Using the localizer laser beam of the CT scanner assists in surface marking of the skin (**Fig. 10**). The needle tip can be located by the low-attenuation beam-hardening artifact. Perpendicular insertion of the needle is the simplest approach. For angulated approaches, however, the CT gantry should be tilted to the plane of insertion.

For selected cases, the needle can be held with sponge forceps and inserted under continuous fluoroscopy. The radiation dose to the patient and operator, however, will be increased. For anterior biopsy of cervical lesions (C3 to C7), an anterolateral approach is adopted. The operator's fingers are used to displace the carotid artery/jugular vein bundle laterally and guard the structures from the biopsy needle. The positions of the esophagus and trachea are noted on the image. The needle is directed toward the vertebral body, preferably from the patient's right side, while avoiding the carotid/jugular vascular bundle, trachea, and esophagus (see **Fig. 2**).

For posteriorly located spinal lesions, approaches include transpedicular (**Fig. 11**), transcostovertebral (see **Fig. 1**), and posterolateral paravertebral (see **Fig. 3**). A lateral approach also has been described, to allow access to the vertebral body and the disc. The advantage of this approach is that the needle tip remains away from the nerve roots. If the anterior displacement of abdominal contents is inadequate, however, then this approach should not be used. A transforaminodiskal approach also has been reported. As hematogenous infections usually begin in subchondral bone before involving the intervertebral disk, both the disc and subchondral bone should be sampled together. The needle trajectory chosen is

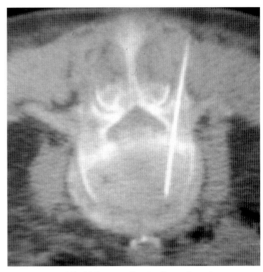

Fig. 11. CT-guided biopsy of L4/5 disc using the transpedicular approach.

perpendicular to the table top,[8] thus making it slightly oblique to the endplates and vertebral discs.

For fine-needle biopsy, multiple small to-and-fro passes are done through the most optimal portion of the lesion to maximize cellular yield. The needle is attached by means of an extension tubing to a 20 mL syringe. 5 mL of air is included in the syringe, and the plunger withdrawn to the 20 mL mark to create a vacuum.[11] The vacuum must be released before withdrawing the needle. For cutting biopsy of soft tissues, the size of the specimen to be obtained should be estimated from images so that the appropriate length of the notched inner stylet can be advanced into the lesion for specimen collection (**Fig. 12**). The outer needle then is released using a spring mechanism (biopsy gun) (see **Fig. 6**) to capture the desired core specimen.

For trephine biopsy, a corkscrew rotating movement is used to advance the serrated needle toward the lesion (**Fig. 13**). Once the proximal end of the anticipated core biopsy specimen is reached, the diamond-tipped inner needle is removed and the outer needle advanced into the lesion using the same corkscrew rotating movement. When the hollow outer needle has traversed the desired length of core specimen, a 10 mL syringe is attached to the needle and the plunger withdrawn to create a vacuum (**Fig. 14**). While maintaining this plunger position, the needle is jiggled gently, with the aim of breaking off the core specimen from the rest of the lesion. The plunger then is released and the needle withdrawn, with the core remaining within the end of the needle (see **Fig. 13C**). A blunt longer inner needle then is

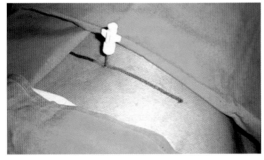

Fig. 10. Photograph shows placement of the biopsy needle at the skin previously marked using a light beam.

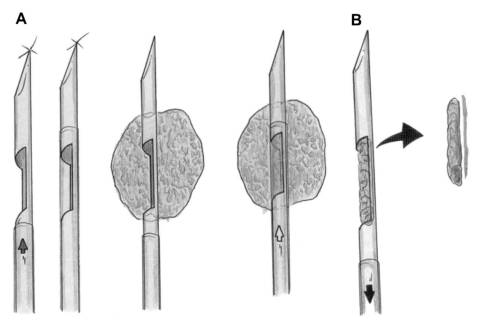

Fig. 12. (*A, B*) Diagrams show cutting biopsy of soft tissues where the specimen is collected within the notched inner stylet that is advanced into the lesion to capture the desired tissue core.

inserted to dislodge the core of tissue. An electric or air-powered drill may be used to facilitate needle insertion, particularly in sclerotic lesions (**Fig. 15**).

Handling of Specimens

FNAC specimens are injected onto glass slides and smeared using a second glass slide. Some slides are air dried and stained with Diff-Quick (Fisher Scientific Biomedical Sciences Incorporated, Swedesboro, New Jersey) for immediate cytologic assessment for adequacy. Other slides are fixed immediately with 95% ethanol for later staining using the Papanicolaou method.[11]

Core biopsy specimens can be placed on wet gauze and sent to the pathology department immediately. Alternatively, they may be placed in 10% formalin. If infection is suspected, additional material should be sent in a sterile container, and/or placed directly into culture material.

Fine-needle material can be applied to rapid staining and preliminary assessment techniques. Imprints or frozen sections also can be obtained from core specimens to enable rapid staining and interpretation.[35] Cytomorphology in technically satisfactory smears is superior even to core biopsy. Double-staining methods allow assessment of nuclear and cytoplasmic detail. For certain cases, FNAC even may yield a microcell block, allowing assessment of tissue architecture. This is rarely obtained in tumors with collagenous matrix, however.[35] The advantage of core specimens is greater tissue volume in general, allowing ancillary tests (eg, cytokeratin, epithelial membrane, CD, light chain, and factor VIII antibody markers) to be performed.[35] For non-Hodgkin lymphoma, consider flushing some aspirate into Hank's solution for flow cytometric immunophenotyping.[35]

Specimens obtained should be divided for histopathology, cytology, and culture, especially when infection is suspected. Michel and colleagues[8] obtained positive microbiological findings in 11 of 18 patients who had spondylodiskitis, and false-negative results in the remaining seven. Sixteen of 18 patients, however, had abnormal histology. The two types of tests were found to be complementary, as some lesions that were negative on microbiology were positive for spondylodiskitis on histology, and vice versa. Imprint cytology has been advocated to improve biopsy outcome.[81] Akerman and colleagues[82] noted that FNAC specimens permitted flow cytometric DNA analysis.

Tips for Successful Biopsy

If possible, osteolytic or soft tissue component of the lesion should be targeted (**Fig. 16**). Sampling only the sclerotic areas may result in a poor yield, comprising crushed bony fragments.[73] In a study of 222 patients who had 38 inadequate biopsies, the most common cause for failure was the sclerotic nature of the lesion, especially osteosarcoma.[83] To

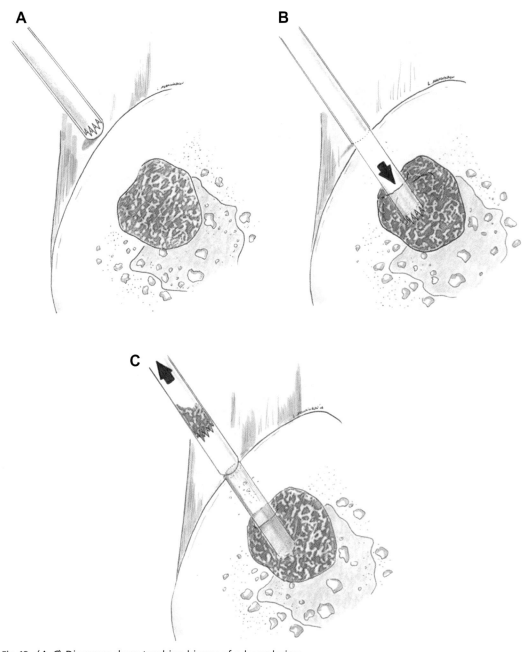

Fig. 13. (*A–C*) Diagrams show trephine biopsy of a bony lesion.

avoid clearly cystic or necrotic areas that are prone to nondiagnostic biopsies, evaluation of contrast CT or MR images may be useful to show the solid and more viable tumor tissue (**Fig. 17**).

Adequate samples should be obtained. Most authors recommend at least three to four good cores of specimen, if possible. For lymphoma, up to eight cores are recommended. False-positive histologic results can have serious therapeutic implications, accounting for a generally conservative approach. Having a cytopathologist or cytotechnologist on standby to ensure adequacy of sample is advantageous. The presence of spindle cells from a tumor biopsy shows that a sarcoma has been targeted correctly. Many practitioners, however, the present authors included, feel that FNAC is generally adequate for sarcomas and lymphoma because of low amounts of tissue obtained and limited expertise in interpretation of aspirated specimens.

For suspected infections, specimens should be sent routinely for histopathological and

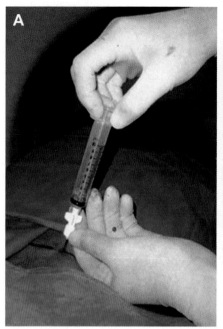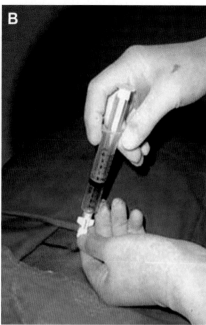

Fig.14. (*A, B*) Photograph shows application of the vacuum through plunger withdraw during the jiggling motion with the aim to dislodge the bony specimen.

microbiological assessment (see **Fig. 16**), because 40% to 60% of histologically proven infections turn out to be culture-negative.[8,53,54] Wu and colleagues[54] found that aspiration of at least 2 mL of fluid from large abscess cavities increased fluid culture positivity to 83%, compared with 29% when no fluid was aspirated. Antibiotics should be discontinued for at least 24 to 48 hours before the biopsy, to decrease possible negative cultures.[43,54] Excessive local bleeding after biopsy can be controlled by instilling gel foam through the needle.

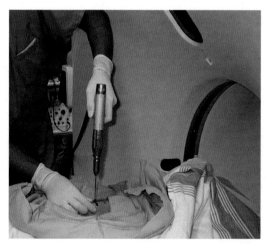

Fig. 15. Use of an air-powered drill attached to the biopsy needle.

Expected Results

Tumors may be classified into (1) malignant versus benign, (2) specific histotype of malignancy, or (3) grade of malignancy (for sarcoma—low [grade 1, 2], high [grade 3, 4], or ungradable).

Recommendations on reporting of bone and soft tissue sarcoma biopsies have been published.[84,85] Histologic subtyping of high-grade adult soft tissue sarcomas is not usually necessary for surgical treatment purposes, but rather when chemotherapy or radiotherapy is needed for advanced lesions.[35]

Several studies have found increased diagnostic accuracy with core biopsy compared with FNAC.[13,14,86–88] Combination techniques[89] usually show increased diagnostic accuracy. Although lesions not well-demonstrated on FNAC can be assessed better with core biopsies, there have been cases described in many series where FNAC resulted in diagnoses that would have been missed with core biopsy. It is therefore prudent to send specimens for both cytologic and histologic assessments. Accuracy rates of malignant lesions are consistently greater than for benign lesions. Distinguishing between benign and malignant lesions also is done more accurately than subtyping a particular malignancy.

Postprocedure Routines

The patient should be monitored in a recovery area for 2 to 4 hours for any deterioration in vital signs

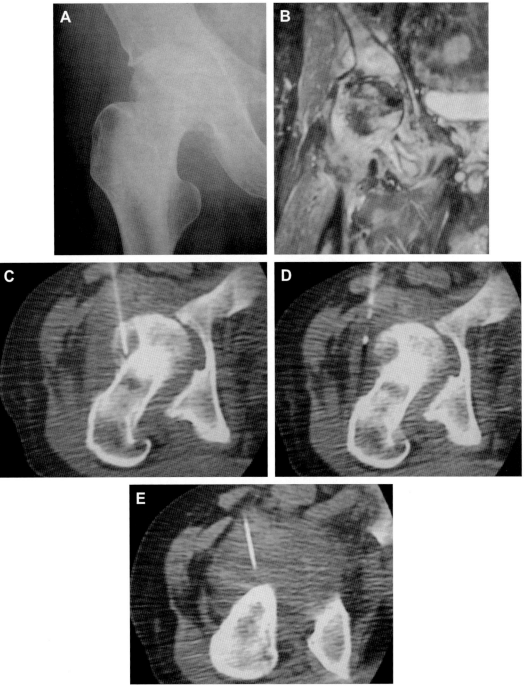

Fig. 16. Maximization of specimen collection in septic arthritis. (*A*) Radiograph shows right hip joint space narrowing and ill-defined osteolytic lesions in the femoral head. (*B*) Coronal T2-W MR image shows patchy hyperintense signal changes in the bones and soft tissue around the right hip joint. Biopsies of the (*C*) femoral head osteolytic lesion, (*D*) thickened synovium, and (*E*) aspiration of joint effusion were performed. Note that different needles were used, tailored according to specimen type.

and puncture site hematoma. Vital signs should be charted every 15 minutes for the first hour, 30 minutes for the next 2 hours, and hourly thereafter. For thoracic spine biopsies, doing a chest radiograph is advisable to exclude pneumothorax, but this is usually not necessary if biopsy had been done under CT guidance. If there are no complications, and the vital signs are stable, the patient is

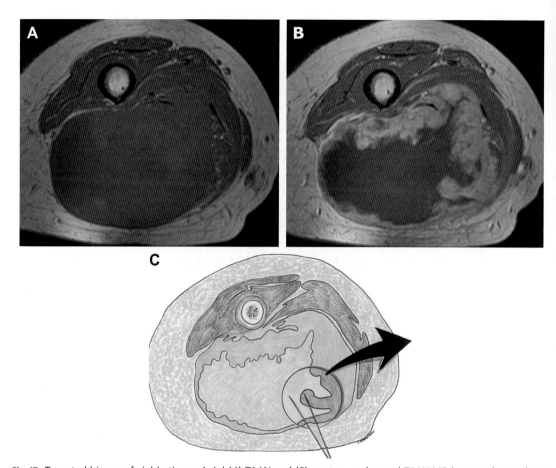

Fig. 17. Targeted biopsy of viable tissue. Axial (*A*) T1-W and (*B*) contrast-enhanced T1-W MR images show a large intramuscular tumor in the thigh with a prominent area of central necrosis. (*C*) Diagram shows planned biopsy route to sample viable tumor and to avoid the necrotic area.

discharged with printed advice regarding potential late complications and instructions on how to proceed and whom to contact if signs or symptoms occur. A follow-up appointment then is scheduled with the referring clinician to discuss the biopsy findings.

Complications

The risk of complications with percutaneous biopsy is lower than for open surgical biopsy. Reported complication rates are between 0% and 10%,[27] with serious complications occurring in less than 1% of patients. This compares favorably against the up to 16% reported complication rate of open biopsy.[63] The most frequently reported complications are:

- Bleeding. This usually responds to compression alone, but in severe cases, may require transfusion.
- Needle breakage

- Infection
- Neurologic injury including paralysis and cord compression (eg, from vertebral hemangioma or metastatic renal cell carcinoma)
- Pneumothorax. For thoracic spine biopsy, reported rates are between 4% and 11%
- Tumor seeding the needle track. Estimated risk of tumor seeding by FNAC is three to nine cases per 100,000 patients. The minimally invasive nature of percutaneous biopsy translates to minimal contamination of adjacent tissues, unlike open biopsy, which potentially can lead to gross contamination. This is minimized further by careful planning of the biopsy track in conjunction with the operating surgeon and excision of the biopsy track during definitive surgery. This can be facilitated by tattooing the skin with indelible ink.
- Diagnostic errors are possible related to sampling factors, tumor type, sample fixation/handling methods, and pathologist experience.

SUMMARY

Image-guided percutaneous biopsy of musculo-skeletal lesions is a safe and useful procedure for diagnosing and managing patients who have suspected bone and soft tissue lesions. Preprocedural careful planning is required, however, including completion of staging before biopsy and being absolutely certain of the biopsy track. Employment of the appropriate imaging technique to guide biopsy, needle selection, specimen handling, adopting a meticulous approach, and being aware of potential complications are advocated.

ACKNOWLEDGMENTS

The authors thank Lorie Marchinkow for providing the line diagrams.

REFERENCES

1. Parapia LA. Trepanning or trephines: a history of bone marrow biopsy. Br J Haematol 2007;139:14–9.
2. Coley Bl SG, Ellis EB. Diagnosis of bone tumors by aspiration. Am J Surg 1931;13:215–24.
3. deSantos LA, Lukeman JM, Wallace S, et al. Percutaneous needle biopsy of bone in the cancer patient. AJR Am J Roentgenol 1978;130:641–9.
4. Lalli AF. Roentgen-guided aspiration biopsies of skeletal lesions. J Can Assoc Radiol 1970;21:71–3.
5. deSantos LA, Murray JA, Ayala AG. The value of percutaneous needle biopsy in the management of primary bone tumors. Cancer 1979;43:735–44.
6. Palombini L, Marino D, Vetrani A, et al. Fine-needle aspiration biopsy in primary malignant and metastatic bone tumors. Appl Pathol 1983;1:76–81.
7. Masood S. Diagnosis of tuberculosis of bone and soft tissue by fine-needle aspiration biopsy. Diagn Cytopathol 1992;8:451–5.
8. Michel SC, Pfirrmann CW, Boos N, et al. CT-guided core biopsy of subchondral bone and intervertebral space in suspected spondylodiskitis. AJR Am J Roentgenol 2006;186:977–80.
9. Akerman M, Berg NO, Persson BM. Fine-needle aspiration biopsy in the evaluation of tumor-like lesions of bone. Acta Orthop Scand 1976;47:129–36.
10. Thommesen P, Frederiksen P. Fine needle aspiration biopsy of bone lesions: clinical value. Acta Orthop Scand 1976;47:137–43.
11. Ward WG Sr, Kilpatrick S. Fine-needle aspiration biopsy of primary bone tumors. Clin Orthop Relat Res 2000;(373):80–7.
12. Appelbaum AH, Kamba TT, Cohen AS, et al. Effectiveness and safety of image-directed biopsies: coaxial technique versus conventional fine-needle aspiration. South Med J 2002;95:212–7.
13. Dupuy DE, Rosenberg AE, Punyaratabandhu T, et al. Accuracy of CT-guided needle biopsy of musculoskeletal neoplasms. AJR Am J Roentgenol 1998;171:759–62.
14. Hau A, Kim I, Kattapuram S, et al. Accuracy of CT-guided biopsies in 359 patients with musculoskeletal lesions. Skeletal Radiol 2002;31:349–53.
15. Bommer KK, Ramzy I, Mody D. Fine-needle aspiration biopsy in the diagnosis and management of bone lesions: a study of 450 cases. Cancer 1997;81:148–56.
16. Kattapuram SV, Rosenthal DI. Percutaneous biopsy of the cervical spine using CT guidance. AJR Am J Roentgenol 1987;149:539–41.
17. Kattapuram SV, Rosenthal DI. Percutaneous biopsy of skeletal lesions. AJR Am J Roentgenol 1991;157:935–42.
18. Khuu H, Moore D, Young S, et al. Examination of tumor and tumor-like conditions of bone. Ann Diagn Pathol 1999;3:364–9.
19. Leffler SG, Chew FS. CT-guided percutaneous biopsy of sclerotic bone lesions: diagnostic yield and accuracy. AJR Am J Roentgenol 1999;172:1389–92.
20. Logan PM, Connell DG, O'Connell JX, et al. Image-guided percutaneous biopsy of musculoskeletal tumors: an algorithm for selection of specific biopsy techniques. AJR Am J Roentgenol 1996;166:137–41.
21. Yao L, Nelson SD, Seeger LL, et al. Primary musculoskeletal neoplasms: effectiveness of core-needle biopsy. Radiology 1999;212:682–6.
22. Vieillard MH, Boutry N, Chastanet P, et al. Contribution of percutaneous biopsy to the definite diagnosis in patients with suspected bone tumor. Joint Bone Spine 2005;72:53–60.
23. Madhavan VP, Smile SR, Chandra SS, et al. Value of core-needle biopsy in the diagnosis of soft tissue tumors. Indian J Pathol Microbiol 2002;45:165–8.
24. Liu XM, Wang WC, Liu MH, et al. [Application of ultrasound-guided percutaneous biopsy in the preoperative diagnosis and treatment of bone tumors]. Zhong Nan Da Xue Xue Bao Yi Xue Ban 2005;30:694–6 [in Chinese].
25. Konermann W, Wuisman P, Hillmann A, et al. [Value of sonographically guided biopsy in the histological diagnosis of benign and malignant soft tissue and bone tumors]. Z Orthop Ihre Grenzgeb 1995;133:411–21 [in German].
26. Kilpatrick SE, Ward WG, Chauvenet AR, et al. The role of fine-needle aspiration biopsy in the initial diagnosis of pediatric bone and soft tissue tumors: an institutional experience. Mod Pathol 1998;11:923–8.
27. Welker JA, Henshaw RM, Jelinek J, et al. The percutaneous-needle biopsy is safe and recommended in the diagnosis of musculoskeletal masses. Cancer 2000;89:2677–86.
28. Samii VF, Nyland TG, Werner LL, et al. Ultrasound-guided fine-needle aspiration biopsy of bone lesions: a preliminary report. Vet Radiol Ultrasound 1999;40:82–6.

29. Vignoli M, Ohlerth S, Rossi F, et al. Computed tomography-guided fine-needle aspiration and tissue-core biopsy of bone lesions in small animals. Vet Radiol Ultrasound 2004;45:125–30.

30. Remagen W. [Pathology and classification of bone tumors. Problems in bone biopsy]. Ther Umsch 1979;36:598–604 [in German].

31. Iezzoni JC, Fechner RE. The biopsy. The pathologist's point of view. Surg Oncol Clin N Am 1995;4: 1–14.

32. Kilpatrick SE, Pike EJ, Geisinger KR, et al. Chondroblastoma of bone: use of fine-needle aspiration biopsy and potential diagnostic pitfalls. Diagn Cytopathol 1997;16:65–71.

33. Domanski HA. Fine-needle aspiration cytology of soft tissue lesions: diagnostic challenges. Diagn Cytopathol 2007;35:768–73.

34. Rinas AC, Ward WG, Kilpatrick SE. Potential sampling error in fine-needle aspiration biopsy of dedifferentiated chondrosarcoma: a report of 4 cases. Acta Cytol 2005;49:554–9.

35. Domanski HA, Akerman M, Carlen B, et al. Coreneedle biopsy performed by the cytopathologist: a technique to complement fine-needle aspiration of soft tissue and bone lesions. Cancer 2005;105: 229–39.

36. Powers CN, Berardo MD, Frable WJ. Fine-needle aspiration biopsy: pitfalls in the diagnosis of spindle-cell lesions. Diagn Cytopathol 1994;10:232–40 [discussion: 241].

37. Garland DE. A clinical perspective on common forms of acquired heterotopic ossification. Clin Orthop Relat Res 1991;(263):13–29.

38. Greenspan A. Benign bone-forming lesions: osteoma, osteoid osteoma, and osteoblastoma. Clinical, imaging, pathologic, and differential considerations. Skeletal Radiol 1993;22:485–500.

39. Greenspan A. Bone island (enostosis): current concept—a review. Skeletal Radiol 1995;24:111–5.

40. Lambiase RE, Levine SM, Terek RM, et al. Long bone surface osteomas: imaging features that may help avoid unnecessary biopsies. AJR Am J Roentgenol 1998;171:775–8.

41. Chew FS, Richardson ML. Radiological reasoning: a benign-appearing bone mass. AJR Am J Roentgenol 2005;184:S169–74.

42. Resnick D, Kransdorf MJ. Bone and joint imaging. 3rd edition. Philadelphia: Elsevier Saunders; 2005. p. 1522.

43. Peh WCG. Imaging-guided bone biopsy. Ann Acad Med Singapore 2003;32:557–61.

44. Peh WCG. The role of imaging in the staging of bone tumors. Crit Rev Oncol Hematol 1999;31: 147–67.

45. Destombe C, Botton E, Le Gal G, et al. Investigations for bone metastasis from an unknown primary. Joint Bone Spine 2007;74:85–9.

46. Ledermann HP, Schweitzer ME, Morrison WB, et al. MR imaging findings in spinal infections: rules or myths? Radiology 2003;228:506–14.

47. Turpin S, Lambert R. Role of scintigraphy in musculoskeletal and spinal infections. Radiol Clin North Am 2001;39:169–89.

48. Ruhs SA, el-Khoury GY, Chrischilles EA. A cost minimization approach to the diagnosis of skeletal neoplasms. Skeletal Radiol 1996;25:449–54.

49. Ashford RU, McCarthy SW, Scolyer RA, et al. Surgical biopsy with intraoperative frozen section. An accurate and cost-effective method for diagnosis of musculoskeletal sarcomas. J Bone Joint Surg Br 2006;88:1207–11.

50. Fraser-Hill MA, Renfrew DL, Hilsenrath PE. Percutaneous needle biopsy of musculoskeletal lesions. 2. Cost-effectiveness. AJR Am J Roentgenol 1992; 158:813–8.

51. Howard CB, Einhorn M, Dagan R, et al. Fine-needle bone biopsy to diagnose osteomyelitis. J Bone Joint Surg Br 1994;76:311–4.

52. Schweitzer ME, Deely DM, Beavis K, et al. Does the use of lidocaine affect the culture of percutaneous bone biopsy specimens obtained to diagnose osteomyelitis? An in vitro and in vivo study. AJR Am J Roentgenol 1995;164:1201–3.

53. White LM, Schweitzer ME, Deely DM, et al. Study of osteomyelitis: utility of combined histologic and microbiologic evaluation of percutaneous biopsy samples. Radiology 1995;197:840–2.

54. Wu JS, Gorbachova T, Morrison WB, et al. Imaging-guided bone biopsy for osteomyelitis: are there factors associated with positive or negative cultures? AJR Am J Roentgenol 2007;188:1529–34.

55. Chew FS, Kline MJ. Diagnostic yield of CT-guided percutaneous aspiration procedures in suspected spontaneous infectious diskitis. Radiology 2001; 218:211–4.

56. Dich VQ, Nelson JD, Haltalin KC. Osteomyelitis in infants and children. A review of 163 cases. Am J Dis Child 1975;129:1273–8.

57. Peh WCG. CT-guided percutaneous biopsy of spinal lesions. Biomedical Imaging and Interventional Journal 2006;2:e25.

58. Kandarpa K, Aruny JE. Handbook of interventional radiologic procedures. 3rd edition. Philadelphia: Lippincott Williams & Wilkins; 2002. p. 765.

59. Barth KH, Matsumoto AH. Patient care in interventional radiology: a perspective. Radiology 1991; 178:11–7.

60. Davies NM, Livesley PJ, Cannon SR. Recurrence of an osteosarcoma in a needle biopsy track. J Bone Joint Surg Br 1993;75:977–8.

61. Schwartz HS, Spengler DM. Needle tract recurrences after closed biopsy for sarcoma: three cases and review of the literature. Ann Surg Oncol 1997;4: 228–36.

62. Wafa H, Grimer RJ. Surgical options and outcomes in bone sarcoma. Expert Rev Anticancer Ther 2006;6:239–48.

63. Mankin HJ, Mankin CJ, Simon MA. The hazards of the biopsy, revisited. Members of the Musculoskeletal Tumor Society. J Bone Joint Surg Am 1996;78: 656–63.

64. Liu PT, Valadez SD, Chivers FS, et al. Anatomically based guidelines for core needle biopsy of bone tumors: implications for limb-sparing surgery. Radiographics 2007;27:189–205 [discussion: 206].

65. Anderson MW, Temple HT, Dussault RG, et al. Compartmental anatomy: relevance to staging and biopsy of musculoskeletal tumors. AJR Am J Roentgenol 1999;173:1663–71.

66. Toomayan GA, Robertson F, Major NM. Lower extremity compartmental anatomy: clinical relevance to radiologists. Skeletal Radiol 2005;34: 307–13.

67. Toomayan GA, Robertson F, Major NM, et al. Upper extremity compartmental anatomy: clinical relevance to radiologists. Skeletal Radiol 2006;35:195–201.

68. Haaga JR, LiPuma JP, Bryan PJ, et al. Clinical comparison of small- and large-caliber cutting needles for biopsy. Radiology 1983;146:665–7.

69. Coucher JR, Dimmick SJ. Coaxial cutting needle biopsies: how important is it to rotate the cutting needle between passes? Clin Radiol 2007;62:808–11.

70. Bickels J, Jelinek JS, Shmookler BM, et al. Biopsy of musculoskeletal tumors. Current concepts. Clin Orthop Relat Res 1999;(368):212–9.

71. Yang YJ, Damron TA. Comparison of needle core biopsy and fine-needle aspiration for diagnostic accuracy in musculoskeletal lesions. Arch Pathol Lab Med 2004;128:759–64.

72. Roberts CC, Morrison WB, Leslie KO, et al. Assessment of bone biopsy needles for sample size, specimen quality, and ease of use. Skeletal Radiol 2005; 34:329–35.

73. Ahrar K, Himmerich JU, Herzog CE, et al. Percutaneous ultrasound-guided biopsy in the definitive diagnosis of osteosarcoma. J Vasc Interv Radiol 2004;15:1329–33.

74. Gupta S, Takhtani D, Gulati M, et al. Sonographically guided fine-needle aspiration biopsy of lytic lesions of the spine: technique and indications. J Clin Ultrasound 1999;27:123–9.

75. Civardi G, Livraghi T, Colombo P, et al. Lytic bone lesions suspected for metastasis: ultrasonically guided fine-needle aspiration biopsy. J Clin Ultrasound 1994;22:307–11.

76. Konermann W, Wuisman P, Ellermann A, et al. Ultrasonographically guided needle biopsy of benign and malignant soft tissue and bone tumors. J Ultrasound Med 2000;19:465–71.

77. Saifuddin A, Mitchell R, Burnett SJ, et al. Ultrasound-guided needle biopsy of primary bone tumors. J Bone Joint Surg Br 2000;82:50–4.

78. Saifuddin A, Burnett SJ, Mitchell R. Pictorial review: ultrasonography of primary bone tumors. Clin Radiol 1998;53:239–46.

79. Daly B, Templeton PA. Real-time CT fluoroscopy: evolution of an interventional tool. Radiology 1999; 211:309–15.

80. Paulson EK, Sheafor DH, Enterline DS, et al. CT fluoroscopy–guided interventional procedures: techniques and radiation dose to radiologists. Radiology 2001;220:161–7.

81. Chang YC, Yu CJ, Lee WJ, et al. Imprint cytology improves accuracy of computed tomography-guided percutaneous transthoracic needle biopsy. Eur Respir J 2008;31:54–61.

82. Akerman M, Killander D, Rydholm A, et al. Aspiration of musculoskeletal tumors for cytodiagnosis and DNA analysis. Acta Orthop Scand 1987;58: 523–8.

83. Ayala AG, Zornosa J. Primary bone tumors: percutaneous needle biopsy. Radiologic–pathologic study of 222 biopsies. Radiology 1983;149:675–9.

84. Abdul-Karim FW, Bauer TW, Kilpatrick SE, et al. Recommendations for the reporting of bone tumors. Association of Directors of Anatomic and Surgical Pathology. Hum Pathol 2004;35:1173–8.

85. Association of Directors of Anatomic and Surgical Pathology. Recommendations for reporting soft tissue sarcomas. Am J Clin Pathol 1999;111: 594–8.

86. Altuntas AO, Slavin J, Smith PJ, et al. Accuracy of computed tomography-guided core-needle biopsy of musculoskeletal tumors. ANZ J Surg 2005;75: 187–91.

87. Ayala AG, Ro JY, Fanning CV, et al. Core-needle biopsy and fine-needle aspiration in the diagnosis of bone and soft tissue lesions. Hematol Oncol Clin North Am 1995;9:633–51.

88. Bennert KW, Abdul-Karim FW. Fine-needle aspiration cytology vs. needle core biopsy of soft tissue tumors. A comparison. Acta Cytol 1994;38:381–4.

89. Schweitzer ME, Gannon FH, Deely DM, et al. Percutaneous skeletal aspiration and core biopsy: complementary techniques. AJR Am J Roentgenol 1996;166:415–8.

Positron Emission Tomography–CT Imaging in Guiding Musculoskeletal Biopsy

Paul J. O'Sullivan, FFRRCSI, MRCPI[a],*, Eric M. Rohren, MD, PhD[b],
John E. Madewell, MD, BS[a]

KEYWORDS
- PET-CT • Musculoskeletal • Biopsy

Bone and soft tissue sarcomas are uncommon neoplasms. The overall incidence of soft tissue sarcomas in children is 0.8/100,000/year.[1] The incidence of primary bone tumors is also low with a rate of 0.9/100,000/year for osteosarcoma alone.[2] In adults, primary bone neoplasms are equally rare; chondrosarcoma has an incidence of 0.8/100,000/year.[2] The survival rates for bone sarcomas are still variable, depending on the histologic subclass. The relative 5-year survival rate is 53.9% for osteosarcoma, 75.2% for chondrosarcoma, and 50.6% for Ewing's sarcoma.[3] Because of this rare incidence, and still often poor survival rates, diagnostic imaging plays a key role in management of these tumors.

Sarcomas, primarily because of their infrequent nature, often represent a difficult diagnostic problem for clinicians. Traditionally, the diagnosis of such tumors depended highly on clinical symptoms, signs, and plain radiography. Although plain radiography is still central to diagnosis of bone tumors, newer modalities have added greatly to diagnosis and particularly staging of sarcomas. Computed tomography (CT) now readily provides detailed imaging of subtle cortical or medullary lesions identified with plain radiography, such as a periosteal reaction, erosion or lytic lesion seen in osseous sarcomas. Magnetic resonance (MR) imaging uses excellent spatial and contrast resolution to provide detailed imaging of soft tissue and bone sarcomas. In particular, MR imaging has greatly improved the accuracy of local and regional staging in sarcomas, identifying different muscle and fascial planes often transgressed by such malignancies.

The fusion of positron emission tomography (PET) and CT to provide PET-CT has become the next progression in tumor imaging. The use of PET (currently most often with F-18 fluorodeoxyglucose [FDG] as the emitting radiopharmaceutical) has provided a diagnostic modality that identifies metabolically active disease in a number of malignancies.[4,5] The integration of PET with CT has provided accurate disease localization. The activity of disease and potential response to chemotherapeutic agents can be assessed with PET-CT.[6] Bone and soft tissue sarcomas frequently are assessed with PET-CT. This is done to identify the extent of local disease and the presence of regional and distant metastatic disease and assess tumor response to ongoing therapy. In this way, PET can improve the staging accuracy and management of patients with sarcomas.

Typically, sites of malignant involvement are visualized on FDG-PET as regions of increased tracer localization (often termed "hypermetabolism"). Such activity is not diagnostic of tumor; however, and abnormalities on PET can

[a] Diagnostic Imaging, University of Texas MD Anderson Cancer Center, 1515 Holcombe Boulevard, Houston, TX 77030, USA
[b] Positron Emission Tomography, University of Texas MD Anderson Cancer Center, 1515 Holcombe Boulevard, Houston, TX 77030, USA
* Corresponding author.
E-mail address: sullypos@yahoo.com (P.J. O'Sullivan).

Radiol Clin N Am 46 (2008) 475–486
doi:10.1016/j.rcl.2008.02.004
0033-8389/08/$ – see front matter © 2008 Elsevier Inc. All rights reserved.

sometimes be caused by benign processes or image artifacts.[7] PET-CT is a highly sensitive technique in identifying metabolically active lesions; however, the resolution is limited especially for small lesions (less than 6–7 mm). It often is not possible to accurately characterize a lesion just by its appearance on PET-CT or other imaging studies. In oncology patients, the presence of local or distal metastases must always be considered, and the presence or absence of such disease can have a large impact on clinical management. The biopsy of a metabolically active lesion often is required in these incidences. The purpose of this article is to discuss musculoskeletal tumors, when biopsy is warranted, when biopsy should be avoided, and the role that PET-CT may have in directing biopsy.

THE PRIMARY LESION

When a primary musculoskeletal malignancy is identified with CT or MR imaging, a PET-CT may be performed to assess the primary lesion, in addition to searching for locoregional metastases and distant disease. A biopsy of all primary sarcomas is required to determine the histologic subtype and to direct appropriate surgery or chemoradiotherapy.

Primary malignant tumors often have higher rates of cellular metabolism when compared with normal tissues. There is an increased metabolic rate in tumor tissue and hence higher glucose use. An increase in the number of glucose membrane transporters has been seen in cells that preferentially uptake FDG.[8] This increased glucose use is thought to be the basis on which FDG is taken up in malignant tissue, which subsequently appears "hot" on an FDG-PET study. This "hot" or FDG-avid focus with CT localization can provide a biopsy target in a suspected malignant tumor. This is process is illustrated in **Fig. 1**. A 28-year-

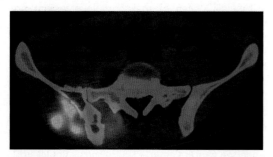

Fig. 1. PET-CT directs biopsy of FDG-avid tumor site: 28-year-old man with FDG-avid osteosarcoma of the pelvis. The FDG-avid tumor and surrounding soft tissue component are readily seen on the fused PET-CT image.

old man was diagnosed with an osteosarcoma within the right side of the pelvis. The fused PET-CT images in this patient showed marked increased FDG uptake seen within the tumor and the extensive surrounding soft-tissue component.

Tumor Heterogeneity

Many primary sarcomas are not uniform in their histologic architecture and have varying degrees of differentiation. Within a tumor, the tissue present may vary from near-normal tissue histology, to gross malignant tumor formation, which may be well-, moderately, or poorly differentiated. This heterogeneity often is seen in retroperitoneal liposarcomas.[9] Using conventional imaging methods, it can be difficult to direct biopsies to sample the regions of highest histologic grade. Often several biopsies of different regions in the tumor will be required, providing an increasing technical challenge for the operator, longer procedure duration, and the potential of increased morbidity to the patient.

PET-CT can be of benefit in directing a biopsy in such patients.[10] When a PET-CT is performed, the varying degree of tumor differentiation often becomes evident because of the varying degrees of FDG accumulation. More metabolically active regions of tumor typically are more aggressive and poorly differentiated. The degree of tracer uptake on PET typically is expressed by the "standardized uptake value" or SUV, which is a semiquantitative measure of radiotracer accumulation within a region of interest. Sites of intense tracer uptake will have higher standardized uptake values[11] and appear brighter on the PET images produced. This is shown in **Fig. 2**. A 64-year-old man had a retroperitoneal liposarcoma. The varying degrees of tumor differentiation are suspected from the PET image (see **Fig. 2**A), which shows marked increased SUV uptake in the posterior aspect of the tumor, corresponding to the poorly differentiated, more aggressive part of the lesion. The corresponding CT image (see **Fig. 2**B) shows higher soft tissue attenuation in the posterior aspect of the tumor and lower attenuation "fat-like" tissue in the anterior aspect of the lesion. A biopsy of the posterior component was performed showing a high-grade dedifferentiated liposarcoma. A prior biopsy had been performed in the anterior aspect of the lesion, producing an "intermediate grade" liposarcoma. The patient's subsequent treatment was directed by the high-grade dedifferentiated component, with surgery and postoperative chemotherapy.

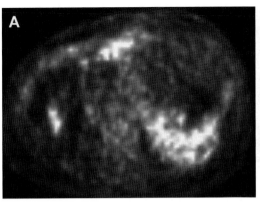 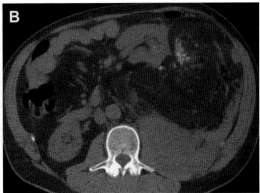

Fig. 2. PET-CT directs biopsy site of heterogeneous tumor: 64-year-old man with retroperitoneal liposarcoma. (A) Unfused PET image shows marked hypermetabolic activity in the posterior aspect of tumor, directing biopsy site. (B) Corresponding CT shows intermediate grade (fatlike) tumor anteriorly, and high-grade (soft tissue) dedifferentiated tumor posteriorly.

Tumor Necrosis and Biopsy Site

Primary sarcoma tumors of the bone and soft tissue often grow to a large size, occasionally greater than 20 cm as in the case of malignant fibrous histiocytoma. The central portion of these tumors often outgrows the blood supply, and the mass becomes centrally necrotic. Some sarcomas can have a large myxomatous component, eg, myxomatous leiomyosarcoma and myxoid malignant peripheral nerve sheath tumors.[12] Using the traditional ultrasound-guided biopsy technique, it is not uncommon to yield a nondiagnostic sample in such tumors with a large necrotic or myxomatous component. The use of PET-CT in this regard can be helpful. The more viable component of the tumor will possess greater metabolic activity and hence a higher SUV, appearing "hotter" on the PET component[13] of the study. The knowledge of this fact is useful in directing the biopsy of primary tumors and increasing the likelihood of attaining a diagnostic sample.

The CT component of the examination provides detailed information about the tumor anatomic location and images adjacent organs or vasculature that should be avoided during the biopsy procedure. This is illustrated in **Fig. 3**. An 18-year-old man presented with a lower extremity osseous malignancy. The fused PET-CT images eloquently identify the hypermetabolic periphery of the lesion. A subsequent biopsy of the tumor periphery showed a high-grade osteoblastic osteosarcoma. The final pathologic resected specimen confirmed the high-grade osteosarcoma with 70% to 75% tumor necrosis.

The utility of PET-CT in directing tumor site biopsy and avoiding adjacent organs and vascular structures is illustrated in **Fig. 4**. A 64-year-old man presented with a right upper quadrant mass and left side pelvic pain. The fused PET-CT images (see **Fig. 4**A) show a mass medial to the liver, with peripheral FDG hypermetabolism. The lesion is intimately related to a number of adjacent small bowel loops (which show normal luminal background FDG activity). The fused PET-CT images of the pelvis (see **Fig. 4**B) show a large destructive mass in the left side of the pelvis, with diffuse FDG hypermetabolism. The femoral vessels are seen to lie anterior to the tumor. The upper abdominal

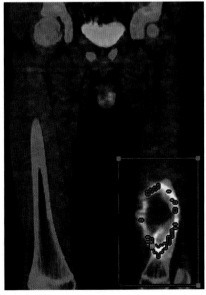

Fig. 3. PET-CT directs biopsy of peripheral tumor hypermetabolism: 18-year-old man with osteoblastic osteosarcoma distal left femur. The fused PET-CT image shows the peripheral tumor hypermetabolism and central tumor necrosis with no FDG activity.

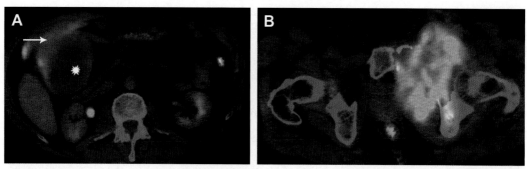

Fig. 4. PET-CT aids inappropriate biopsy of adjacent structures: 64-year-old man with a hemiangiopericytoma of the left side of the pelvis. (*A*) The fused PET-CT image of the abdomen shows an oval-shaped mass (*star*) medial to the liver, with peripheral hypermetabolism, intimately related to the small bowel (*arrow*). (*B*) Fused PET-CT of the pelvis shows a large destructive pelvis mass with diffuse FDG hypermetabolism. Biopsy of this lesion was performed successfully under ultrasound guidance, avoiding the femoral vessels.

lesion did not undergo biopsy because of its intimate relationship to small bowel and extensive necrotic appearance. The pelvic lesion underwent successful biopsy under ultrasound guidance avoiding the femoral vasculature, identifying a metastatic hemiangiopericytoma.

Tumor Upstaging

One of the primary utilities of PET-CT in guiding biopsies of malignancy has been the "upstaging" of malignant tumors. This has been seen in esophageal and lung malignancies[4,5] and has a similar role in musculoskeletal tumors. Previously unidentified locoregional or distant metastases are now not infrequently discovered on PET-CT. Biopsy of these lesions often identifies a previously unsuspected distant metastases. This results in upstaging of the malignancy. This upstaging does place the patient in a group with a poorer prognostic outcome. However, importantly, it more accurately directs appropriate therapy, eg, chemoradiotherapy versus surgery, and prevents unnecessary surgical procedures and decreases potential patient morbidity.

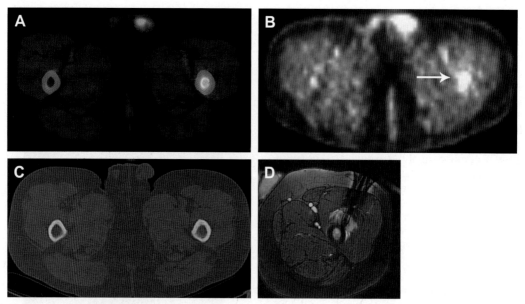

Fig. 5. Unsuspected lesions identified may require biopsy: 48-year-old man with mucinous adenocarcinoma of the anus. (*A*) The fused PET-CT image of the pelvis identifies the hypermetabolic metastases in the left femur. Normal increased FDG activity is noted in the left testis. (*B*) The unfused PET image shows a focus of increased activity in the left femur (*arrow*). (*C*) There is no definite abnormality seen in the femur on the CT study. (*D*) An image of the MR imaging–guided biopsy shows increased signal in the femoral metastases and signal void from the contours of the core biopsy needle.

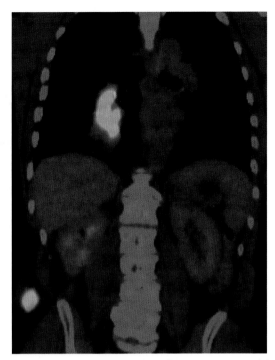

Fig. 6. PET-CT may upstage a malignancy: 63-year-old man diagnosed with non–small cell lung cancer. The fused PET-CT image shows the FDG-avid lung cancer primary and identifies an unsuspected hypermetabolic metastases in the adipose tissue of the right flank.

The ability of PET-CT to direct such biopsies is illustrated in **Figs. 5 and 6**. The first patient is a 48-year-old man with a biopsy-proven poorly differentiated mucinous adenocarcinoma of the anus with extension into the seminal vesicles. A PET-CT was performed for further evaluation. The fused PET-CT images clearly show a hypermetabolic focus within the medullary cavity of the left femur (see **Fig. 5A**). This FDG-avid focus is also seen on the unfused PET images (see **Fig. 5B**) but not visualized on the CT component (see **Fig. 5C**). A MR imaging–guided core biopsy of this lesion (see **Fig. 5D**) identified metastatic mucinous adenocarcinoma consistent with the patient's primary anal adenocarcinoma. The staging of this patient's disease was then upstaged from stage 3A anal cancer to stage 4.

The imaging in this patient also illustrates the benefits of using "fused" PET-CT images. The lesion is not seen on the unfused CT study and is potentially difficult to identify on the unfused PET study alone. The combination of the two modalities provides excellent anatomic localization of this hypermetabolic focus, improves conspicuity, and clearly identifies a lesion requiring biopsy.

The utility of PET-CT in upstaging malignancy is also readily seen in **Fig. 6**. This solitary fused PET-CT image of a 63-year-old man with non–small cell lung cancer (NSCLC), eloquently shows the hypermetabolic right infrahilar lung primary. The same image shows a right flank hypermetabolic soft tissue lesion. A fine-needle aspiration biopsy was performed on the basis of the PET-CT and produced metastatic tissue consistent with NSCLC. This metastatic lesion would have been outside the typical CT thorax field of view performed in most institutions for evaluation of NSCLC, and thus this lesion would not have been identified. The tumor staging in this patient increased from stage 2 to stage 4, with the PET-CT identification and subsequent biopsy of this distal metastasis.

METASTASES
Field of View

PET-CT is now used frequently in the re-assessment of patients who have had a primary malignancy treated. It has been shown to be a useful modality in the identification of occult metastases in sarcomas.[14] Similarly new, occult, or unsuspected metastases may be discovered during the subsequent follow-up period after definitive treatment with surgery or radiochemotherapy. PET-CT not infrequently identifies lesions requiring biopsy because of the wider field of view used. On PET-CT, a primary sarcoma in the thorax or abdomen is typically assessed with an imaging field-of-view extending from the skull vertex to the lesser trochanter. A lower extremity sarcoma would be assessed with the above field-of-view plus complete imaging of the entire lower extremities.

The utility of PET-CT in directing biopsies in this regard is illustrated in **Fig. 7**. A 54-year-old man with a history of melanoma in the left calf 4 years previously was evaluated with PET-CT. A prior inguinal lymph node dissection had been performed, and there was no clinical evidence of recurrence. The fused PET-CT image (see **Fig. 7**) shows an FDG-avid focus in the left humeral head. A biopsy of this lesion was performed, identifying metastatic melanoma in bone. Surgical resection of this lesion was undertaken, followed by postoperative radiotherapy.

Melanoma is a disease process that often spreads via the lymphatic system, and widely dispersed cutaneous lesions are not infrequent. These patients often are followed up with clinically because complete imaging of the entire body is not practical or sensitive. PET-CT enables imaging of most or all of the entire body and is a useful tool

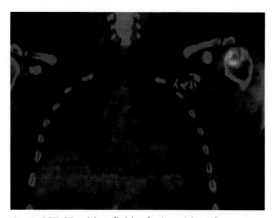

Fig. 7. PET-CT wider field of view identifies unsuspected metastases: 54-year-old man with a prior diagnosis of melanoma in the left forearm. The fused PET-CT image identified an FDG-avid lesion in the left humerus. A core bone biopsy produced metastatic melanoma in bone.

in identifying lesions that require biopsy in melanoma and other malignancies.[10]

F-18 Fluorodeoxyglucose Activity of Lesions

Many different sarcomas produce metastases that have increased FDG uptake. Like the primary tumor, these metastases have higher glucose use than normal tissues (see **Fig. 7**) and appear hypermetabolic on the PET component. Sarcomas are known to frequently produce metastases in the lung parenchyma. Unfortunately, not all pulmonary metastases are seen to possess increased FDG activity on PET imaging. In particular, the identification of small lung nodules (<1 cm in size) can be problematic on PET alone.[15] One investigator has stated that the sensitivity for PET in identifying

pulmonary metastases is as low as 68.3%, whereas the sensitivity for CT in the same study was 95%. The same investigator further stated that a significant number of known pulmonary metastases were not visualized on PET.[15] Therefore, the lack of visible FDG uptake in otherwise suspicious pulmonary nodules does not exclude the possibility of metastatic disease and should not preclude further workup. Comparison with prior imaging, or a fine-needle aspiration biopsy (FNAB) of these pulmonary nodules often is necessary for definitive diagnosis.

An illustration of the necessity to biopsy such PET negative pulmonary nodules is illustrated in **Fig. 8**. A 14-year-old girl with a previously resected distal femur high-grade osteosarcoma had a 13-mm pulmonary nodule identified on PET-CT (see **Fig.** 8A). This nodule clearly has no increased FDG activity compared with the highly FDG-avid adjacent myocardium. In addition, a focus of calcification can be seen centrally in this nodule. An FNAB of this lesion performed under CT guidance (see **Fig.** 8b) found metastatic high-grade osteosarcoma with osteoblastic and chondroblastic differentiation.

There are other limitations of PET-CT in directing the biopsy of suspicious lesions. FDG is not only accumulated by malignant tumors, but it is also accumulated by a number of benign processes.[16] Benign tumors that have been demonstrated to show increased FDG uptake and appear hot on PET-CT include thyroid adenomas, Warthin tumors, neurofibromas, and adenomatous colonic polyps.[16]

This is illustrated in **Fig. 9**. A 53-year-old man with a diagnosis of cystic squamous cell carcinoma of the tongue underwent a PET-CT for evaluation of potential metastatic disease. An expansile lytic

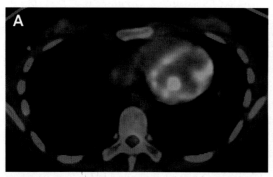
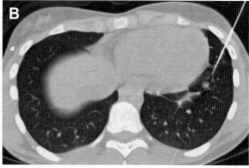

Fig. 8. Pulmonary metastases often not FDG avid and require biopsy: 14-year-old girl with a previously resected high-grade distal femur osteosarcoma. (A) Fused PET-CT of the thorax shows the non–FDG-avid 13- to14-mm (short-axis) metastatic pulmonary nodule adjacent the normal markedly FDG-avid myocardium. Central nodular calcification is present. Incidental note is made of a second calcified nodule in the adipose tissue lateral to the right breast, presumed metastases in this patient with osteosarcoma. (B) A CT image of the FNAB of this FDG-negative pulmonary osteosarcoma metastases.

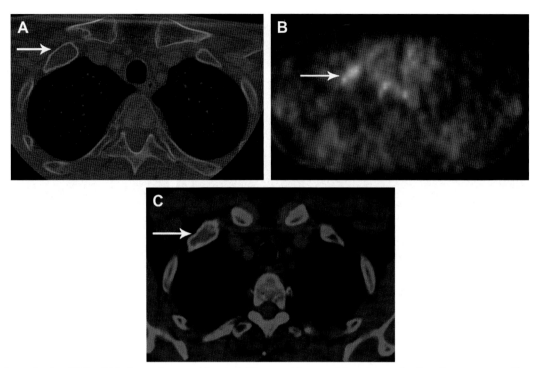

Fig. 9. Benign FDG-avid lesions often are biopsied: 53-year-old man with a diagnosis of cystic squamous cell carcinoma of the tongue. (*A*) The CT image shows an expansile, lytic lesion in the anterior aspect of the right first rib (*arrow*). (*B*) The unfused PET images show increased metabolic activity in this lesion (*arrow*). (*C*) The fused PET-CT images confirm the increased focus of FDG activity in the lytic lesion with the first rib (*arrow*). Note the other imaged ribs do not show any hypermetabolic activity.

lesion is seen on the CT component in the anterior aspect of the right first rib (see **Fig. 9**A). The PET component shows increased FDG uptake in this lesion (see **Fig. 9**B), and the fused PET-CT images (see **Fig. 9**C) confirm the hypermetabolic activity within this lesion in the right first rib. A subsequent CT-guided biopsy was performed that produced fragments of bland hyaline cartilage. The lesion was diagnosed as an enchondroma.

As stated, identification of metastases is based on their hypermetabolic activity and increased uptake of FDG when compared with surrounding tissues. However, not all metastases avidly trap FDG. Well-differentiated metastases may not have high expression of cell surface glucose transporter molecules and may not be hypermetabolic, such as in prostate cancer.[17] One investigator has recently compared the utility of PET-CT to combined CT, MR imaging and bone scan (BS) in detecting distal metastases in pediatric sarcomas. PET-CT detected distal metastases in 10 of 13 patients (77%). Combined CT/BS also failed to identify distal metastases in three patients.[17] Although PET-CT is certainly a useful modality in the detection of distant metastases, further work is still required to assess its true sensitivity.

The potential lack of increased FDG uptake in distal metastases is illustrated in **Fig. 10**. A 34-year-old woman had with high-grade osteosarcoma of the left upper extremity. The coronal fused PET-CT of the thorax shows a densely calcified osteosarcoma in the left humerus. A peripheral hypermetabolic active rim of tumor is readily seen (see **Fig. 10**A). A coronal fused PET-CT of the thorax and abdomen shows a 2-cm densely calcified mass within the adipose tissue of the right flank (see **Fig. 10**B). Minimal background FDG activity is seen in this lesion. An excision biopsy proved this densely calcified lesion to be high-grade metastatic osteosarcoma. This patient's imaging shows that even in the absence of increased FDG uptake, biopsy of a suspicious lesion may still be warranted.

Resolution

One of the known limitations of PET imaging is the relatively low spatial resolution, typically on the order of 5 to 6 mm.[18] This, coupled with the fact that increased FDG activity is seen in a range of benign and malignant processes, can result in FDG-avid foci being identified but without further

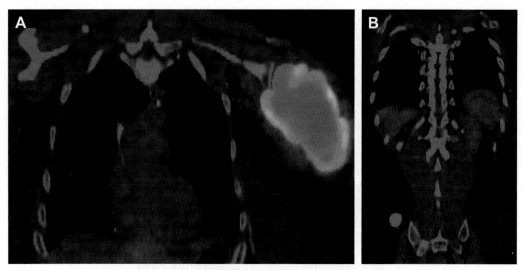

Fig. 10. Non–FDG-avid metastases require biopsy: 34-year-old woman with high-grade osteosarcoma of the left upper extremity. (*A*) Fused PET-CT shows osteosarcoma of the left humerus with peripheral hypermetabolic rim. (*B*) Fused coronal abdominal PET-CT show a 2-cm densely calcified metastases within the adipose tissue of the right flank.

differentiation of the likely histologic nature of the lesion. The addition of CT to the PET component has improved spatial resolution, but additional imaging with MRI or a tissue biopsy often is still required.

An illustration of this potential issue is seen in **Fig. 11**. A 57-year-old woman who had a prior excision of a liposarcoma of the left ankle re-presented with a painful mass in the left calf. The fused PET-CT images show a markedly FDG-avid focus within the muscle of the left calf (see **Fig. 11**A). This could easily represent regional metastases from the excised liposarcoma. MR imaging was performed for further evaluation. The axial T1, fat-saturated,

postgadolinium image shows a rim-enhancing collection in the calf periphery and enhancing lateral gastrocnemius muscle but no discrete mass. A biopsy of this collection under ultrasound guidance produced frank purulent fluid from an abscess. This again shows the potential need for a biopsy in the presence of an FDG-avid lesion.

SPECIFIC ISSUES

PET-CT has shown itself to be a useful modality in identifying lesions of high FDG uptake concerning metastases that require a biopsy. It has also been

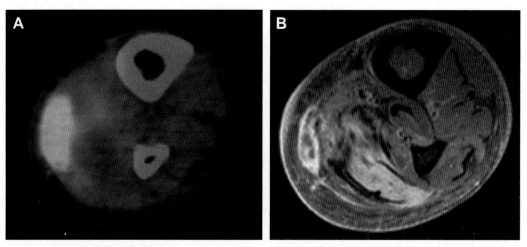

Fig. 11. Low resolution of PET-CT may necessitate biopsy: A 57-year-old woman with a prior liposarcoma of the left ankle, re-presents with calf pain. (*A*) Fused PET-CT of the calf shows a hypermetabolic mass in the soft tissues medially. (*B*) Axial T1 postgadolinium image shows the rim-enhancing abscess in the soft tissues.

useful in monitoring therapeutic interventions such as chemoradiotherapy. Changes in the maximum standardized uptake values (SUV) as a response to therapy can be seen in lesions at PET-CT imaging before any morphologic change in the appearance of a lesion.[19] A decrease in the maximum SUV represents a favorable response to ongoing chemotherapy. This affords the treating clinician earlier knowledge of a beneficial response to potentially toxic ongoing therapeutic regimes or provides useful information on the potential need for selection for an alternative therapeutic regime. This is particularly seen in lymphoma.[20]

Repeat Biopsy

With a favorable chemotherapeutic response, the tumor should decrease progressively in size and

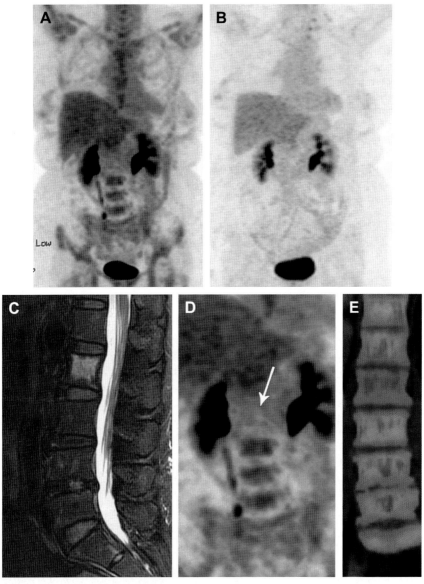

Fig. 12. AVN may mimic metastases on MR imaging but has little to no activity on PET-CT: 54-year-old woman with large B-cell lymphoma stage 4 with extensive bone involvement. (*A*) An unfused coronal PET image shows the diffuse heterogeneous marrow pattern in this patient with extensive osseous lymphoma. There is some superimposed marrow activity caused by a chemotherapy response. (*B*) A complete therapeutic response with no residual increased FDG activity. A physiologic background FDG distribution is seen. (*C*) Sagittal T2 MR imaging of the lumbar spine shows diffuse high T2 signal in the second lumbar vertebrae. (*D*) Coronal cropped PET image of the lumbar spine shows an absence of FDG uptake in the L2 vertebra (*arrow*). Normal excretion of FDG is seen in the renal calyces. (*E*) Coronal cropped PET-CT confirms the absence of increased FDG uptake in the L2 vertebra.

intensity on PET-CT. A complete therapeutic response is a frequently used phrase in the PET-CT report to indicate that there is either no residual activity in the mass or the degree of uptake is equivalent to background soft tissues (**Fig. 12**A,B). In these patients, even though it is not possible to exclude potential microscopic residual disease at the tumor site, a repeat biopsy usually is not performed to assess for residual disease. A biopsy at these sites would likely have a low diagnostic yield, produce unnecessary patient discomfort, and would unlikely affect patient management.

Current practice involves ongoing follow-up of these treated tumor sites with PET-CT to assess for potential tumor recurrence and performing a biopsy when a suspicious FDG-avid lesion with an increasing maximum SUV is seen.[21] The importance of the need for performing a repeat biopsy is evident in patients being treated for Hodgkin's disease. One investigator recently reviewed 27 patients with positive PET-CT studies suggestive of recurrence of Hodgkin's disease. Four patients (4 of 27, 14.8%) had a false-positive result, the subsequent biopsy revealing only inflammatory changes. This illustrates the need for repeat biopsy to avoid unnecessary toxic chemotherapeutic regimes.[22]

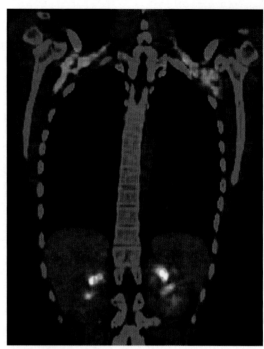

Fig. 13. Typical brown fat distribution does not require biopsy: 24-year-old woman with marked increased FDG uptake in a typical brown-fat distribution around the shoulders on a fused coronal PET-CT image.

Avascular Necrosis

PET-CT has been identified as a useful modality in assessing treatment response in patients with soft tissue[20] and osseous lymphoma.[23] A hypermetabolic FDG-avid lesion should be appreciated at a site of local tumor, recurrence, or metastatic disease. In patients who undergo chemoradiotherapy, potential osseous side affects such as avascular necrosis (AVN) may be observed. The appearance of these lesions at MRI can be unusual. The typical peripheral serpiginous border of AVN may not be seen. Patchy regions of high signal are seen in acute edematous areas of AVN, and potential MRI features mimicking those of metastatic disease may be observed. PET-CT can be of benefit in evaluating these lesions and directing if a biopsy is required.

This is also illustrated in **Fig. 12**. A 54-year-old woman with a history of large B-cell lymphoma stage 4 with extensive bone involvement had acute low back pain. MR imaging of the lumbar spine was performed for evaluation. High signal on the T2 images was seen throughout the L2 vertebra, which is concerning for metastatic disease (see **Fig. 12**C). The corresponding unfused PET lumbar spine images show an absence of increased FDG activity in this vertebra, with

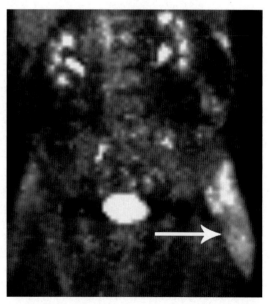

Fig. 14. FDG-avid muscle activity does not necessitate biopsy: 56-year-old man with unilateral increased FDG uptake (*arrow*) in the distribution of the left glutei muscle groups on an unfused coronal PET image.

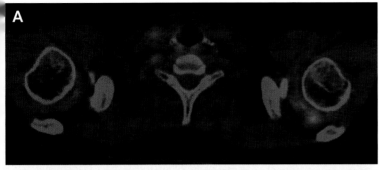

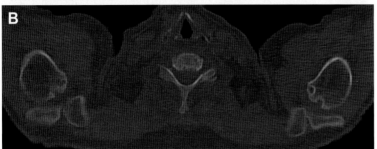

Fig. 15. FDG-avid osteoarthritis does not necessitate biopsy: 64-year-old man with shoulder pain. (*A*) Increased periarticular FDG uptake is seen in the left shoulder on the fused PET-CT. (*B*) Changes of articular surface sclerosis and subchondral cyst formation are seen on the unfused CT component.

increased activity in all adjacent vertebrae (see **Fig. 12**D). The fused PET-CT confirms the absence of activity in the L2 vertebra (see **Fig. 12**E). A diagnosis of avascular necrosis was made, and a biopsy was not performed.

Avoid Biopsy

As previously stated, there are a number of benign lesions (eg, neurofibromas) that can take up FDG and appear hypermetabolic. There are also a number of physiologic and nonmalignant processes that can also appear hypermetabolic on PET-CT.[7] These physiologic and nonmalignant processes often have a typical pattern at PET-CT that enables them to be identified and hence do not warrant biopsy.

Brown fat is commonly identified at PET-CT. It is typically seen in young female patients in the neck, shoulders (**Fig. 13**), and paravertebral regions or within the mediastinum and retroperitoneum.[24] It can be confidently identified by its characteristic distribution, the absence of a focal mass, and the presence of fat on the CT component of the examination. Another commonly encountered FDG-avid physiologic process is muscle activity. The patient is required to remain still before and during the PET-CT examination to prevent a focal increase in glucose use by moving muscle groups. The focal increased FDG uptake that occurs can be misleading, because it often is a unilateral process. However linear FDG uptake in a known muscle group position should suggest the diagnosis (**Fig. 14**). Other inflammatory conditions

such as osteoarthritis and rheumatoid arthritis frequently produce foci of increased FDG uptake. The periarticular distribution of FDG (**Fig. 15**A) and the presence of erosions or sclerosis on the CT component (**Fig. 15**B) should suggest the diagnosis.

Future Directions

The real-time use of PET-CT guidance for direction of biopsies is not yet performed as far as the authors are aware. However, it should be potentially feasible. The initial image acquisition would take longer to acquire (3–4 minutes) and obtain a static PET-CT of the region of interest. After that the biopsy would be performed purely by CT guidance.

A high-resolution positron emission mammography imaging and biopsy device (PEM) has been developed to detect and guide the biopsy of suspicious breast lesions.[25] This can potentially improve diagnosis of cancer in women with radiodense or fibrocystic breasts. PET images are acquired to detect suspicious focal uptake of the radiotracer and guide biopsy of the area. Limited-angle PEM images could then be used to verify the biopsy needle position before tissue sampling.

SUMMARY

PET-CT is a useful device in identifying musculoskeletal lesions that require biopsy. It can be used to localize the primary lesion, identify a site to biopsy, and evaluate metastatic lesions that require follow-up biopsies. Not all malignant tumors have hypermetabolic activity, and there are many benign lesions and physiologic processes that do have increased FDG uptake. Knowledge of these issues is important when reviewing PET-CT and directing subsequent musculoskeletal biopsies.

REFERENCES

1. Weihkopf T, Blettner M, Dantonello T, et al. Incidence and time trends of soft tissue sarcomas in German children 1985–2004–a report from the population-based German Childhood Cancer Registry. Eur J Cancer 2008;44(3):432–40.

2. Larsson SE, Lorentzon R. The incidence of malignant primary bone tumors in relation to age, sex and site. A study of osteogenic sarcoma, chondrosarcoma and Ewing's sarcoma diagnosed in Sweden from 1958 to 1968. J Bone Joint Surg Br 1974;56:534–40.

3. Damron TA, Ward WG, Stewart A. Osteosarcoma, chondrosarcoma, and Ewing's sarcoma: national cancer data base report. Clin Orthop Relat Res 2007;459:40–7.

4. Bruzzi JF, Munden RF. PET/CT imaging of lung cancer. J Thorac Imaging 2006;21:123–36.

5. Bruzzi JF, Munden RF, Truong MT, et al. PET/CT of esophageal cancer: its role in clinical management. Radiographics 2007;27:1635–52.

6. Konski AA, Cheng JD, Goldberg M, et al. Correlation of molecular response as measured by 18-FDG positron emission tomography with outcome after chemoradiotherapy in patients with esophageal carcinoma. Int J Radiat Oncol Biol Phys 2007;69: 358–63.

7. Truong MT, Erasmus JJ, Macapinlac HA, et al. Integrated positron emission tomography/computed tomography in patients with non-small cell lung cancer: normal variants and pitfalls. J Comput Assist Tomogr 2005;29:205–9.

8. de Geus-Oei LF, van Krieken JH, Aliredjo RP, et al. Biological correlates of FDG uptake in non-small cell lung cancer. Lung Cancer 2007;55:79–87.

9. Tomonaga T, Okuyama K, Nagao K, et al. [Retroperitoneal liposarcoma with various histological figures]. Gan No Rinsho 1986;32:927–32 [in Japanese].

10. Nguyen NC, Chaar BT, Osman MM. Prevalence and patterns of soft tissue metastasis: detection with true whole-body F-18 FDG PET/CT. BMC Med Imaging 2007;12:7–8.

11. Suzuki R, Watanabe H, Yanagawa T, et al. PET evaluation of fatty tumors in the extremity: possibility of using the standardized uptake value (SUV) to differentiate benign tumors from liposarcoma. Ann Nucl Med 2005;19:661–70.

12. Graadt van Roggen JF, Hogendoorn PC, Fletcher CD. Myxoid tumors of soft tissue. Histopathology 1999;35:291–312.

13. Park HS, Chung JW, Jae HJ, et al. FDG-PET for evaluating the antitumor effect of intraarterial 3-bromopyruvate administration in a rabbit VX2 liver tumor model. Korean J Radiol 2007;8:216–24.

14. Kobayashi E, Kawai A, Seki K, et al. Bilateral adrenal gland metastasis from malignant fibrous histiocytoma: value of [F-18] FDG PET-CT for diagnosis of occult metastases. Ann Nucl Med 2006;20:695–8.

15. Iagaru A, Chawla S, Menendez L, et al. 18F-FDG PET and PET/CT for detection of pulmonary metastases from musculoskeletal sarcomas. Nucl Med Commun 2006;27:795–802.

16. Metser U, Miller E, Lerman H, et al. Benign nonphysiologic lesions with increased 18F-FDG uptake on PET/CT: characterization and incidence. AJR Am J Roentgenol 2007;189:1203–10.

17. Takahashi N, Inoue T, Lee J, et al. The roles of PET and PET/CT in the diagnosis and management of prostate cancer. Oncology 2008;72:226–33.

18. Surti S, Karp JS. Imaging characteristics of a 3-dimensional GSO whole-body PET camera. J Nucl Med 2004;45:1040–9.

19. Beresford M, Lyburn I, Sanghera B, et al. Serial integrated (18) F-fluorodeoxythymidine PET/CT monitoring neoadjuvant chemotherapeutic response in invasive ductal carcinoma. Breast J 2007;13: 424–5.

20. Hutchings M, Mikhaeel NG, Fields PA, et al. Prognostic value of interim FDG-PET after two or three cycles of chemotherapy in Hodgkin lymphoma. Ann Oncol 2005;16:1160–8.

21. Soudack M, Shalom RB, Israel O, et al. Utility of sonographically guided biopsy in metabolically suspected recurrent lymphoma. J Ultrasound Med 2008;27:225–31.

22. Schaefer NG, Taverna C, Strobel K, et al. Hodgkin disease: diagnostic value of FDG PET/CT after first-line therapy–is biopsy of FDG-avid lesions still needed? Radiology 2007;244:257–62.

23. Schaefer NG, Strobel K, Taverna C, et al. Bone involvement in patients with lymphoma: the role of FDG-PET/CT. Eur J Nucl Med Mol Imaging 2007; 34:60–7.

24. Clarke JR, Brglevska S, Lau EW, et al. Atypical brown fat distribution in young males demonstrated on PET/CT. Clin Nucl Med 2007;32:679–82.

25. Raylman RR, Majewski S, Smith MF, et al. The positron emission mammography/tomography breast imaging and biopsy system (PEM/PET): design, construction and phantom-based measurements. Phys Med Biol 2008;53:637–53.

Spinal Injection Procedures: A Review of Concepts, Controversies, and Complications

Manraj K.S. Heran, MD, FRCPC[a,b,*],
Andrew D. Smith, MBChB, FRANZCR[a], Gerald M. Legiehn, MD, FRCPC[c]

KEYWORDS

- Spinal injections • Complications • Steroids • Epidural
- Facet • Nerve • Synovial cyst • Fluoroscopy

The field of spinal injection procedures is growing at a tremendous rate. Many disciplines are involved, including radiology, anesthesiology, orthopedics, physiatry and rehabilitation medicine, as well as other specialties. However, there remains tremendous variability in the assessment of patients receiving these therapies, methods for evaluation of outcome, and in the understanding of where these procedures belong in the triaging of those who require surgery. In this article, we attempt to highlight the biologic concepts on which these therapies are based, controversies that have arisen with their increasing use, and a description of complications that have been reported. We will not discuss the specific techniques of performing the various spinal injection procedures, because these have been well described by many authors.

Spinal pain and radiculopathy are very common conditions. Acute spine pain of a nontraumatic origin has a good prognosis for spontaneous recovery when it is not associated with significant neurologic deficits. One third of patients typically recover within 1 week, whereas two thirds recover within 2 months. With respect to those with disc herniations and spinal pain, only 10% have pain beyond 6 weeks. Most patients can be treated successfully with conservative measures, including appropriate rest, physical and chiropractic therapy, and graded rehabilitation. Maneuvers, such as improving aerobic fitness and flexibility, strengthening core muscles, and weight loss are advocated.[1,2] Analgesic and anti-inflammatory medications often are instituted, with no studies identifying superiority of one class of drugs over another. Medical therapy is tailored to the individual's type of discomfort, age, concurrent medical illnesses, and compliance issues. However, a small proportion of patients with neck and back pain will not respond to these conservative measures and will continue to experience discomfort beyond 3 months.

Numerous textbooks and review articles have been written on nonsurgical percutaneous interventions used to diagnose and treat patients with pain of spinal origin.[3–10] The challenge does not lie in performing these procedures. Rather, it is in identifying the source of the patient's pain.[11] Kuslich and colleagues[12] point to several potential causes for pain of spinal origin, including the facet joints, intervertebral disks, nerve roots, ligaments, and associated fascial structures. Many

[a] Division of Neuroradiology, Vancouver General Hospital, University of British Columbia, 899 West 12th Avenue, Vancouver, BC V5Z 1M9, Canada
[b] Department of Radiology, British Columbia's Children's Hospital, University of British Columbia, 4480 Oak Street, Vancouver, BC V6H 3V4, Canada
[c] Division of Interventional Radiology, Vancouver General Hospital, University of British Columbia, 899 West 12th Avenue, Vancouver, BC V5Z 1M9, Canada
* Corresponding author. Department of Radiology, Vancouver General Hospital, 899 W. 12th Avenue, Vancouver, BC V5Z 1M9, Canada.
E-mail address: manraj.heran@vch.ca (M.K.S. Heran).

Radiol Clin N Am 46 (2008) 487–514
doi:10.1016/j.rcl.2008.02.005
0033-8389/08/$ – see front matter © 2008 Elsevier Inc. All rights reserved.

investigators have commented on the relative contributions of these structures to pain in the cervical, thoracic, and lumbar spine, with no causative etiology in up to 19% of patients.[13–15] Clinical history, physical examination, and imaging studies may not be that helpful in determining the source of pain.[16–23] The origin of spinal pain can be quite complex, and morphologic alterations as seen on imaging studies correlate weakly with patient pain. Innumerable reports exist in the literature regarding the value and limitations of imaging in accurately assessing the source of spinal pain.[24–58] Plain films are of limited value and are rarely used for the initial evaluation.[59,60] Many imaging findings in patients with spinal symptoms can also be found in asymptomatic individuals.[7,61–77] More refined imaging-procedure-clinical correlations may show increasing value of radiologic tools for assessing spinal disease.[78]

This distinction becomes particularly important because there has been a clearly documented increase in the number of spinal surgical procedures that are being performed. The yearly growth rate of cases requiring spinal instrumentation has been estimated at 6% to 8%, with a 3% to 5% increase in the number of cases not requiring instrumentation.[79,80] The rate of back surgery is even higher in the United States, where it is at least 40% greater than in any other country, and more than five times that of countries like Scotland and England.[81,82] As the prevalence of pain after lumbar spinal surgery ("postlumbar laminectomy syndrome" or "failed back syndrome") ranges from 5% to 40%, surgery may not provide patients with the symptom relief they are seeking.[81–88] Clearly, a more accurate pinpointing of the causative etiology of a person's spinal pain would allow for better decision making regarding the type of therapy required for its alleviation.

Spinal injection procedures comprise a less-invasive and relatively conservative treatment option for those with neck or back pain. They are thought to be more effective than oral medications because they deliver the active medication directly to the anatomic site implicated in generating the pain. Their use has increased as patients and referring physicians become more aware of the nonsurgical options available to alleviate pain and improve function. Such techniques have been used for many decades yet remain controversial. Criticisms include the lack of standardized guidelines or substantive reviews on this topic, variability in defining short-term and long-term success, associated costs of interventional therapy, and the variable use of image guidance in performing these procedures.[61,89] It has been reported that, even in experienced hands, blind epidural steroid injections (ESIs) result in inaccurate needle placement in up to 30% of cases.[90] The use of fluoroscopy and computed tomography (CT) has become widely accepted because these modalities significantly improve the technical accuracy of drug delivery. Injection of iodinated contrast aids in confirming correct needle-tip position and avoiding potential complications. In patients allergic to iodinated contrast media, other agents, such as gadolinium, may be used.[91]

The application of percutaneous interventional techniques is highly variable among the multiple specialties involved, even for the most commonly performed procedures.[81] In fact, most of these procedures are performed by nonradiologists. Societies, such as the American Society of Interventional Pain Physicians, have attempted to develop guidelines and an ongoing process of evidence synthesis to bring some consensus to these procedures.[13,92–94] A series of systemic reviews of these procedures was performed recently.[11,81,95–99] Interestingly, there is minimal reference to reports published by radiologists, despite some very large series reported. This omission reflects the lack of a multidisciplinary approach to this difficult diagnostic and management problem and criticism that data reported in radiology series are not rigorous with respect to accumulation, assessment, and follow-up. These criticisms are interesting, because the technical ability of interventional radiologists in performing image-guided spinal procedures is extremely high. Issues other than patient care may contribute to this lack of cohesiveness and teamwork among the different disciplines involved.

Spinal injection procedures can be separated into those being performed for diagnostic purposes and those done to provide therapeutic benefit. Given the lack of specificity of existing imaging and clinical tools to elucidate the source of a person's spinal pain, targeted diagnostic injections have been touted to potentially aid in making this determination. However, many investigators challenge this notion.[2,7,100–104] Pain is subjective. It may be influenced by psychologic, social, financial, and legal factors, as well as by placebo and the efficacy of concurrent therapies, such as physical therapy and medications. The literature is quite conflicted on the efficacy of these diagnostic and therapeutic spinal injections; however, patients appreciate having a nonsurgical option and do not mind coming at regular intervals to obtain the desired pain relief and functional improvement. We attempt to address some of these controversies as they specifically relate to commonly performed spinal injection procedures. Sacroiliac joint injections, discography, or procedures in the setting of oncology will not be discussed. Vertebroplasty, kypoplasty, and other spinal cement augmentation procedures are addressed in other chapters of this issue. Though adhesiolysis, intradiscal therapies, placement of intrathecal infusion pumps, and spinal cord stimulators may also be of benefit in these patients, their scope is too wide to be adequately covered in this chapter.

MEDICATIONS FOR SPINAL INJECTION THERAPY

The objective of percutaneous spinal injection procedures is to diagnose the causative etiology of spinal pain and, if possible, offer therapy. Because it often is difficult to determine the origin of spinal pain, patients typically are advised that targeted diagnostic procedures may not be effective if the pain generator is elsewhere. Through a series of targeted injections, there is a greater likelihood of determining the correct source of pain. Injections should not affect more than one target area to avoid confusion and misdiagnosis. This potentially avoids offering incorrect percutaneous therapeutic procedures or surgery, thereby improving patient selection for appropriate procedures. There is no consensus among interventional pain management specialists regarding the type, dosage, or frequency of injections. No clear answer exists as to the total number of injections a patient may have or the efficacy of combining different injections or medications.

The mainstay of diagnostic procedures is the administration of local anesthetic medications. Their mechanism of action is through dampening of C-fiber activity and via interruption of the nociceptive input and reflex mechanisms of the afferent limb of local pain fibers, thereby interrupting the pain–spasm cycle.[11] Some investigators even suggest that the anesthetic works on free glutamate released by herniated disc material.[105,106] The injectate may have local physical effects, including clearing adhesions or inflammatory exudates from the target neural structure. Local anesthetic administration allows testing of the hypothesis that the target structure is the source of the patient's pain. Optimally, all controlled blocks would include placebo injections; however, this often is not practical in the clinical setting. As an alternative, investigators have injected local anesthetics with different durations of action on two separate visits.[11] Ideally, the interval between these two procedures is approximately 2 weeks, with a minimum of 1 week advocated. Interestingly, the only study that assessed validity of the block response comparing a short-acting local anesthetic (lidocaine)

with a long-acting local anesthetic (bupivacaine) in selective nerve root blocks showed no difference between these to anesthetics.[57]

The administration of corticosteroids typically is to offer therapeutic benefit. Corticosteroids work by membrane stabilization, inhibition of synthesis or action of neural peptides, phospholipase A2 activity blockade, suppression of sensitization of dorsal horn neurons, and prolonged suppression of ongoing neuronal discharge.[11] Local physical effects as described for anesthetics may also play a role. The most commonly used formulations of long-acting steroids are listed in **Table 1**. All have been shown to be safe and effective for this use.[11] Controversy remains as to the minimal effective dose required to achieve a therapeutic response, the frequency with which corticosteroids can be administered, and the safety profile of particulate and nonparticulate steroids.[107–111] As far as efficacy, Dreyfuss and colleagues[112] did not show a difference between particulate and nonparticulate steroids in their comparative effectiveness of cervical transforaminal injections for cervical radicular pain. However, Stanczak and colleagues[113] reported a statistically significant greater efficacy using Kenalog versus Celestone in ESI performed on 597 patients 71% improvement versus 54%, 14 days after the procedure. Owlia and colleagues[114] compared 80 mg versus 40 mg of methylprednisolone in lumbar ESI and found no difference in efficacy with a reduced adverse profile with the lower dose. Although there appear to be no gender differences in response to these medications, specific sex-dependent dimensions of pain coping were associated with treatment responses. Inman and colleagues[115] also found that men reported significantly greater pain intensity and unpleasantness than women for the first injection, with no differences thereafter.

NERVE ROOT INJECTIONS
Controversy

Nerve root injections are of limited use in the evaluation of spinal disorders with radicular features. The variability in their technique and the heterogeneity in causative etiologies does not allow for critical appraisal of the existing data.

Spinal pain can be a result of neural dysfunction. The pathophysiology of spinal radicular pain is a subject of ongoing research and controversy. Pathogenic mechanisms that have been implicated include direct physical contact and compression of a nerve root by disc material or encroaching osteophytes. This compression can lead to dysfunction and vascular compromise of

Table 1
Commonly used corticosteroid preparations for spinal injections

Corticosteroid	Brand Name	Description	Common Dose[a]
Methylprednisolone acetate	Depo-Medrol	Particles densely packed; smaller than red blood cells; not prone to aggregation; contains benzyl alcohol (potentially neurotoxic); may not completely dissolve	20–80 mg
Triamcinolone diacetate	Aristocort	Particles vary greatly in size; form aggregations	40–120 mg
Triamcinolone acetonide	Kenalog	Particles vary greatly in size; form aggregations	40–80 mg (ESI) 20–40 mg (other sites)
Triamcinolone hexacetonide	Aristospan	Similar to triamcinolone acetonide, with less intense but more sustained action	20–40 mg
Betamethasone acetate/ phosphate mixture	Celestone Soluspan	Particles vary greatly in size; form aggregations but is soluble	12–18 mg (ESI)
Dexamethasone	Decadron	Particles 5–10 times smaller than red blood cells; can aggregate	variable

[a] Dosage for spinal injection procedures is highly variable, with no formal consensus reached. The lowest effective dose is recommended to avoid potential for systemic adverse reactions.

the target nerve.[11] However, Mixter and Ayers showed that radicular pain can also occur without disc herniation.[42] Subsequently, nerve root inflammation has become the central unifying concept behind spinal radicular pain with numerous proinflammatory cytokines implicated in causing chemical irritation, including phospholipase A2, metalloproteinases, interleukin-6, prostaglandin E2, and tumor necrosis factor.[7,11] The rationale for nerve root blocks, therefore, is to address this inflammatory component and test the hypothesis that the target nerve root is the source of a patient's pain.

Despite their frequent use in the care of patients with spinal pain, the validity and value of diagnostic nerve blocks has been frequently debated.[13,92,98,102,116–120] The goal of the procedure is to allow the injectate to come into contact with the locus of the pain generator, which typically is in the radicular space. This is defined by the fascial planes surrounding the nerve root, dorsal root ganglion, and spinal nerve as they exit the intervertebral foramen.[121] Several investigators have described their efficacy in both diagnosis and therapy.[7,104,122–127] These and other investigators tout the merits of spinal nerve root injections and suggest that long-term relief of symptoms can be provided in a correctly selected population. A variety of names have been given to this procedure: selective nerve root block, selective nerve root sleeve injection,

selective epidural, selective spinal nerve block, selective ventral ramus block, and periradicular injection. In the last year, a systematic review of image-guided selective nerve root injections was done by Datta and colleagues[98], attempting to address issues such as nomenclature, performance, and benefit of these procedures.

Although selective nerve root blocks and transforaminal injections often are considered the same procedure, purists insist on describing these as separate and distinct techniques. This is based largely on the premise that the injectate may come in contact with adjacent dorsal rami, spinal nerves, or sinuvertebral nerves if the needle tip is too medial, thereby possibly resulting in a false-positive benefit.[123,128] Indeed, Castro and colleagues and Wolff and colleagues both showed significant epidural spread and spread to an adjacent nerve root (up to 48% and 27%, respectively), even with as little as 0.5 mL of anesthetic or the use of electrostimulation. Anomalies of the nerve roots are not uncommon, a specific example being the furcal nerve.[129,130] This usually arises from the L4 root level and contributes to both the lumbar and sacral plexuses. Neurologic symptoms suggestive of two-root involvement frequently are a result of furcal nerve compression. The term "transforaminal" is considered to be a misnomer by some, giving a false sense of the needle traversing the foramen when the needle tip is essentially paraforaminal.[131] A "safe triangle" for injection has been proposed for minimizing complications associated with nerve root injections.[132] However, no comment is made as to the ideal depth of the needle tip in the anterior-posterior position. Crall and colleagues[133] studied the effect of various needle tip positions on immediate postinjection pain in selective lumbar nerve blocks in 1202 procedures and found that there was no difference on immediate pain reduction regardless of whether the needle tip was within or adjacent to the intervertebral foramen. This would suggest that false-positive results caused by the above-described mechanisms could be minimized by injections performed adjacent to the foramen. Although contrast does not necessarily need to be injected when computed tomography (CT) guidance is used, it is mandatory for fluoroscopic procedures to appropriately characterize needle position and potential distribution of the injectate (**Figs. 1–4**).

Efficacy of selective nerve root blocks is also dependent on the type of pathology causing spinal radicular pain. Strobel and colleagues[58] found that patients with cervical foraminal disc herniation and resultant foraminal nerve root compromise had better pain relief than those with superimposed spinal stenosis. Similar findings were seen in selective nerve root injections in the lumbar spine for radicular pain caused by disc herniation versus spinal stenosis.[134] Lutz and colleagues[125]

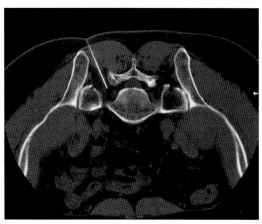

Fig. 2. CT-guided selective right S1 nerve root block, using 22-gauge spinal needle.

found that patients with moderate to severe lateral recess stenosis responded less favorably to selective nerve root injections and were more likely to require subsequent surgery. Previous reports of the lack of therapeutic efficacy of selective nerve root blocks may be contaminated by cases of epidural or intraneural fibrosis or posttraumatic neural injury.[104]

Datta and colleagues[98] found there to be moderate evidence for the effectiveness of selective nerve root injections as a diagnostic tool in spinal pain with radicular features. They also support use of these injections for evaluating equivocal radicular pain. Selective nerve root injections are useful in the diagnostic evaluation of spinal radicular pain as well as for providing therapeutic benefit. Much of the controversy revolves around the complex pathophysiology of radicular pain and the inability of past studies to accurately assess the causative etiology as well as accurately categorize the location of administration of the injectate. Although no ideal position probably exists, it seems reasonable to assume that injections adjacent to the foramen are adequate, while minimizing false-positive procedures and potential for complications.

EPIDURAL STEROID INJECTIONS
Controversy

Long-term efficacy of ESIs has not been shown, with lack of a preferred method for administration of medications.

The number and frequency of ESIs is arbitrary. Patients should not receive more than three injections in total.

Epidural injections have been around for many decades. 1930 marked the first time an intrasacral epidural injection was performed for the treatment

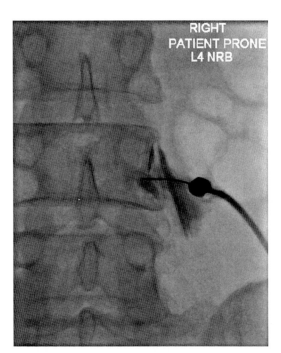

RIGHT
PATIENT PRONE
L4 NRB

Fig. 1. Prone, postero-anterior projection shows selective sensory nerve root block with contrast outlining the right L4 nerve root, after placement of 22-gauge spinal needle.

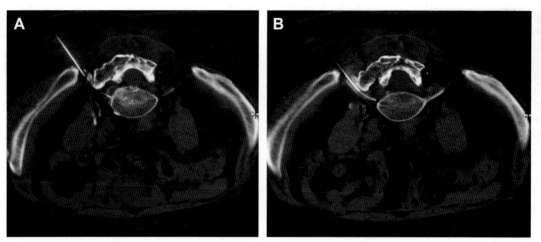

Fig. 3. (*A,B*) CT-guided right L5 nerve root block using coaxial needle technique. Because of postsurgical fusion changes, a transforaminal approach was not possible. Therefore, using a more lateral approach, a coaxial technique was used, with a 22-gauge curved needle placed through an 18-gauge guiding needle. Iodinated contrast medium then was administered to confirm needle tip adjacent to the L5 nerve root.

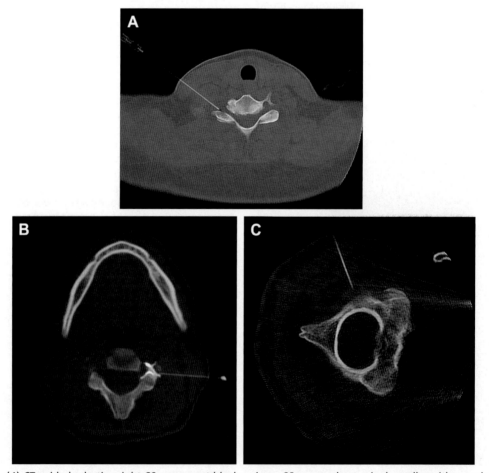

Fig. 4. (*A*) CT-guided selective right C6 nerve root block, using a 22-gauge short spinal needle, without administration of contrast medium. (*B*) CT-guided left C4 nerve root block, using a 25-gauge needle, with administration of iodinated contrast medium to exclude intravascular positioning of needle tip. (*C*) CT-guided right occipital nerve root block, without administration of contrast medium, using a 22-gauge short spinal needle.

of sciatica.[135] Direct epidural injection of cortico-steroids for treatment of cervical and lumbar spinal pain syndromes was first described in 1952.[136] The first cervical ESI was performed in 1972.[137] Since then, these injection techniques have become commonplace for treatment of multilevel nerve root compromise (polyradiculopathy), central spinal stenosis, or equivocal cases of radicular-type symptomatology.[7,138] ESI treatment of symptomatic lumbar spinal stenosis associated with epidural lipomatosis has also been reported, as has treatment of phantom lumbar radiculopathy.[139,140] Several different routes have been developed to deliver medications to the epidural space: interlaminar, transforaminal, and caudal (**Figs. 5 and 6**). Although a valuable technique, the caudal approach has the lowest likelihood of being positioned correctly.[141–143] Investigators have reported that the transforaminal route may be more effective than interlaminar or caudal techniques, possibly because of a higher incidence of steroid placement in the ventral epidural space[144,145] Vad and colleagues[146] reported an 84% success rate after an average follow-up period of 1.4 years in those receiving transforaminal ESI. A national survey conducted by Cluff and colleagues[147] polling academic and private practice anesthesia programs found no clear-cut consensus as to the ideal method for performing ESI. The investigators also found a startling lack of imaging used to guide needle placement, with only 39% of academic practices using it in the cervical region. Similarly, a wide discrepancy was seen between private practice and academic centers for using a transforaminal

route for ESI in postlaminectomy patients (61% versus 15%).

Advocates of ESI point to its ability to shorten the clinical course of the disease process, provide symptomatic relief translating into improvement in quality of life and potential reduction of oral medications, and potentially keep patients out of the hospital.[148–150] Kwon and colleagues[151] recently reported significant pain relief in patients treated with cervical interlaminar ESIs. They suggested that the most important outcome predictor was whether cervical pain was caused by disc herniation or spinal stenosis, with those with disc herniations fairing better. In their retrospective analysis of 140 patients, Delport and colleagues[152] concluded that one third of their patient population had sustained symptomatic relief, 53% showed improvement in their functional abilities, and 74% were satisfied with ESI as a form of treatment. It is important to note that these investigators varied their steroid dose (60–100 mg of triamcinolone) and method of drug administration (transforaminal versus caudal approach) and that 30% of their patient population reported no relief from the ESI. The "WEST" Study Group also concluded that ESI did not improve physical function, reduce the need for surgery, or allow earlier return to work when compared with a placebo group.[153] They found no benefit of repeated ESI versus single injection. A 2003 audit of the use of epidural injections for back pain and sciatica published in the *Australian Health Review* concluded that more than 80% of injections were used for conditions that were not indicated.[154]

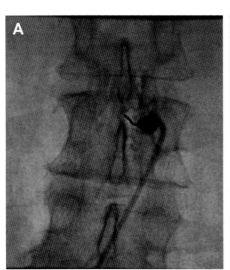
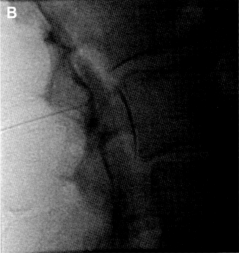

Fig. 5. (*A*) Antero-posterior and (*B*) lateral projections show L3/4 interlaminar epidural steroid injection under fluoroscopic guidance, using a 22-gauge Touhy needle. Iodinated contrast medium confirms needle tip positioning within the epidural space, with the lateral projection showing anterior epidural extension of contrast.

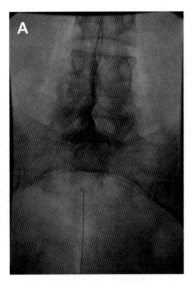 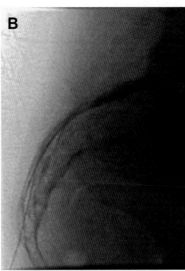

Fig. 6. (*A*) Antero-posterior and (*B*) lateral fluoroscopic projections of an ESI via the caudal/sacral hiatal approach. Using a 22-gauge spinal needle, iodinated contrast medium has been injected to ensure appropriate positioning of needle tip within the epidural space.

Critical reviews of the literature have been performed by several investigators.[11,149,150,154–157] Several efforts have been made to perform randomized controlled trials evaluating the efficacy of ESI.[153,158,159] These have been conflicted, especially regarding long-term efficacy. A review performed by Young and colleagues[160] determined that there were few prospective, randomized, controlled trials showing efficacy of ESIs, with many showing conflicting results. Several of the studies they reviewed showed favorable short-term outcomes; however, there were fewer conclusive results for benefit beyond 6 months. Young and colleagues did state that ESI was a useful tool for predicting surgical outcome, having a sensitivity between 65% and 100%, a specificity of 71% to 95%, and a positive predictive value as high as 95% for 1-year surgical outcome. A systemic review by Abdi and colleagues[95] found that evidence was strong and limited for short-term and long-term relief, respectively, in management of lumbar radicular pain with interlaminar or transforaminal lumbar ESI. Moderate evidence was present for managing lumbar radicular pain in postlaminectomy syndrome, with strong and moderate evidence for short-term and long-term relief, respectively, for caudal ESIs in the management of chronic lumbar radiculopathy or postlumbar laminectomy syndrome. There was moderate evidence for cervical interlaminar or transforaminal ESI in managing cervical radiculopathy. In contrast, the Therapeutics and Technology Assessment Subcommittee of the American Academy of Neurology was much less enthusiastic, stating that, in general, ESI for radicular lumbosacral pain did not impact functional impairment, change

need for surgery, or provide long-term pain relief beyond 3 months.[157] Although there may be some short-term benefit derived from these procedures, they could not recommend their routine use. Additionally, Armon and colleagues[157] stated that there was insufficient evidence to make any recommendations for the use of ESI in treating cervical radicular pain.

The mechanism by which ESI works is uncertain. There is likely a physical property at work in which the volume of injectate aids in lysis of adhesions or clearing inflammatory exudates from the target neural structures. This aspect of ESI is difficult to account for, especially with the differences in volumes injected by different proceduralists. Valat and colleagues[159] allude to this in their randomized, double-blind, controlled trial in which similar short-term efficacy was seen comparing isotonic saline and prednisolone acetate injected epidurally for sciatica. ESIs also rely in part on the premise that they will diffuse to the site of inflammation for their pharmacologic effects. There is no guarantee of this, and this may be a reason for procedural failure, such as in the setting of an injection performed several levels away from the target site or when there is known epidural scarring/adhesions. In addition, specific anatomic boundaries to free dispersal of injectate can be present, such as the plica medianis, a midline dural reflection. If not recognized, this can confine injected medications to one side of the epidural space. As a result, epidurography is considered an important part of ESIs.[90,161,162]

The volume of the injectate is mainly dictated by the approach used and the location being injected. Smaller volumes typically are instilled in the cervical and thoracic spine, with 1.5 to 2 mL for transforaminal ESI, and 3 to 5 mL for interlaminar procedures. Lumbar procedures use even higher volumes, with 3 to 4 mL for transforaminal ESI, 6 to 10 mL for interlaminar ESI, and up to 20 mL for caudal ESI.[163] However, even these injection volumes are not based on any scientific merit. CT-guided procedures, in which technical ability to visualize the needle is optimized, often use smaller volumes, especially for interlaminar lumbar ESI (**Fig. 7**). There does not appear to be any difference in therapeutic efficacy, and the difference in volumes may be based on the modality of imaging guidance used rather than a biologic effect. Because the systemic effects of corticosteroids, such as on the hypothalamus–pituitary axis, may persist for up to 2 weeks, repeat injections are advocated with at least 2-week intervals. Patients not showing response to an initial ESI may still show improvement after one or two additional injections. As such, it is classically advocated to perform a "series" of three ESI procedures. However, no medical outcome studies have been done to support this regimen. It is prudent to evaluate the patient after each injection and determine the benefit, both in terms of degree and duration. Although there is no limit on the number of ESIs a patient may receive, the overall constitution of the patient, the causative etiology of his or her spinal-mediated pain, and his or her perspective on long-term therapy and surgery are extremely important in planning future therapy.

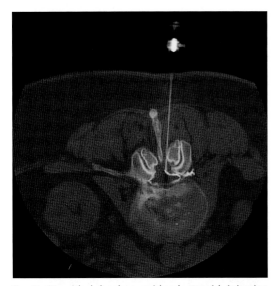

Fig. 7. CT-guided lumbar epidural steroid injection using a 22-gauge needle. Iodinated contrast medium outlines the epidural space with some contrast spillage into the left neural foramen.

PERCUTANEOUS PROCEDURES FOR FACET-MEDIATED SPINAL PAIN
Controversy

Intra-articular facet blocks and medial branch blocks are equivalent when assessing a patient for facet denervation procedures. However, the false-positive rates for both procedures are too high for them to be useful.

Rhizotomy procedures for facet-mediated pain do not provide sufficient long-term relief to justify their use. The methods for evaluating which patients will benefit from these procedures are flawed, with no uniformity in how these procedures are performed.

The zygapophyseal joints (commonly referred to as facet joints) often are implicated as an important source of spinal pain. They may account for 34% to 48% of those with persistent upper back and mid back pain, 15% to 45% of those with low back pain, 36% to 67% of patients with neck pain, and 16% of those with lumbar pain from failed back surgery.[96,97,164] This is thought to be caused by segmental instability, degenerative osteoarthritis, and superimposed inflammatory synovitis.[165,166] In a rabbit model, Cavanaugh and colleagues[167] showed the importance of sensitization and excitation of the nerve fibers of the medial branches of the dorsal rami, which heavily innervate the facet joints upon inflammation or repetitive trauma. They also showed the beneficial effects of hydrocortisone and lidocaine infiltrated locally, with marked reduction in this nerve activity. However, it often is difficult to clinically assess for this, because there typically are other associated etiologies for spine pain. Investigators recently have suggested several clinical features that may be useful in determining if pain is originating from the facet joints.[61,168,169] These are listed in **Box 1**. Careful history taking and physical examination can suggest facet disease as a contributor to spinal pain.[169]

Imaging often is not helpful. Although Houseni and colleagues[68] recently showed the potential of fluorodeoxyglucose (FDG) positron emission tomography (FDG-PET) in the diagnosis of facet joint arthropathy, this has limited availability and is expensive. A study by Pneumaticos and colleagues suggesting a role for single photon emission computed tomography (SPECT) in selecting those benefiting from facet joint injections was deemed to have significant methodologic flaws.[97,170] Kim and Wang[67] assessed the value of magnetic resonance imaging (MRI) and SPECT in studying 230 facet joints in patients with facet-mediated axial back pain and found that synovial abnormalities, not facet hypertrophy, correlated with positive

---

Box 1
Clinical features suggestive of facet-mediated spinal pain

Low back stiffness (typically most marked in the morning)

Unilateral low back pain

Tenderness on unilateral palpation of the facet joint or ipsilateral transverse process

Lack of radicular features

Pain eased by flexion or worsened by hyperextension, rotation, or lateral bending

Absence of root tension signs

Hip, buttock, or back pain with straight leg raising

Referred pain above the knee

SPECT findings. Schwarzer and colleagues[66] also showed that the degree of degenerative change as identified on CT was a poor indicator of facet-mediated spinal pain. The current consensus remains that there is no association between results of facet blocks and clinical findings, including radiologic assessment.[7,97]

The main facet joint procedures include intra-articular and periarticular injections, medial branch blocks, and denervation procedures of the medial branches (using radiofrequency or cryoneurolysis techniques).[96] The choice between intra-articular blocks and medial branch blocks is a point of controversy between those performing these procedures and serves to contaminate the literature with respect to patient evaluation for additional percutaneous or surgical therapies. Intra-articular injections often are more difficult and time consuming than medial branch blocks because they require access to the joint space (which may be extremely difficult or impossible in a badly degenerated facet joint) and an injection that does not rupture or overly distend the joint (**Figs. 8 and 9**). Sarazin and colleagues[171] have described a fluoroscopic-guided technique for injecting the inferior articular recess of a facet joint without requiring profiling of the joint. In the past, there has been disagreement as to whether intra-articular injections are preferable to periarticular injections (**Fig. 10**).[172,173] However, leak of injectate around the facet joint can result in local epidural effects as well as other factors that may confound the assessment of the efficacy of intra-articular therapy. Although it was traditionally thought that only intra-articular injections offered a therapeutic response, investigators have shown

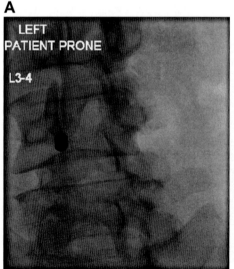
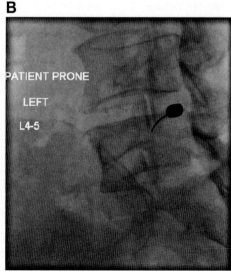

Fig. 8. Prone, obliqued views of (*A*) left L3/4 and left (*B*) L4/5 facet joint steroid injections, using a 22-gauge spinal needle.

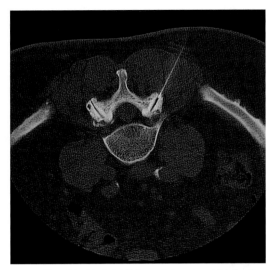

Fig. 9. CT-guided left L4/5 facet joint steroid injection using a 22-gauge spinal needle. Note the intra-articular position of the needle, with gas injected to confirm it position.

similar, and possibly better, efficacy with medial branch blocks.[96,174] Investigators also have tried to compare intra-articular injections directly with medial branch blocks.[175] However, these studies did not use control diagnostic blocks, had poor assessment tools, and did not have blinded evaluations by an independent observer.[96]

The superior portion of each lumbar zygapophyseal joint receives innervation from the medial branch originating from one level above, whereas the medial branch originating at the same level provides innervation to the inferior portion. Medial branch blocks can be performed effectively using

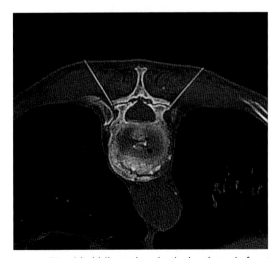

Fig. 10. CT-guided bilateral periarticular thoracic facet joint steroid injections, using 22-gauge spinal needles.

a single-needle technique (Fig. 11).[176] Their main objective is to confirm facet-mediated spinal pain. However, they are also used to select those patients who may benefit from facet denervation procedures, because history, physical examination, and imaging are not considered valid procedures. Birkenmaier and colleagues[177] compared medial branch blocks with pericapsular blocks in patient selection and found that uncontrolled medial branch blocks were superior, although both seemed effective. The false-negative response rate of medial branch blocks has been reported to be 11%.[178] Although diagnostic blocks are associated with a false-positive rate reported to vary between 25% and 45%, most investigators believe that a positive response of at least 50% improvement on previous diagnostic medial branch blocks is mandatory.[7,97,179] Some investigators prefer a response of at least 80% improvement. Repeating blocks with either placebo control or using anesthetic agents of different durations can aid in minimizing false-positive responses.[97] Repeated medial branch blocks also have been advocated to increase the likelihood of durable facet-mediated spinal pain.[180] The power of placebo cannot be discounted, especially in the short-term assessment of procedural efficacy. Carette and colleagues[181] showed equal immediate average pain reduction in those receiving intra-articular methylprednisolone versus isotonic saline, with longer sustained efficacy in the steroid group. However, when adjuvant therapies, such as oral medications and physiotherapy were taken into account, this difference was not that significant. In addition, inclusion of corticosteroid in the injectate used for medial branch blocks may not provide additional benefit. A study by Manchikanti and colleagues found that local anesthetic administration was sufficient to obtain the same benefit previously reported for combination anesthetic–steroid injectates.[182,183] This would suggest that breaking the pain–spasm cycle may be sufficient for providing sustained pain relief rather than the anti-inflammatory actions of corticosteroid therapy.

Facet denervation is a procedure by which a discrete lesion is created of the medial branches of the dorsal rami that innervate a facet joint. Although techniques such as cryoneurolysis and laser denervation have been performed, radiofrequency thermal-mediated ablation of the medial branch is the mainstay of facet denervation techniques. Fluoroscopy remains the main imaging modality for guiding needle placement (Fig. 12). Facet denervation has been advocated as a minimally invasive method of dealing with facet-mediated pain when conservative treatment has

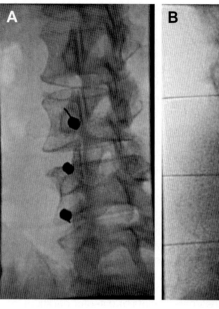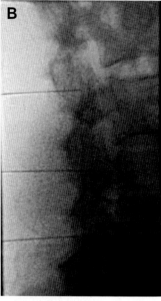

Fig. 11. (*A*) Prone postero-anterior and (*B*) lateral fluoroscopic images during 22-gauge spinal needle placement for Left L3/4 and L4/5 medial branch blocks. Note positioning of needle tips at the junction of the transverse process and the base of the superior facet, at the superolateral margin of the pedicle. The lateral projection confirms needle positions at the posterior aspect of the superior articular process at each level.

failed, and has strong representation on both sides of the argument of whether it is effective in providing durable pain relief.[96,169,179,184–187] Investigators have reported sustained pain relief at 12 months in 63% of patients.[179,188] In the cervical region, because of the anatomic differences in innervation, multiple lesions of target nerves are required to optimize long-term pain relief.[96] Data suggesting lack of efficacy of radiofrequency neurotomy has been criticized for methodologic flaws.[96,169]

The procedure is performed with minimal or no sedation because sensory and motor stimulation maneuvers typically are conducted to increase lesional specificity while reducing injury to the dorsal root ganglion or motor branches. Despite claims that it can shorten procedure time and reduce patient discomfort, the use of general anesthesia significantly limits access to facet denervation while profoundly increasing the procedural cost, as well as introducing the potential morbidity of a general anesthetic.[189] Use of general anesthesia, therefore, is strongly discouraged. Continuous radiofrequency application is the most commonly performed technique, although some

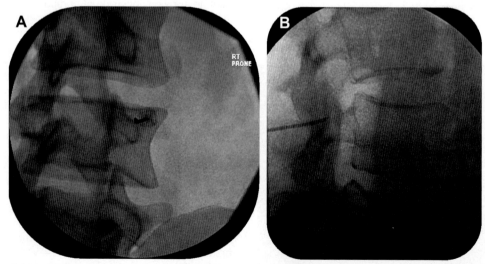

Fig. 12. (*A*) Prone postero-anterior and (*B*) lateral fluoroscopic images during right L3/4 rhizotomy. The positioning of the rhizotomy needle is at the same location as for a medial branch block. Lateral view shows the tip of a radio-opaque 18-gauge radiofrequency cannula (with coaxial radiofrequency needle, 145 mm in length, 10 mm active tip not shown) at the level of the facet joint, just posterior to the superior facet of L4. The bevel has been deliberately directed inferiorly.

have used pulsed radiofrequency with reported success.[190,191] Although several technical variations exist, Gofeld and Faclier recently compared these techniques with respect to cannula size, location, approach, and size of thermal lesion created.[188] Their suggestions attempt to consolidate previous approaches and make the performance of radiofrequency ablation more uniform.

Intra-articular facet, perifacet, and medial branch blocks are not equivalent. The evidence-based practice guidelines by Boswell and colleagues[11] suggest the current belief is that accuracy of facet joint nerve blocks is strong in the diagnosis of facet-mediated pain in the cervical and lumbar spine and moderate in the thoracic region. Medial branch blocks are considerably better in determining who may benefit from facet denervation. Although intra-articular injections still may be useful in the lumbar spine, evidence is limited in the cervical region. Although false-positive results can occur, these can likely be reduced through meticulous technique and repeated diagnostic injections. Evidence for facet denervation supports its use in this setting. Despite the many studies and reviews that have been published on percutaneous therapies for facet-mediated pain, larger, prospective, randomized controlled trials are still needed. There is considerable heterogeneity in the data published on this topic. However, uniform inclusion and exclusion criteria are necessary, and more recent studies and investigators have aimed at reducing variability in workup and procedural approach, with better long-term follow-up.

COMPUTED TOMOGRAPHY FLUOROSCOPY
Controversy

CT fluoroscopy adds nothing to percutaneous spinal injection procedures and only increases radiation exposure to the patient and operator.

Radiation exposure during the performance of spinal injection procedures is a very real concern. Although there are interesting reports of sonographically guided needle procedures in the spine,[192–194] injection procedures typically use CT or fluoroscopy for guidance. Fluoroscopy is often preferred to CT because of its increased availability, dynamic range of assessment, and speed of procedure performance. ALARA ("as low as reasonably achievable") radiation principles are important, with use of last image hold and grid-controlled pulsed fluoroscopy, and minimization of image magnification and obliqued views. Schmid and colleagues[195] compared different modes of fluoroscopy and showed that 1 minute of continuous fluoroscopy resulted in an effective dose of 0.43 mSv, whereas use of pulsed fluoroscopy reduced this to less than 0.1 mSv (for 3 pulses per second). Botwin and colleagues[196] evaluated the radiation exposure to the operator and radiography technologist, and confirmed a low dose exposure, although cumulative exposure to the operator's hands must be remembered. Investigators favoring CT cite the excellent visualization of the target structure, thereby allowing precise placement of the needle tip and improved technical success. Some suggest that injection of iodinated contrast may not be necessary for certain procedures when performed under CT.[122,197,198] Disadvantages often raised are the increased physician time and increased radiation exposure that CT has in comparison with fluoroscopy. Schmid and colleagues[195], however, were able to show significant reduction in dose exposure achievable in CT through minimizing mAs and limited scanning. Using their methods, 0.22 to 0.43 mSv were achievable for 4 to 10 scans.

Advances in CT technology have led to the development of CT fluoroscopy (CTF). CTF allows the operator to stand by the patient and manipulate the needle, with acquisition of low-dose images in near real time through the use of partial reconstruction algorithms. It was first described for use in guiding biopsies and drainage procedures.[199,200] As the technology has improved, CTF has been increasingly used to perform biopsies of almost all organ systems, proving especially useful for procedures on deeper structures or on those that are difficult to localize because of motion.[199,201,202]

Initially, techniques using continuous CTF were used; however, radiation exposure to the patient and operator proved to be prohibitively high. Proceduralists have adopted a "quick-check method," whereby images are acquired intermittently throughout the procedure, typically after manipulation of the needle, and with the operator away from the patient during acquisitions. Carlson and colleagues[203] reported a 94% reduction in median calculated patient-absorbed dose per procedure by using this method. Appropriate lead shielding of the patient can reduce scatter radiation, with standard radiation protection protocols followed by the operator (thyroid shield, lead apron, inverse square law, floor shield).[204] Through use of the laser function of the CT scanner and correlating this with the target structure and existing position of the needle (as seen on the last acquisition), images are only acquired through the level of interest, rather than spanning through a volume of tissue. This can minimize the number of images required to perform the procedure. Lowering the mAs (10–60 mAs, often under

20 mAs) while performing CTF can result in a significant reduction in radiation dose, with little impact on precision of needle placement.[205] Though measured radiation doses to the operator vary with procedure, values as low as 0.1 mrem/procedure are possible.[205]

The main advantage of CTF is that it combines the precise localization possible in CT with improvements in speed offered through its fluoroscopic component. Several investigators have written on the potential benefits of CTF in performing spinal injection procedures.[205–209] CTF has been shown to offer significant improvements in the time taken to perform a procedure compared with conventional CT.[210] Carlson and colleagues[203] showed a 32% decrease in overall procedure time using CTF, with Wagner reporting 100% success rate for performing selective lumbar nerve root blocks, with an average physician room time of 7 minutes, four images per procedure, and an average of 2 seconds of CT fluoroscopy time.[206] CTF in cervical injection procedures has also been reported.[205,207,208] Bartynski and colleagues showed the benefit of CTF in performing lower cervical nerve root blocks in patients with large body habitus through use of the swimmer's position, whereas Wagner describes limited use of continuous CTF while injecting contrast to ensure nonvascular placement of needles during foraminal nerve root blocks.[205,208] In his series of more than 200 cervical nerve root blocks performed in this manner, Wagner showed five cases in which CTF demonstrated intravascular positioning of the needle tip requiring repositioning before administration of the steroid and local anesthetic.

CTF is a powerful tool for performing spinal procedures. With appropriate scanning parameters and using the "quick-check method," the radiation dose associated with CTF can be reduced dramatically, while maintaining the superior localization possible in CT. CTF shortens procedure time in comparison with standard CT guidance and may allow a dynamic assessment of possible intravascular needle positions not possible in conventional CT and sometimes difficult to visualize using fluoroscopy.

SYNOVIAL CYSTS
Controversy

Symptomatic synovial cysts are best managed surgically.

Juxtafacet cysts are uncommon causes of spinal pain, with two types of cystic alteration occurring in the zygapophyseal joints of the spine.[211,212] Ganglion cysts have a collagen capsule or fibrous wall without a synovial lining and typically contain myxoid material. Synovial cysts are lined by synovial cells and typically contain thin, straw-colored fluid. Although they can occur after trauma, these cysts tend to develop in the setting of advanced facet degenerative disease and, although rare, typically occur at the L4/5 level. Pirotte and colleagues[213] reported an incidence of 61% at this level in their study of 46 patients. Less frequently, they can occur at the L5/S1 level, followed by the L3/4 and L2/3 levels.[211,214,215] Most patients present in their sixth or seventh decades, with a slight predominance of men versus women affected.[215] Usually they are incidental findings on spine imaging studies.[216] When symptomatic, patients can present with lumbar pain, with or without motor or sensory impairment. The presentation may mimic a variety of other spinal pathologies, including neurogenic claudication/spinal stenosis and disc herniation. Some believe the radicular features are caused by the cyst, whereas back pain is caused by the osteoarthritis of the adjacent facet joint. When motor or sensory findings are present, they usually reflect the anatomic location of the compressive synovial cyst and the level of maximal stenosis. Spinal instability can be associated, and Epstein suggests that up to 40% of patients can have an associated degenerative spondylolisthesis.[215,216] Rarely, they can become large enough to present as a cauda equina syndrome.

The diagnosis of synovial cysts can be made readily by either CT or MRI, although MRI may be the preferred modality.[213,217] They typically contain fluid of variable consistency but may show internal vacuum phenomenon, especially if the adjacent joint contains gas. Up to 30% may have wall calcifications. Concomitant osteoarthritic changes of the adjacent joint usually are present and often severe. Although considered rare, improved spinal imaging techniques may actually result in identifying more incidental synovial cysts than previously thought.[218] Although little is known about their natural history, and there have been case reports of spontaneous resolution, conservative therapy for symptomatic cysts often is unsuccessful.[216,219–223] Surgical management for patients with symptomatic cysts traditionally has been advocated.[213–216,224–226] However, percutaneous therapies have been attempted, with the first report on percutaneous imaged-guided facet joint steroid injection in a symptomatic facet joint synovial cyst by Casselman in 1985.[227] Since then, several studies have shown acceptable outcomes of facet joint steroid administration for synovial cyst therapy.[211,217,218,228–232] Bureau and colleagues[218] evaluated 12 patients and reported a 75% success rate with respect to clinical pain relief. Sauvage and colleagues[217] showed 50% of their study group to have sustained clinical benefit at 6 months after therapy. Fluoroscopic and CT-guided approaches have been used, with most series and case reports describing access to the ipsilateral facet joint, intra-articular confirmation with iodinated contrast, and subsequent injection of corticosteroids. Some investigators have deliberately attempted to rupture the synovial cyst through progressive distension (**Fig. 13**).[218] Some investigators attempt to aspirate the contents of the cyst before steroid administration, with Lutz and Shen advocating using larger access needles (20 gauge versus 22 gauge)

because they believe that this may aid in ease of aspiration.[211,233] Melfi and Aprill[234] describe a technique of direct synovial cyst puncture via an interlaminar intraspinal approach, with fenestration of the cyst using the 18-gauge access needle. Interestingly, they chose a combination of CT and fluoroscopic guidance in their case report and did not instill any corticosteroids as part of the therapeutic procedure.

Controversy remains regarding the efficacy of percutaneous synovial cyst therapy. Investigators advocating percutaneous therapy report the need for repeat procedures in some patients to have sustained benefit. Also, it has been suggested that it may be the act of fenestration/rupture that

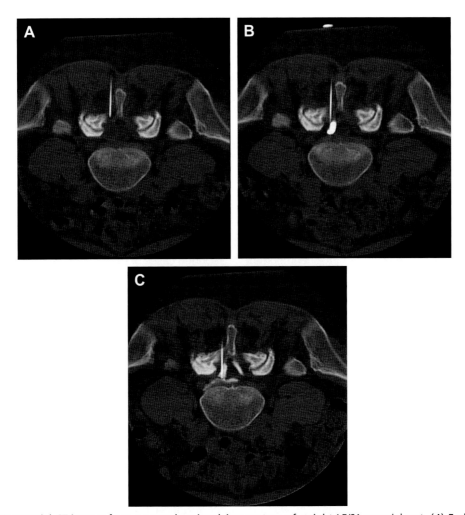

Fig. 13. Sequential CT images from a procedure involving rupture of a right L5/S1 synovial cyst. (*A*) Early image shows the 22-gauge spinal needle being directed toward the synovial cyst using an interlaminar approach. Note the moderate-sized synovial cyst arising from the right L5/S1 facet joint, projecting medially and compressing the thecal sac. (*B*) Confirmation of needle tip within the synovial cyst via administration of iodinated contrast medium. (*C*) Subsequent rupture of the cyst upon progressive distension with a Kenalog/buvicaine mixture, with demonstration of contrast spillage into the epidural space. It should be noted that a right S1 nerve root block was performed immediately before the above cyst procedure (not shown).

predicts long-term efficacy rather than just simple intra-articular facet joint corticosteroid injection. One cannot argue with a minimally invasive approach used to treat this rare entity. It is compelling to think that surgery can be avoided in selected patients with symptomatic synovial cysts. which patients remains the question.

COMPLICATIONS
Controversy

Spinal injection procedures can be associated with potentially devastating complications and should not be performed because there are limited data to support their efficacy as diagnostic and therapeutic procedures.

When performing spinal injection procedures, one must weigh the benefit of the procedure against the potential for complications. However, the risk profile is not the same for all spinal procedures. Likelihood of complications is also related to the use and quality of imaging being used. What about the type of corticosteroid? Needle position? Needle size? How about the approach used for performing a specific spinal injection procedure? These and other questions serve as the basis for reviewing the current literature regarding the incidence, type, and severity of complications that have been reported in the setting of spinal injection procedures.

Spinal injection procedures typically are performed using aseptic technique and image guidance. Patients are almost always awake for the procedure, thereby able to provide important feedback, such as expressing pain when a needle may be in contact with the target nerve, as well as minimizing the confounding influences of conscious sedation on diagnostic injections.[164,235,236] In fact, it is strongly discouraged to have anyone sedated for a spinal injection procedure, unless there are case-specific reasons for doing so.[90] Hodges and colleagues[237] reported two cases of permanent cervical spinal cord injury in patients who had received intravenous sedation for cervical ESIs.

Bleeding complications are not common. The use of small needles (most commonly 22 gauge) and meticulous image-guided techniques make this a rare occurrence. However, there are case reports of patients with epidural hematomas after epidural corticosteroid injections as well as a report of a patient requiring surgery for a cervical spinal subdural hematoma causing quadriparesis after a cervical ESI.[238–240] Although institutions differ greatly, for those patients coming for an ESI or a cervical procedure who currently are taking antiplatelet medications, we will ask them to not take these medications for at least 5 days. Patients on anticoagulants are considered to be at even higher risk and must be reviewed on a case-by-case basis regarding their management. Thankfully, bleeding complications from facet injections or noncervical nerve root injections are exceedingly rare.

Infection is a rare complication. Most large series do not report infection among their complications. However, several case reports have been published.[241–243] Inadvertent disc entry can occur during certain types of spinal injection procedures, such as transforaminal epidural injections.[244] Hooten and colleagues[245] reported an L5/S1 discitis after a lumbar epidural corticosteroid injection in a 64-year-old man presenting 6 weeks after the procedure with a 4-week history of worsening right-sided paraspinous pain. It is notable that their patient had experienced recurrent pulmonary infections before his procedure, although he did not have a pneumonia at the time of his presentation. Gaul and colleagues[246] describe 8 of 128 patients (6.25%) having meningitis and iatrogenic (para)spinal abscesses after spinal injection procedures. These procedures were performed 2 to 21 days before admission to the hospital, with six having an identified organism in their cerebrospinal fluid (CSF) (*Staphylococcus aureus* in four and coagulase-negative staphylococcus in two). One patient died, whereas three survived with neurologic sequelae. Hooten and colleagues identified 27 case reports of infectious complications and reviewed the literature, finding 11 reported cases of epidural abscess, two of epidural abscess with meningitis, and one of meningitis, all of which were attributed to epidural corticosteroid injections.[245,247] They found that many of the patients were immunocompromised, with the dominant infective organism being *S aureus*. Their recommendation was that antibiotic prophylaxis should be considered for immunocompromised patients before undergoing this procedure. Yue and Tan describe an elderly woman who had a caudal ESI who returned 1 month later with L2/3 and L4/5 discitis/osteomyelitis.[248] The causative organism was *Pseudomonas aeruginosa*.

Selective lumbar nerve blocks are performed extremely frequently. Fortunately, complications associated with these procedures are quite uncommon. Stalcup and colleagues[249] examined the relationship between needle-tip position and complications in a retrospective cohort of 2217 procedures. They concluded that the overall minor complication rate was approximately 5%, with no statistical difference between needle-tip position within or adjacent to the lumbar neural foramen. Medial branch block and intra-articular facet injections are considered quite safe. Potential complications of rhizotomy procedures are rare and are listed in **Box 2**. Unintentional damage to a spinal nerve can be prevented through appropriate motor and sensory stimulation before the denervation procedure. Complications after image-guided transforaminal lumbar epidural injections also are rare. In 207 patients receiving 322 injections, Botwin and colleagues[250] reported 3% incidence of transient nonpositional headache that resolved within 24 hours, 2.4% incidence of increased back pain, and 1% incidence of facial flushing. Their incidence of minor complications was 9.6% per injection. No major complications were noted, and there were no dural punctures. However, inadvertent dural puncture is of concern and is a known complication of translaminar epidural injection procedures. Because loss of air pressure resistance can result in up to 30% inaccurate needle-tip placement, adequate imaging guidance and the performance of an epidurogram are considered essential for confident identification of the lumbar epidural space before administration of medications.[90,251,252] Though many proceduralists rely on loss-of-resistance technique and imaging guidance, a large series by Shetty and colleagues[253] showed this still occurred in 0.5% of cases. Patient age over 70 years and male sex are suggested as predictors of poor reliability of the loss-of-resistance technique.[252] Huston and colleagues[254] reported an incidence of 0.33% when performing cervical and lumbosacral selective nerve root injections. Dural puncture can result in CSF leak with possible intracranial hypotension, arachnoiditis, and transient paraparesis/cauda equina symptomatology in the setting of inadvertent intrathecal injection of medications, and even pneumocephalus with resultant severe headache.[255–258] The most extreme complication reported is an intramedullary injection resulting in paralysis.[259] As well, Saigal and colleagues[260] report an extremely unusual complication of a thoracic intradural *Aspergillus* abscess in an immunocompetent individual after an ESI.

The most feared complication of spinal injection procedures is stroke. Although once considered exceedingly rare, there are an increasing number of reports of this potentially devastating complication in both the brain and spinal cord.[257,261–268] Although the etiology remains unclear, several mechanisms have been implicated, with the main one being injury to or injection into a spinal radiculomedullary artery or vertebral artery. This may lead to direct injection of medication into this circulation, or spasm or dissection of the contacted artery, with consequent ischemic or embolic complications. Houten and Errico[257] reported on three patients with low thoracic spinal cord infarctions from lumbar spinal injection procedures, with two being transforaminal ESIs at L3/4, and one selective S1 nerve root injection. No bleed-back or aspiration of CSF was noted before corticosteroid administration, and all needle positions were verified with injection of contrast under imaging surveillance. The investigators implicate injury to the artery of Adamkiewicz as the likely explanation for these infarcts. It is important to remember that radiculomedullary arteries other than the artery of Adamkiewicz may also be present, including the artery of the conus. These may also be prone to inadvertent puncture. An anatomic study found that the deep cervical artery lies adjacent to the upper cervical facets and may give off the artery of the cervical expansion in approximately 10% of individuals.[269] Investigators have described vascular uptake of contrast despite negative aspiration on the needle, raising considerable concern regarding safety of needle placement.[205,270] And, although contrast injection may not demonstrate initial intra-arterial needle position, this may still occur if the needle is moved upon connection of the medication syringe.

The majority of stroke complications occur with cervical spinal injection procedures, most

---

Box 2
Potential complications from facet-denervation procedures

Infection

Bleeding

Painful cutaneous dysesthesia

Pain "flare" caused by neurogenic inflammation (short term)

Pneumothorax (for thoracic procedures)

Deafferentation pain

Damage to spinal nerve or motor branches

commonly transforaminal ESIs. Rozin and colleagues report a death resulting from perforation of the left vertebral artery during a C7 transforaminal ESI, whereas Beckman and colleagues describe a 31-year-old man having a cerebellar infarction associated with brainstem herniation after a similar procedure performed for right C8 radicular symptoms.[261,268] Ludwig and Burns[266] describe a cervical spinal cord infarction resulting in motor-incomplete tetraplegia after a fluoroscopic-guided left transforaminal C6 ESI. Scanlon and colleagues[263] asked all US physician members of the American Pain Society to complete an anonymous survey to better characterize these complications. Despite a low overall response rate (21.4%), 78 complications were reported, including 16 posterior circulation infarcts of the brain, 12 cervical spinal cord infarcts, and two combined brain-spinal cord infarcts. Thirteen of these ultimately proved fatal. The investigators implicate a mechanism of inadvertent intra-arterial injection of particulate corticosteroids with resultant distal embolic infarct, because particulate steroids (methylprednisolone) were used in many of these cases. Similarly, Tiso and colleagues[267] also implicate particulate steroids in their report of a massive cerebellar infarction after a right C5/6 transforaminal ESI. In their analysis of 1036 patients undergoing fluoroscopically guided extraforaminal cervical nerve blocks, Ma and colleagues[271] describe an overall minor complication rate of 1.7% and highlight the increased rate of complication (6% versus 1.5%) when needle positioning was more anterior than desired. They list minor complications as headache, temporary pain, nausea, numbness, and weakness. They also showed that the complication rate associated with deep versus superficial (medial foraminal versus lateral extraforaminal) needle position was not statistically different (1.9% versus 0.8%). Botwin and colleagues[272] reviewed 157 consecutive patients in whom they performed fluoroscopically guided interlaminar cervical epidural injections, and found an incidence of all complications of 16.8%, the most common of which were increased neck pain and transient nonpositional headache, which together accounted for 11%.

Very rare complications have been reported, such as epidural lipomatosis after lumbar ESIs.[273] This resolved after discontinuation of the steroid injections. A case of bilateral retinal detachment after ESIs has also been reported as has documented gas embolism after spinal epidural injection.[274,275] Young describes a patient experiencing temporary blindness from retinal hemorrhages occurring after a lumbar ESI and reviews the literature on this bizarre complication, whereas Slipman and colleagues report a patient experiencing dysphonia after an ESI procedure.[276,277] There also has been a report of persistent hiccups as a consequence of a thoracic ESI for discogenic pain.[278] Theoretically, delayed hypersensitivity reactions to intra-articular corticosteroid injections also may occur.[279]

The potential for locally injected corticosteroids to harm adjacent bone and cartilage is controversial. It is now felt that the occurrence of avascular necrosis is more related to the severity of the associated disease or systemic steroid use, rather than local corticosteroid therapy. Although earlier animal studies suggested that normal cartilage could be injured, similar studies in primate joints failed to show any negative effects from intra-articular injections.

A unique complication that must be considered is the systemic effect of injected corticosteroid preparations.[280] Systemic absorption invariably occurs with locally injected depot corticosteroids, with a transient deleterious effect on the hypothalamus-pituitary-adrenal axis.[281–283] Ward and colleagues[282] designed a study to investigate the effect of epidural glucocorticosteroid administration on insulin sensitivity. Ten healthy patients with sciatica were treated with 80 mg of triamcinoline administered via a caudal epidural technique. They underwent insulin tolerance testing immediately before the procedure, and 24 hours and 1 week after the procedure. Fasting glucose, insulin, and cortisol levels also were measured. The investigators found a potent suppression of insulin action by the injected steroid medication, with significantly raised fasting insulin and glucose levels immediately after the procedure. Whereas the rate of glucose disappearance after insulin administration returned to normal at 1 week after the procedure, morning cortisol levels remained significantly suppressed. Tuncer and colleagues[283] also found similar transient adrenal suppression after a single epidural injection of betamethasone, with adrenocorticotropic hormone and cortisol remaining significantly suppressed at 7 days and returning to normal at 3 weeks. Maximal glucose elevation appears to occur within the first 48 hours. These studies clearly show the considerable transient systemic impact of corticosteroids used in spinal injection procedures. Such effects should be taken into account when performing these procedures on patients with diabetes. As it may take up to 2 weeks for this suppression of the hypothalamus–pituitary axis to resolve, the frequency with which steroid medications are taken should take this into account.[284]

Complications can occur in any procedure. Percutaneous interventions for spinal pain are no exception. Thankfully, their frequency is quite low, with the majority being minor and transient. Specific procedures, however, such as those in the cervical region, carry with them a possibility for rare but potentially devastating complications and require extreme vigilance. Fortunately, stroke is extremely rare. Still, these and other spinal injection procedures require careful consideration regarding indications, technique, and imaging to be used, as well as the goals of the procedure. A good understanding of the medications being used is mandatory, as is their potential for local and systemic concerns. With the above considerations, spinal injection procedures remain a safe and minimally invasive way to diagnose and treat those with spinal pain syndromes.

THE FUTURE

Controversy will continue to surround the topic of image-guided spinal injection procedures. The importance of good clinical assessment and long-term follow-up cannot be understated, as well as understanding the natural history of the spinal disease being investigated or treated. Current state-of-the-art imaging techniques may improve the accuracy of detection of sources of pain, and large double-blinded studies hopefully will provide answers to questions currently not addressed through the heterogeneous data that have been published thus far.[170] Until then, a practical approach to their use seems justified.

REFERENCES

1. Mazanec DJ, Podichetty VK, Hsia A. Lumbar canal stenosis: start with nonsurgical therapy. Cleve Clin J Med 2002;69(11):909–17.
2. DePalma MJ, Bhargava A, Slipman CW. A critical appraisal of the evidence for selective nerve root injection in the treatment of lumbosacral radiculopathy. Arch Phys Med Rehabil 2005;86(7):1477–83.
3. Deen HG, Fenton DS, Lamer TJ. Minimally invasive procedures for disorders of the lumbar spine. Mayo Clin Proc 2003;78(10):1249–56.
4. Levin KH. Nonsurgical interventions for spine pain. Neurol Clin 2007;25(2):495–505.
5. Malanga G, Nadler S. Nonoperative treatment of low back pain. Mayo Clin Proc 1999;74:1135–48.
6. Fenton DS, Czervionke LF. Image-guided spine intervention. Philadelphia: WB Saunders Co; 2003. p. 298.
7. Leonardi M, Pfirrmann CW, Boos N. Injection studies in spinal disorders. Clin Orthop Relat Res 2006;443:168–82.
8. Hodge J. Facet, nerve root, and epidural block. Semin Ultrasound CT MR 2005;26(2):98–102.
9. Peloso PM, Gross AR, Haines TA, et al. Medicinal and injection therapies for mechanical neck disorders: a Cochrane systematic review. J Rheumatol 2006;33(5):957–67.
10. Saal JA, Saal JS, Herzog RJ. The natural history of lumbar intervertebral disc extrusions treated nonoperatively. Spine 1990;15(7):683–6.
11. Boswell MV, Trescot AM, Datta S, et al. Interventional techniques: evidence-based practice guidelines in the management of chronic spinal pain. Pain Physician 2007;10(1):7–111.
12. Kuslich SD, Ulstrom CL, Michael CJ. The tissue origin of low back pain and sciatica: a report of pain response to tissue stimulation during operations on the lumbar spine using local anesthesia. Orthop Clin North Am 1991;22(2):181–7.
13. Boswell MV, Shah RV, Everett CR, et al. Interventional techniques in the management of chronic spinal pain: evidence-based practice guidelines. Pain Physician 2005;8(1):1–47.
14. Pang WW, Mok MS, Lin ML, et al. Application of spinal pain mapping in the diagnosis of low back pain–analysis of 104 cases. Acta Anaesthesiol Sin 1998;36(2):71–4.
15. Manchikanti L, Singh V, Pampati V, et al. Evaluation of the relative contributions of various structures in chronic low back pain. Pain Physician 2001;4(4):308–16.
16. Sandmark H, Nisell R. Validity of five common manual neck pain provoking tests. Scand J Rehabil Med 1995;27(3):131–6.
17. Seffinger MA, Najm WI, Mishra SI, et al. Reliability of spinal palpation for diagnosis of back and neck pain: a systematic review of the literature. Spine 2004;29(19):E413–25.
18. Young S, Aprill C, Laslett M. Correlation of clinical examination characteristics with three sources of chronic low back pain. Spine J 2003;3(6):460–5.
19. Revel M, Poiraudeau S, Auleley GR, et al. Capacity of the clinical picture to characterize low back pain relieved by facet joint anesthesia. Proposed criteria to identify patients with painful facet joints. Spine 1998;23(18):1972–6 [discussion: 1977].
20. Schwarzer AC, Derby R, Aprill CN, et al. The value of the provocation response in lumbar zygapophyseal joint injections. Clin J Pain 1994;10(4):309–13.
21. Tong HC, Haig AJ, Geisser ME, et al. Comparing pain severity and functional status of older adults without spinal symptoms, with lumbar spinal stenosis, and with axial low back pain. Gerontology 2007;53(2):111–5.
22. Laslett M, McDonald B, Aprill CN, et al. Clinical predictors of screening lumbar zygapophyseal joint blocks: development of clinical prediction rules. Spine J 2006;6(4):370–9.
23. Laslett M, McDonald B, Tropp H, et al. Agreement between diagnoses reached by clinical examination

and available reference standards: a prospective study of 216 patients with lumbopelvic pain. BMC Musculoskelet Disord 2005;6:28.

24. Andersson GB, Mekhail NA, Block JE. Treatment of intractable discogenic low back pain. A systematic review of spinal fusion and intradiscal electrothermal therapy (IDET). Pain Physician 2006;9(3):237–48.

25. Appleby D, Andersson G, Totta M. Meta-analysis of the efficacy and safety of intradiscal electrothermal therapy (IDET). Pain Med 2006;7(4):308–16.

26. Gibson JN, Waddell G. Surgery for degenerative lumbar spondylosis: updated Cochrane Review. Spine 2005;30(20):2312–20.

27. Gibson JN, Grant IC, Waddell G. The Cochrane review of surgery for lumbar disc prolapse and degenerative lumbar spondylosis. Spine 1999;24(17):1820–32.

28. Schwarzer AC, Aprill CN, Derby R, et al. Clinical features of patients with pain stemming from the lumbar zygapophysial joints. Is the lumbar facet syndrome a clinical entity? Spine 1994;19(10):1132–7.

29. Schwarzer AC, Wang SC, Bogduk N, et al. Prevalence and clinical features of lumbar zygapophysial joint pain: a study in an Australian population with chronic low back pain. Ann Rheum Dis 1995;54(2):100–6.

30. Manchikanti L, Pampati V, Fellows B, et al. Prevalence of lumbar facet joint pain in chronic low back pain. Pain Physician 1999;2(3):59–64.

31. Manchikanti L, Pampati V, Fellows B, et al. The diagnostic validity and therapeutic value of lumbar facet joint nerve blocks with or without adjuvant agents. Curr Rev Pain 2000;4(5):337–44.

32. Manchikanti L, Pampati V, Fellows B, et al. The inability of the clinical picture to characterize pain from facet joints. Pain Physician 2000;3(2):158–66.

33. Manchikanti L, Hirsch JA, Pampati V. Chronic low back pain of facet (zygapophysial) joint origin: is there a difference based on involvement of single or multiple spinal regions? Pain Physician 2003;6(4):399–405.

34. Manchikanti L, Singh V, Pampati V, et al. Is there correlation of facet joint pain in lumbar and cervical spine? An evaluation of prevalence in combined chronic low back and neck pain. Pain Physician 2002;5(4):365–71.

35. Manchikanti L, Manchukonda R, Pampati V, et al. Prevalence of facet joint pain in chronic low back pain in postsurgical patients by controlled comparative local anesthetic blocks. Arch Phys Med Rehabil 2007;88(4):449–55.

36. Barnsley L, et al. The prevalence of chronic cervical zygapophysial joint pain after whiplash. Spine 1995;20(1):20–5 [discussion: 26].

37. Lord SM, Lord SM, Wallis BJ, et al. Chronic cervical zygapophysial joint pain after whiplash. A placebo-controlled prevalence study. Spine 1996;21(15):1737–44 [discussion: 1744–5].

38. O'Neill CW, Kurgansky ME, Derby R, et al. Disc stimulation and patterns of referred pain. Spine 2002;27(24):2776–81.

39. Derby R, Eek B, Lee SH, et al. Comparison of intradiscal restorative injections and intradiscal electrothermal treatment (IDET) in the treatment of low back pain. Pain Physician 2004;7(1):63–6.

40. Mixter WJ, Barr JS. Rupture of the intervertebral disc with involvement of the spinal canal. N Engl J Med 1934;211:210–5.

41. Rosen S, Falco F. Radiofrequency stimulation of intervertebral discs. Pain Physician 2003;6(4):435–8.

42. Mixter WJ, Ayers JB. Herniation or rupture of the intervertebral disc into the spinal canal. N Engl J Med 1935;213:385–95.

43. Crock HV. A reappraisal of intervertebral disc lesions. Med J Aust 1970;1(20):983–9.

44. Wheeler AH, Murrey DB. Chronic lumbar spine and radicular pain: pathophysiology and treatment. Curr Pain Headache Rep 2002;6(2):97–105.

45. Ebraheim NA, Elgafy H, Semaan HB. Computed tomographic findings in patients with persistent sacroiliac pain after posterior iliac graft harvesting. Spine 2000;25(16):2047–51.

46. Katz V, Schofferman J, Reynolds J. The sacroiliac joint: a potential cause of pain after lumbar fusion to the sacrum. J Spinal Disord Tech 2003;16(1):96–9.

47. Maigne JY, Planchon CA. Sacroiliac joint pain after lumbar fusion. A study with anesthetic blocks. Eur Spine J 2005;14(7):654–8.

48. Schofferman J, Reynolds J, Herzog R, et al. Failed back surgery: etiology and diagnostic evaluation. Spine J 2003;3(5):400–3.

49. Slipman CW, et al. Etiologies of failed back surgery syndrome. Pain Med 2002;3(3):200–14 [discussion: 214–7].

50. Waguespack A, Schofferman J, Slosar P, et al. Etiology of long-term failures of lumbar spine surgery. Pain Med 2002;3(1):18–22.

51. Sampath P, Bendebba M, Davis JD, et al. Outcome in patients with cervical radiculopathy. Prospective, multicenter study with independent clinical review. Spine 1999;24(6):591–7.

52. Waddell G, Kummel EG, Lotto WN, et al. Failed lumbar disc surgery and repeat surgery following industrial injuries. J Bone Joint Surg Am 1979;61(2):201–7.

53. Lieberman IH. Disc bulge bubble: spine economics 101. Spine J 2004;4(6):609–13.

54. Deyo RA, Mirza SK. Trends and variations in the use of spine surgery. Clin Orthop Relat Res 2006;443:139–46.

55. Deyo RA, Nachemson A, Mirza SK. Spinal-fusion surgery—the case for restraint. N Engl J Med 2004;350(7):722–6.

56. Haig AJ, Tong HC, Yamakawa KS, et al. Predictors of pain and function in persons with spinal stenosis, low back pain, and no back pain. Spine 2006; 31(25):2950–7.

57. Anderberg L, Annertz M, Brandt L, et al. Selective diagnostic cervical nerve root block–correlation with clinical symptoms and MRI-pathology. Acta Neurochir (Wien) 2004;146(6):559–65 [discussion: 565].

58. Strobel K, Pfirrmann CW, Schmid M, et al. Cervical nerve root blocks: indications and role of MR imaging. Radiology 2004;233(1):87–92.

59. Scavone JG, Latshaw RF, Weidner WA. Anteroposterior and lateral radiographs: an adequate lumbar spine examination. AJR Am J Roentgenol 1981; 136(4):715–7.

60. Scavone JG, Latshaw RF, Rohrer GV. Use of lumbar spine films. Statistical evaluation at a university teaching hospital. JAMA 1981;246(10):1105–8.

61. Silbergleit R, Mehta BA, Sanders WP, et al. Imaging-guided injection techniques with fluoroscopy and CT for spinal pain management. Radiographics 2001;21(4):927–39 [discussion: 940–2].

62. Haldeman S. North American Spine Society: failure of the pathology model to predict back pain. Spine 1990;15(7):718–24.

63. Wiesel SW, Tsourmas N, Feffer HL, et al. A study of computer-assisted tomography. I. The incidence of positive CAT scans in an asymptomatic group of patients. Spine 1984;9(6):549–51.

64. Boden SD, Davis DO, Dina TS, et al. Abnormal magnetic-resonance scans of the lumbar spine in asymptomatic subjects. A prospective investigation. J Bone Joint Surg Am 1990;72(3):403–8.

65. Boden SD, McCowin PR, Davis DO, et al. Abnormal magnetic-resonance scans of the cervical spine in asymptomatic subjects. A prospective investigation. J Bone Joint Surg Am 1990;72(8):1178–84.

66. Schwarzer AC, Wang SC, O'Driscoll D, et al. The ability of computed tomography to identify a painful zygapophysial joint in patients with chronic low back pain. Spine 1995;20(8):907–12.

67. Kim KY, Wang MY. Magnetic resonance image-based morphological predictors of single photon emission computed tomography-positive facet arthropathy in patients with axial back pain. Neurosurgery 2006;59(1):147–56 [discussion: 147–56].

68. Houseni M, Chamroonrat W, Zhuang H, et al. Facet joint arthropathy demonstrated on FDG-PET. Clin Nucl Med 2006;31(7):418–9.

69. Borenstein DG, O'Mara JW Jr, Boden SD, et al. The value of magnetic resonance imaging of the lumbar spine to predict low-back pain in asymptomatic subjects: a seven-year follow-up study. J Bone Joint Surg Am 2001;83(9):1306–11.

70. Wood KB, Garvey TA, Gundry C, et al. Magnetic resonance imaging of the thoracic spine. Evaluation of asymptomatic individuals. J Bone Joint Surg Am 1995;77(11):1631–8.

71. Matsumoto M, Fujimura Y, Suzuki N, et al. MRI of cervical intervertebral discs in asymptomatic subjects. J Bone Joint Surg Br 1998;80(1):19–24.

72. Jensen MC, Brant-Zawadzki MN, Obuchowski N, et al. Magnetic resonance imaging of the lumbar spine in people without back pain. N Engl J Med 1994;331(2):69–73.

73. Magora A, Bigos SJ, Stoloy WC, et al. The significance of medical imaging findings in low back pain. Pain Clinic 1994;7:99–105.

74. Videman T, Battie MC, Gibbons LE, et al. Associations between back pain history and lumbar MRI findings. Spine 2003;28(6):582–8.

75. Kleinstuck F, Dvorak J, Mannion AF. Are "structural abnormalities" on magnetic resonance imaging a contraindication to the successful conservative treatment of chronic nonspecific low back pain? Spine 2006;31(19):2250–7.

76. Haig AJ, Tong HC, Yamakawa KS, et al. Spinal stenosis, back pain, or no symptoms at all? A masked study comparing radiologic and electrodiagnostic diagnoses to the clinical impression. Arch Phys Med Rehabil 2006;87(7):897–903.

77. Yang SC, Yang PH. Significance of the bright facet sign on T2W MRI of the lumbar facet joint. Mid-Taiwan J Med 2005;10:150–4.

78. Kapural L, Mekhail N, Bena J, et al. Value of the magnetic resonance imaging in patients with painful lumbar spinal stenosis (LSS) undergoing lumbar epidural steroid injections. Clin J Pain 2007;23(7): 571–5.

79. Goffin J, Van Calenbergh F, van Loon J, et al. Intermediate follow-up after treatment of degenerative disc disease with the Bryan Cervical Disc Prosthesis: single-level and bi-level. Spine 2003;28(24): 2673–8.

80. Cherkin DC, Deyo RA, Loeser JD, et al. An international comparison of back surgery rates. Spine 1994;19(11):1201–6.

81. Trescot AM, Chopra P, Abdi S, et al. Systematic review of effectiveness and complications of adhesiolysis in the management of chronic spinal pain: an update. Pain Physician 2007;10(1):129–46.

82. Weinstein JN, Lurie JD, Olson PR, et al. United States' trends and regional variations in lumbar spine surgery: 1992–2003. Spine 2006;31(23):2707–14.

83. Ross JS, Robertson JT, Frederickson RC, et al. Association between peridural scar and recurrent radicular pain after lumbar discectomy: magnetic resonance evaluation. ADCON-L European Study Group. Neurosurgery 1996;38(4):855–61 [discussion: 861–3].

84. Bono CM, Lee CK. Critical analysis of trends in fusion for degenerative disc disease over the past 20 years: influence of technique on fusion rate

and clinical outcome. Spine 2004;29(4):455–63 [discussion: Z5].

85. North RB, Campbell JN, James CS, et al. Failed back surgery syndrome: 5-year follow-up in 102 patients undergoing repeated operation. Neurosurgery 1991;28(5):685–90 [discussion: 690–1].

86. Fritsch EW, Heisel J, Rupp S. The failed back surgery syndrome: reasons, intraoperative findings, and long-term results: a report of 182 operative treatments. Spine 1996;21(5):626–33.

87. Weinstein JN, Tosteson TD, Lurie JD, et al. Surgical vs nonoperative treatment for lumbar disk herniation: the Spine Patient Outcomes Research Trial (SPORT): a randomized trial. JAMA 2006;296(20): 2441–50.

88. Weinstein JN, Lurie JD, Tosteson TD, et al. Surgical vs nonoperative treatment for lumbar disk herniation: the Spine Patient Outcomes Research Trial (SPORT) observational cohort. JAMA 2006; 296(20):2451–9.

89. Straus BN. Chronic pain of spinal origin: the costs of intervention. Spine 2002;27(22):2614–9 [discussion: 2620].

90. Johnson BA, Schellhas KP, Pollei SR. Epidurography and therapeutic epidural injections: technical considerations and experience with 5334 cases. AJNR Am J Neuroradiol 1999;20(4):697–705.

91. Safriel Y, Ali M, Hayt M, et al. Gadolinium use in spine procedures for patients with allergy to iodinated contrast–experience of 127 procedures. AJNR Am J Neuroradiol 2006;27(6):1194–7.

92. Manchikanti L, Staats PS, Singh V, et al. Evidence-based practice guidelines for interventional techniques in the management of chronic spinal pain. Pain Physician 2003;6(1):3–81.

93. Manchikanti L, Singh V, Kloth D, et al. Interventional techniques in the management of chronic pain: part 2.0. Pain Physician 2001;4(1):24–96.

94. Manchikanti L, Singh V, Bakhit CE, et al. Interventional techniques in the management of chronic pain: part 1.0. Pain Physician 2000;3(1):7–42.

95. Abdi S, Datta S, Trescot AM, et al. Epidural steroids in the management of chronic spinal pain: a systematic review. Pain Physician 2007;10(1): 185–212.

96. Boswell MV, Colson JD, Sehgal N, et al. A systematic review of therapeutic facet joint interventions in chronic spinal pain. Pain Physician 2007;10(1): 229–53.

97. Sehgal N, Dunbar EE, Shah RV, et al. Systematic review of diagnostic utility of facet (zygapophysial) joint injections in chronic spinal pain: an update. Pain Physician 2007;10(1):213–28.

98. Datta S, Everett CR, Trescot AM, et al. An updated systematic review of the diagnostic utility of selective nerve root blocks. Pain Physician 2007;10(1): 113–28.

99. Buenaventura RM, Shah RV, Patel V, et al. Systematic review of discography as a diagnostic test for spinal pain: an update. Pain Physician 2007; 10(1):147–64.

100. van Tulder MW, Koes B, Seitsalo S, et al. Outcome of invasive treatment modalities on back pain and sciatica: an evidence-based review. Eur Spine J 2006;15(Suppl 1):S82–92.

101. Nelemans PJ, de Bie RA, de Vet HC, et al. Injection therapy for subacute and chronic benign low back pain. Cochrane Database Syst Rev 2000;(2): CD001824.

102. North RB, Kidd DH, Zahurak M, et al. Specificity of diagnostic nerve blocks: a prospective, randomized study of sciatica due to lumbosacral spine disease. Pain 1996;65(1):77–85.

103. Cohen SP, Hurley RW. The ability of diagnostic spinal injections to predict surgical outcomes. Anesth Analg 2007;105(6):1756–75 [table of contents].

104. Slipman CW, Chow DW. Therapeutic spinal corticosteroid injections for the management of radiculopathies. Phys Med Rehabil Clin N Am 2002;13(3): 697–711.

105. Harrington JF, Messier AA, Bereiter D, et al. Herniated lumbar disc material as a source of free glutamate available to affect pain signals through the dorsal root ganglion. Spine 2000;25(8):929–36.

106. Harrington JF, Messier AA, Hoffman L, et al. Physiological and behavioral evidence for focal nociception induced by epidural glutamate infusion in rats. Spine 2005;30(6):606–12.

107. Gangi A, Dietemann JL, Mortazavi R, et al. CT-guided interventional procedures for pain management in the lumbosacral spine. Radiographics 1998;18(3):621–33.

108. White AH. Injection techniques for the diagnosis and treatment of low back pain. Orthop Clin North Am 1983;14:553–67.

109. Bush K, Hillier S. A controlled study of caudal epidural injections of triamcinolone plus procaine for the management of intractable sciatica. Spine 1991;16(5):572–5.

110. Nelson DA. Intraspinal therapy using methylprednisolone acetate. Twenty-three years of clinical controversy. Spine 1993;18(2):278–86.

111. Abram SE, O'Connor TC. Complications associated with epidural steroid injections. Reg Anesth 1996;21(2):149–62.

112. Dreyfuss P, Baker R, Bogduk N. Comparative effectiveness of cervical transforaminal injections with particulate and nonparticulate corticosteroid preparations for cervical radicular pain. Pain Med 2006;7(3):237–42.

113. Stanczak J, Blankenbaker DG, De Smet AA, et al. Efficacy of epidural injections of Kenalog and Celestone in the treatment of lower back pain. AJR Am J Roentgenol 2003;181(5):1255–8.

114. Owlia MB, Salimzadeh A, Alishiri G, et al. Comparison of two doses of corticosteroid in epidural steroid injection for lumbar radicular pain. Singapore Med J 2007;48(3):241–5.

115. Inman SL, Faut-Callahan M, Swanson BA, et al. Sex differences in responses to epidural steroid injection for low back pain. J Pain 2004;5(8):450–7.

116. Hogan QH, Abram SE. Neural blockade for diagnosis and prognosis. A review. Anesthesiology 1997; 86(1):216–41.

117. Hildebrandt J. Relevance of nerve blocks in treating and diagnosing low back pain–is the quality decisive? Schmerz 2001;15(6):474–83 [in German].

118. Nachemson A, Vingard E. Assessment of patients with neck and back pain: a best-evidence synthesis. In: Nachemson A, Jonsson E, editors. Neck and back pain. The scientific evidence of causes, diagnosis, and treatment. Philadelphia: Lippincott Williams & Wilkins; 2000. p. 189–236.

119. Jaeschke R, Guyatt G, Lijmer J. Diagnostic tests. In: Guyatt G, Rennie D, editors. Users' guides to the medical literature: a manual for evidence-based clinical practice. Chicago: AMA Press; 2002. p. 121–40.

120. Everett CR, Shah RV, Sehgal N, et al. A systematic review of diagnostic utility of selective nerve root blocks. Pain Physician 2005;8(2):225–33.

121. Hasue M, Kunogi J, Kikuchi S. Imaging methods of the dorsal root ganglion. Diagnostic aids in lumbar spine disease: a preliminary report. Neuro-Orthopedics 1989;8:23–7.

122. Zennaro H, Dousset V, Viaud B, et al. Periganglionic foraminal steroid injections performed under CT control. AJNR Am J Neuroradiol 1998; 19(2):349–52.

123. Castro WH, Gronemeyer D, Jerosch J, et al. How reliable is lumbar nerve root sheath infiltration? Eur Spine J 1994;3(5):255–7.

124. van Akkerveeken PF. The diagnostic value of nerve root sheath infiltration. Acta Orthop Scand Suppl 1993;251:61–3.

125. Lutz GE, Vad VB, Wisneski RJ. Fluoroscopic transforaminal lumbar epidural steroids: an outcome study. Arch Phys Med Rehabil 1998;79(11): 1362–6.

126. Riew KD, Yin Y, Gilula L, et al. The effect of nerve-root injections on the need for operative treatment of lumbar radicular pain. A prospective, randomized, controlled, double-blind study. J Bone Joint Surg Am 2000;82(11):1589–93.

127. Vallee JN, Feydy A, Carlier RY, et al. Chronic cervical radiculopathy: lateral-approach periradicular corticosteroid injection. Radiology 2001;218(3): 886–92.

128. Wolff AP, Groen GJ, Crul BJ. Diagnostic lumbosacral segmental nerve blocks with local anesthetics:

a prospective double-blind study on the variability and interpretation of segmental effects. Reg Anesth Pain Med 2001;26(2):147–55.

129. Kadish LJ, Simmons EH. Anomalies of the lumbosacral nerve roots. An anatomical investigation and myelographic study. J Bone Joint Surg Br 1984;66(3):411–6.

130. Kikuchi S, Hasue M, Nishiyama K, et al. Anatomic features of the furcal nerve and its clinical significance. Spine 1986;11(10):1002–7.

131. Datta S, Pai U. Selective nerve root block–is the position of the needle transforaminal or paraforaminal? Call for a need to reevaluate the terminology. Reg Anesth Pain Med 2004;29(6):616–7 [author reply 617].

132. Pauza K, Bogduk N. Lumbar transforaminal injection of corticosteroids. International Spine Injection Society Newsletter 2003;4:4–20.

133. Crall TS, Gilula LA, Kim YJ, et al. The diagnostic effect of various needle tip positions in selective lumbar nerve blocks: an analysis of 1202 injections. Spine 2006;31(8):920–2.

134. Ng LC, Sell P. Outcomes of a prospective cohort study on peri-radicular infiltration for radicular pain in patients with lumbar disc herniation and spinal stenosis. Eur Spine J 2004;13(4):325–9.

135. Evans W. Intrasacral epidural injection therapy in the treatment of sciatica. Lancet 1930;2:1225–9.

136. Robecchi A, Capra R. Hydrocortisone (compound F); first clinical experiments in the field of rheumatology. Minerva Med 1952;43(98):1259–63.

137. Winnie AP, Hartman JT, Meyers HL Jr, et al. Pain clinic. II. Intradural and extradural corticosteroids for sciatica. Anesth Analg 1972;51(6):990–1003.

138. Stafford MA, Peng P, Hill DA. Sciatica: a review of history, epidemiology, pathogenesis, and the role of epidural steroid injection in management. Br J Anaesth 2007;99(4):461–73.

139. Botwin KP, Sakalkale DP. Epidural steroid injections in the treatment of symptomatic lumbar spinal stenosis associated with epidural lipomatosis. Am J Phys Med Rehabil 2004;83(12):926–30.

140. Aydin SM, Zou SP, Varlotta G, et al. Successful treatment of phantom radiculopathy with fluoroscopic epidural steroid injections. Pain Med 2005; 6(3):266–8.

141. Dincer U, Kiralp MZ, Cakar E, et al. Caudal epidural injection versus non-steroidal anti-inflammatory drugs in the treatment of low back pain accompanied with radicular pain. Joint Bone Spine 2007; 74(5):467–71.

142. Botwin K, Brown LA, Fishman M, et al. Fluoroscopically guided caudal epidural steroid injections in degenerative lumbar spine stenosis. Pain Physician 2007;10(4):547–58.

143. Price CM, Rogers PD, Prosser AS, et al. Comparison of the caudal and lumbar approaches to the

epidural space. Ann Rheum Dis 2000;59(11): 879–82.

144. Schaufele MK, Hatch L, Jones W. Interlaminar versus transforaminal epidural injections for the treatment of symptomatic lumbar intervertebral disc herniations. Pain Physician 2006;9(4):361–6.

145. Ackerman WE III, Ahmad M. The efficacy of lumbar epidural steroid injections in patients with lumbar disc herniations. Anesth Analg 2007;104(5): 1217–22.

146. Vad VB, Bhat AL, Lutz GE, et al. Transforaminal epidural steroid injections in lumbosacral radiculopathy: a prospective randomized study. Spine 2002;27(1):11–6.

147. Cluff R, Mehio AK, Cohen SP, et al. The technical aspects of epidural steroid injections: a national survey. Anesth Analg 2002;95(2):403–8.

148. Papagelopoulos PJ, Petrou HG, Triantafyllidis PG, et al. Treatment of lumbosacral radicular pain with epidural steroid injections. Orthopedics 2001; 24(2):145–9.

149. Hession WG, Stanczak JD, Davis KW, et al. Epidural steroid injections. Semin Roentgenol 2004; 39(1):7–23.

150. McLain RF, Kapural L, Mekhail NA. Epidural steroid therapy for back and leg pain: mechanisms of action and efficacy. Spine J 2005;5(2):191–201.

151. Kwon JW, Lee JW, Kim SH, et al. Cervical interlaminar epidural steroid injection for neck pain and cervical radiculopathy: effect and prognostic factors. Skeletal Radiol 2007;36(5):431–6.

152. Delport EG, Cucuzzella AR, Marley JK, et al. Treatment of lumbar spinal stenosis with epidural steroid injections: a retrospective outcome study. Arch Phys Med Rehabil 2004;85(3):479–84.

153. Arden NK, Price C, Reading I, et al. A multicentre randomized controlled trial of epidural corticosteroid injections for sciatica: the WEST study. Rheumatology (Oxford) 2005;44(11):1399–406.

154. Jackson C, Broadhurst N, Bogduk N. An audit of the use of epidural injections for back pain and sciatica. Aust Health Rev 2003;26(1):34–42.

155. Weinstein SM, Herring SA. Lumbar epidural steroid injections. Spine J 2003;3(3 Suppl):37S–44S.

156. Spaccarelli KC. Lumbar and caudal epidural corticosteroid injections. Mayo Clin Proc 1996;71(2): 169–78.

157. Armon C, Argoff CE, Samuels J, et al. Assessment: use of epidural steroid injections to treat radicular lumbosacral pain: report of the therapeutics and technology assessment subcommittee of the American academy of neurology. Neurology 2007; 68(10):723–9.

158. Wilson-MacDonald J, Argoff CE, Samuels J, et al. Epidural steroid injection for nerve root compression. A randomised, controlled trial. J Bone Joint Surg Br 2005;87(3):352–5.

159. Valat JP, Giraudeau B, Rozenberg S, et al. Epidural corticosteroid injections for sciatica: a randomised, double blind, controlled clinical trial. Ann Rheum Dis 2003;62(7):639–43.

160. Young IA, Hyman GS, Packia-Raj LN, et al. The use of lumbar epidural/transforaminal steroids for managing spinal disease. J Am Acad Orthop Surg 2007;15(4):228–38.

161. Johnson BA. Image-guided epidural injections. Neuroimaging Clin N Am 2000;10(3):479–91.

162. Johnson DW. Back to the future: epidurography. AJNR Am J Neuroradiol 1999;20(4):537.

163. Chen B, Foye PM, Castro CP, et al. Epidural steroid injections. Therapeutic modalities 2007 [cited 2007]; Available at: http://www.emedicine.com/pmr/topic223.htm. Accessed December 15, 2007.

164. Manchikanti L, Pampati V, Damron KS, et al. The effect of sedation on diagnostic validity of facet joint nerve blocks: an evaluation to assess similarities in population with involvement in cervical and lumbar regions (ISRCTNo: 76376497). Pain Physician 2006;9(1):47–51.

165. el-Khoury GY, Renfrew DL. Percutaneous procedures for the diagnosis and treatment of lower back pain: diskography, facet-joint injection, and epidural injection. AJR Am J Roentgenol 1991; 157(4):685–91.

166. Lippitt AB. The facet joint and its role in spine pain. Management with facet joint injections. Spine 1984; 9(7):746–50.

167. Cavanaugh JM, Ozaktay AC, Yamashita HT, et al. Lumbar facet pain: biomechanics, neuroanatomy and neurophysiology. J Biomech 1996;29(9): 1117–29.

168. Wilde VE, Ford JJ, McMeeken JM. Indicators of lumbar zygapophyseal joint pain: survey of an expert panel with the Delphi technique. Phys Ther 2007;87(10):1348–61.

169. Hooten WM, Martin DP, Huntoon MA. Radiofrequency neurotomy for low back pain: evidence-based procedural guidelines. Pain Med 2005; 6(2):129–38.

170. Pneumaticos SG, Chatziioannou SN, Hipp JA, et al. Low back pain: prediction of short-term outcome of facet joint injection with bone scintigraphy. Radiology 2006;238(2):693–8.

171. Sarazin L, Chevrot A, Pessis E, et al. Lumbar facet joint arthrography with the posterior approach. Radiographics 1999;19(1):93–104.

172. Lynch MC, Taylor JF. Facet joint injection for low back pain. A clinical study. J Bone Joint Surg Br 1986;68(1):138–41.

173. Lilius G, Laasonen EM, Myllynen P, et al. Lumbar facet joint syndrome. A randomised clinical trial. J Bone Joint Surg Br 1989;71(4):681–4.

174. Boswell MV, Colson JD, Spillane WF. Therapeutic facet joint interventions in chronic spinal pain: a

systematic review of effectiveness and complications. Pain Physician 2005;8(1):101–14.

175. Marks RC, Houston T, Thulbourne T. Facet joint injection and facet nerve block: a randomised comparison in 86 patients with chronic low back pain. Pain 1992;49(3):325–8.

176. Stojanovic MP, Dey D, Hord ED, et al. A prospective crossover comparison study of the single-needle and multiple-needle techniques for facet-joint medial branch block. Reg Anesth Pain Med 2005; 30(5):484–90.

177. Birkenmaier C, Veihelmann A, Trouillier HH, et al. Medial branch blocks versus pericapsular blocks in selecting patients for percutaneous cryodenervation of lumbar facet joints. Reg Anesth Pain Med 2007;32(1):27–33.

178. Kaplan M, Dreyfuss P, Halbrook B, et al. The ability of lumbar medial branch blocks to anesthetize the zygapophysial joint. A physiologic challenge. Spine 1998;23(17):1847–52.

179. Pevsner Y, Shabat S, Catz A, et al. The role of radiofrequency in the treatment of mechanical pain of spinal origin. Eur Spine J 2003;12(6):602–5.

180. Manchikanti L, Manchikanti KN, Manchukonda R, et al. Evaluation of therapeutic thoracic medial branch block effectiveness in chronic thoracic pain: a prospective outcome study with minimum 1-year follow up. Pain Physician 2006;9(2): 97–105.

181. Carette S, Marcoux S, Truchon R, et al. A controlled trial of corticosteroid injections into facet joints for chronic low back pain. N Engl J Med 1991; 325(14):1002–7.

182. Manchikanti L, Damron K, Cash K, et al. Therapeutic cervical medial branch blocks in managing chronic neck pain: a preliminary report of a randomized, double-blind, controlled trial: clinical trial NCT0033272. Pain Physician 2006;9(4):333–46.

183. Manchikanti L, Manchikanti KN, Manchukonda R, et al. Evaluation of lumbar facet joint nerve blocks in the management of chronic low back pain: preliminary report of a randomized, double-blind controlled trial: clinical trial NCT00355914. Pain Physician 2007;10(3):425–40.

184. Slipman CW, Bhat AL, Gilchrist RV, et al. A critical review of the evidence for the use of zygapophysial injections and radiofrequency denervation in the treatment of low back pain. Spine J 2003;3(4): 310–6.

185. Shin WR, Kim HI, Shin DG, et al. Radiofrequency neurotomy of cervical medial branches for chronic cervicobrachialgia. J Korean Med Sci 2006;21(1): 119–25.

186. Curatolo M, Reiz S. Re: Niemisto L, Kalso E, Malmivaara A, et al. Radiofrequency denervation for neck and back pain: a systematic review within the framework of the cochrane collaboration back review group. Spine 2003;28:1877–88. Spine 2005;30(2):263–4 [author reply 264–5].

187. Gofeld M, Jitendra J, Faclier G. Radiofrequency denervation of the lumbar zygapophysial joints: 10-year prospective clinical audit. Pain Physician 2007;10(2):291–300.

188. Gofeld M, Faclier G. Radiofrequency denervation of the lumbar zygapophysial joints—targeting the best practice. Pain Med 2007;9(2):204–11.

189. Tzaan WC, Tasker RR. Percutaneous radiofrequency facet rhizotomy–experience with 118 procedures and reappraisal of its value. Can J Neurol Sci 2000;27(2):125–30.

190. Mikeladze G, Espinal R, Finnegan R, et al. Pulsed radiofrequency application in treatment of chronic zygapophyseal joint pain. Spine J 2003;3(5):360–2.

191. Lindner R, Sluijter ME, Schleinzer W. Pulsed radiofrequency treatment of the lumbar medial branch for facet pain: a retrospective analysis. Pain Med 2006;7(5):435–9.

192. Greher M, Scharbert G, Kamolz LP, et al. Ultrasound-guided lumbar facet nerve block: a sonoanatomic study of a new methodologic approach. Anesthesiology 2004;100(5):1242–8.

193. Shim JK, Moon JC, Yoon KB, et al. Ultrasound-guided lumbar medial-branch block: a clinical study with fluoroscopy control. Reg Anesth Pain Med 2006;31(5):451–4.

194. Klocke R, Jenkinson T, Glew D. Sonographically guided caudal epidural steroid injections. J Ultrasound Med 2003;22(11):1229–32.

195. Schmid G, Schmitz A, Borchardt D, et al. Effective dose of CT- and fluoroscopy-guided perineural/epidural injections of the lumbar spine: a comparative study. Cardiovasc Intervent Radiol 2006;29(1): 84–91.

196. Botwin KP, Thomas S, Gruber RD, et al. Radiation exposure of the spinal interventionalist performing fluoroscopically guided lumbar transforaminal epidural steroid injections. Arch Phys Med Rehabil 2002;83(5):697–701.

197. Quinn SF, Murtagh FR, Chatfield R, et al. CT-guided nerve root block and ablation. AJR Am J Roentgenol 1988;151(6):1213–6.

198. Murtagh R. The art and science of nerve root and facet blocks. Neuroimaging Clin N Am 2000; 10(3):465–77.

199. Katada K, Kato R, Anno H, et al. Guidance with real-time CT fluoroscopy: early clinical experience. Radiology 1996;200(3):851–6.

200. Meyer CA, White CS, Wu J, et al. Real-time CT fluoroscopy: usefulness in thoracic drainage. AJR Am J Roentgenol 1998;171(4):1097–101.

201. Muehlstaedt M, Bruening R, Diebold J, et al. CT/fluoroscopy-guided transthoracic needle biopsy: sensitivity and complication rate in 98 procedures. J Comput Assist Tomogr 2002;26(2):191–6.

202. Paulson EK, Sheafor DH, Enterline DS, et al. CT fluoroscopy–guided interventional procedures: techniques and radiation dose to radiologists. Radiology 2001;220(1):161–7.

203. Carlson SK, Bender CE, Classic KL, et al. Benefits and safety of CT fluoroscopy in interventional radiologic procedures. Radiology 2001;219(2):515–20.

204. Nawfel RD, Judy PF, Silverman SG, et al. Patient and personnel exposure during CT fluoroscopy-guided interventional procedures. Radiology 2000;216(1):180–4.

205. Wagner AL. CT fluoroscopic-guided cervical nerve root blocks. AJNR Am J Neuroradiol 2005;26(1):43–4.

206. Wagner AL. Selective lumbar nerve root blocks with CT fluoroscopic guidance: technique, results, procedure time, and radiation dose. AJNR Am J Neuroradiol 2004;25(9):1592–4.

207. Kim H, Lee SH, Kim MH. Multislice CT fluoroscopy-assisted cervical transforaminal injection of steroids: technical note. J Spinal Disord Tech 2007;20(6):456–61.

208. Bartynski WS, Whitt DS, Sheetz MA, et al. Lower cervical nerve root block using CT fluoroscopy in patients with large body habitus: another benefit of the swimmer's position. AJNR Am J Neuroradiol 2007;28(4):706–8.

209. Wagner AL, Murtagh FR. Selective nerve root blocks. Tech Vasc Interv Radiol 2002;5(4):194–200.

210. Silverman SG, et al. CT fluoroscopy-guided abdominal interventions: techniques, results, and radiation exposure. Radiology 1999;212(3):673–81.

211. Lutz GE, Shen TC. Fluoroscopically guided aspiration of a symptomatic lumbar zygapophyseal joint cyst: a case report. Arch Phys Med Rehabil 2002;83(12):1789–91.

212. Savitz M. Synovial cysts of the lumbar spine: a review. Br J Neurosurg 1998;12(5):465–6.

213. Pirotte B, Gabrovsky N, Massager N, et al. Synovial cysts of the lumbar spine: surgery-related results and outcome. J Neurosurg 2003;99(1 Suppl):14–9.

214. Khan AM, Synnot K, Cammisa FP, et al. Lumbar synovial cysts of the spine: an evaluation of surgical outcome. J Spinal Disord Tech 2005;18(2):127–31.

215. Epstein NE. Lumbar synovial cysts: a review of diagnosis, surgical management, and outcome assessment. J Spinal Disord Tech 2004;17(4):321–5.

216. Choudhri HF, Perling LH. Diagnosis and management of juxtafacet cysts. Neurosurg Focus 2006;20(3):E1.

217. Sauvage P, Grimault L, Ben Salem D, et al. Lumbar intraspinal synovial cysts: imaging and treatment by percutaneous injection. Report of thirteen cases. J Radiol 2000;81(1):33–8 [in French].

218. Bureau NJ, Kaplan PA, Dussault RG. Lumbar facet joint synovial cyst: percutaneous treatment with steroid injections and distention–clinical and imaging follow-up in 12 patients. Radiology 2001;221(1):179–85.

219. Ewald C, Kalff R. Resolution of a synovial cyst of the lumbar spine without surgical therapy—a case report. Zentralbl Neurochir 2005;66(3):147–51.

220. Hemminghytt S, Daniels DL, Williams AL, et al. Intraspinal synovial cysts: natural history and diagnosis by CT. Radiology 1982;145(2):375–6.

221. Lemish W, Apsimon T, Chakera T. Lumbar intraspinal synovial cysts. Recognition and CT diagnosis. Spine 1989;14(12):1378–83.

222. Mercader J, Munoz Gomez J, Cardenal C. Intraspinal synovial cyst: diagnosis by CT. Follow-up and spontaneous remission. Neuroradiology 1985;27(4):346–8.

223. Hsu KY, Zucherman JF, Shea WJ, et al. Lumbar intraspinal synovial and ganglion cysts (facet cysts). Ten-year experience in evaluation and treatment. Spine 1995;20(1):80–9.

224. Shah RV, Lutz GE. Lumbar intraspinal synovial cysts: conservative management and review of the world's literature. Spine J 2003;3(6):479–88.

225. Banning CS, Thorell WE, Leibrock LG. Patient outcome after resection of lumbar juxtafacet cysts. Spine 2001;26(8):969–72.

226. Howington JU, Connolly ES, Voorhies RM. Intraspinal synovial cysts: 10-year experience at the Ochsner Clinic. J Neurosurg 1999;91(2 Suppl):193–9.

227. Casselman ES. Radiologic recognition of symptomatic spinal synovial cysts. AJNR Am J Neuroradiol 1985;6(6):971–3.

228. Bjorkengren AG, Kurz LT, Resnick D, et al. Symptomatic intraspinal synovial cysts: opacification and treatment by percutaneous injection. AJR Am J Roentgenol 1987;149(1):105–7.

229. Finkelstein SD, Sayegh R, Watson P, et al. Juxtafacet cysts. Report of two cases and review of clinicopathologic features. Spine 1993;18(6):779–82.

230. Lim AK, Higgins SJ, Saifuddin A, et al. Symptomatic lumbar synovial cyst: management with direct CT-guided puncture and steroid injection. Clin Radiol 2001;56(12):990–3.

231. Parlier-Cuau C, Wybier M, Nizard R, et al. Symptomatic lumbar facet joint synovial cysts: clinical assessment of facet joint steroid injection after 1 and 6 months and long-term follow-up in 30 patients. Radiology 1999;210(2):509–13.

232. Reust P, Wendling D, Lagier R, et al. Degenerative spondylolisthesis, synovial cyst of the zygapophyseal joints, and sciatic syndrome: report of two cases and review of the literature. Arthritis Rheum 1988;31(2):288–94.

233. Imai K, Nakamura K, Inokuchi K, et al. Aspiration of intraspinal synovial cyst: recurrence after temporal improvement. Arch Orthop Trauma Surg 1998; 118(1–2):103–5.

234. Melfi RS, Aprill CN. Percutaneous puncture of zygapophysial joint synovial cyst with fluoroscopic guidance. Pain Med 2005;6(2):122–8.

235. Manchikanti L, Pampati V, Damron KS, et al. A randomized, prospective, double-blind, placebo-controlled evaluation of the effect of sedation on diagnostic validity of cervical facet joint pain. Pain Physician 2004;7(3):301–9.

236. Manchikanti L, Damron KS, Rivera JJ, et al. Evaluation of the effect of sedation as a confounding factor in the diagnostic validity of lumbar facet joint pain: a prospective, randomized, double-blind, placebo-controlled evaluation. Pain Physician 2004;7(4):411–7.

237. Hodges SD, Castleberg RL, Miller T, et al. Cervical epidural steroid injection with intrinsic spinal cord damage. Two case reports. Spine 1998;23(19): 2137–42 [discussion: 2141–2].

238. LaBan MM, Kasturi G, Wang IM. Epidural corticosteroid injections precipitating epidural hematomas with spinal paresis. Am J Phys Med Rehabil 2007; 86(2):166–7.

239. Snarr J. Risk, benefits and complications of epidural steroid injections: a case report. AANA J 2007; 75(3):183–8.

240. Reitman CA, Watters W III. Subdural hematoma after cervical epidural steroid injection. Spine 2002;27(6):E174–6.

241. O'Brien DP, Rawluk DJ. Iatrogenic Mycobacterium infection after an epidural injection. Spine 1999; 24(12):1257–9.

242. Huang RC, Shapiro GS, Lim M, et al. Cervical epidural abscess after epidural steroid injection. Spine 2004;29(1):E7–9.

243. Puehler W, Brack A, Kopf A. Extensive abscess formation after repeated paravertebral injections for the treatment of chronic back pain. Pain 2005; 113(3):427–9.

244. Finn KP, Case JL. Disk entry: a complication of transforaminal epidural injection–a case report. Arch Phys Med Rehabil 2005;86(7):1489–91.

245. Hooten WM, Mizerak A, Carns PE, et al. Discitis after lumbar epidural corticosteroid injection: a case report and analysis of the case report literature. Pain Med 2006;7(1):46–51.

246. Gaul C, Neundorfer B, Winterholler M. Iatrogenic (para-) spinal abscesses and meningitis following injection therapy for low back pain. Pain 2005; 116(3):407–10.

247. Hooten WM, Kinney MO, Huntoon MA. Epidural abscess and meningitis after epidural corticosteroid injection. Mayo Clin Proc 2004;79(5):682–6.

248. Yue WM, Tan SB. Distant skip level discitis and vertebral osteomyelitis after caudal epidural injection: a case report of a rare complication of epidural injections. Spine 2003;28(11):E209–11.

249. Stalcup ST, Crall TS, Gilula L, et al. Influence of needle-tip position on the incidence of immediate complications in 2,217 selective lumbar nerve root blocks. Spine J 2006;6(2):170–6.

250. Botwin KP, Gruber RD, Bouchlas CG, et al. Complications of fluoroscopically guided transforaminal lumbar epidural injections. Arch Phys Med Rehabil 2000;81(8):1045–50.

251. Bartynski WS, Grahovac SZ, Rothfus WE. Incorrect needle position during lumbar epidural steroid administration: inaccuracy of loss of air pressure resistance and requirement of fluoroscopy and epidurography during needle insertion. AJNR Am J Neuroradiol 2005;26(3):502–5.

252. Liu SS, Melmed AP, Klos JW, et al. Prospective experience with a 20-gauge Tuohy needle for lumbar epidural steroid injections: Is confirmation with fluoroscopy necessary? Reg Anesth Pain Med 2001;26(2):143–6.

253. Shetty SK, Nelson EN, Lawrimore TM, et al. Use of gadolinium chelate to confirm epidural needle placement in patients with an iodinated contrast reaction. Skeletal Radiol 2007;36(4):301–7.

254. Huston CW, Slipman CW, Garvin C. Complications and side effects of cervical and lumbosacral selective nerve root injections. Arch Phys Med Rehabil 2005;86(2):277–83.

255. Ozdemir O, Calisaneller T, Yildirim E, et al. Acute intracranial subdural hematoma after epidural steroid injection: a case report. J Manipulative Physiol Ther 2007;30(7):536–8.

256. Bilir A, Gulec S. Cauda equina syndrome after epidural steroid injection: a case report. J Manipulative Physiol Ther 2006;29(6):492 [e1–3].

257. Houten JK, Errico TJ. Paraplegia after lumbosacral nerve root block: report of three cases. Spine J 2002;2(1):70–5.

258. Hawley JS, Ney JP, Swanberg MM. Subarachnoid pneumocephalus from epidural steroid injection. Headache 2005;45(3):247–8.

259. Tripathi M, Nath SS, Gupta RK. Paraplegia after intracord injection during attempted epidural steroid injection in an awake-patient. Anesth Analg 2005; 101(4):1209–11 [table of contents].

260. Saigal G, Donovan Post MJ, Kozic D. Thoracic intradural Aspergillus abscess formation following epidural steroid injection. AJNR Am J Neuroradiol 2004;25(4):642–4.

261. Beckman WA, Mendez RJ, Paine GF, et al. Cerebellar herniation after cervical transforaminal epidural injection. Reg Anesth Pain Med 2006;31(3): 282–5.

262. Muro K, O'Shaughnessy B, Ganju A. Infarction of the cervical spinal cord following multilevel transforaminal epidural steroid injection: case report and review of the literature. J Spinal Cord Med 2007;30(4):385–8.

263. Scanlon GC, Moeller-Bertram T, Romanowsky SM, et al. Cervical transforaminal epidural steroid injections: more dangerous than we think? Spine 2007; 32(11):1249–56.

264. Ziai WC, Ardelt AA, Llinas RH. Brainstem stroke following uncomplicated cervical epidural steroid injection. Arch Neurol 2006;63(11):1643–6.

265. Bose B. Quadriparesis following cervical epidural steroid injections: case report and review of the literature. Spine J 2005;5(5):558–63.

266. Ludwig MA, Burns SP. Spinal cord infarction following cervical transforaminal epidural injection: a case report. Spine 2005;30(10):E266–8.

267. Tiso RL, Cutler T, Catania JA, et al. Adverse central nervous system sequelae after selective transforaminal block: the role of corticosteroids. Spine J 2004;4(4):468–74.

268. Rozin L, Cutler T, Catania JA, et al. Death during transforaminal epidural steroid nerve root block (C7) due to perforation of the left vertebral artery. Am J Forensic Med Pathol 2003;24(4):351–5.

269. Huntoon MA. Anatomy of the cervical intervertebral foramina: vulnerable arteries and ischemic neurologic injuries after transforaminal epidural injections. Pain 2005;117(1–2):104–11.

270. Ho KY. Vascular uptake of contrast despite negative aspiration in interlaminar cervical epidural injection. Pain Physician 2006;9(3):267–8.

271. Ma DJ, Gilula LA, Riew KD. Complications of fluoroscopically guided extraforaminal cervical nerve blocks. An analysis of 1036 injections. J Bone Joint Surg Am 2005;87(5):1025–30.

272. Botwin KP, Castellanos R, Rao S, et al. Complications of fluoroscopically guided interlaminar cervical epidural injections. Arch Phys Med Rehabil 2003;84(5):627–33.

273. McCullen GM, Spurling GR, Webster JS. Epidural lipomatosis complicating lumbar steroid injections. J Spinal Disord 1999;12(6):526–9.

274. Kao LY. Bilateral serous retinal detachment resembling central serous chorioretinopathy following epidural steroid injection. Retina 1998;18(5):479–81.

275. MacLean CA, Bachman DT. Documented arterial gas embolism after spinal epidural injection. Ann Emerg Med 2001;38(5):592–5.

276. Young WF. Transient blindness after lumbar epidural steroid injection: a case report and literature review. Spine 2002;27(21):E476–7.

277. Slipman CW, Chow DW, Lenrow DA, et al. Dysphonia associated with epidural steroid injection: a case report. Arch Phys Med Rehabil 2002; 83(9):1309–10.

278. Slipman CW, Shin CH, Patel RK, et al. Persistent hiccup associated with thoracic epidural injection. Am J Phys Med Rehabil 2001;80(8):618–21.

279. Amin N, Brancaccio R, Cohen D. Cutaneous reactions to injectable corticosteroids. Dermatitis 2006; 17(3):143–6.

280. Horani MH, Silverberg AB. Secondary Cushing's syndrome after a single epidural injection of a corticosteroid. Endocr Pract 2005;11(6):408–10.

281. Kay J, Findling JW, Raff H. Epidural triamcinolone suppresses the pituitary-adrenal axis in human subjects. Anesth Analg 1994;79(3):501–5.

282. Ward A, Watson J, Wood P, et al. Glucocorticoid epidural for sciatica: metabolic and endocrine sequelae. Rheumatology (Oxford) 2002;41(1):68–71.

283. Tuncer S, Bariskaner H, Yosunkaya A, et al. Systemic effects of epidural betamethasone injection. The Pain Clinic 2004;16(3):311–5.

284. Cicala RS, Westbrook L, Angel JJ. Side effects and complications of cervical epidural steroid injections. J Pain Symptom Manage 1989;4(2):64–6.

Musculoskeletal Ultrasound Intervention: Principles and Advances

Luck J. Louis, MD, FRCPC

KEYWORDS

- Ultrasound • Musculoskeletal intervention
- Prolotherapy • Barbotage • Ganglion cysts • Ganglia

The use of ultrasonography in interventional musculoskeletal radiology is well established[1–3] and is used primarily to guide needle placement for injections, aspirations, and biopsies. The chief advantage of ultrasound imaging is its ability to perform real-time, multiplanar imaging without ionizing radiation. It is relatively inexpensive, is widely available, and permits comparison with the asymptomatic side. Conversely, the modality is operator dependent and requires detailed knowledge of the relevant anatomy, often resulting in a long learning curve. As well, physically deep and osseous lesions may not be visualized readily.

An exhaustive review of ultrasound-guided musculoskeletal intervention is beyond the scope of this section. The foremost goals of this chapter, then, are to present core principles and practical information that can be applied to most procedures. This includes a discussion of guidelines and precautions regarding the use of corticosteroids, a medication that is commonly injected under ultrasound guidance into soft tissues and joints. After this, various aspects of intra-articular intervention will be presented, including suggested routes of access for several major joints. Intratendinous calcium aspiration and intratendinous prolotherapy performed under ultrasound guidance are relatively new variations on old concepts. Both have shown great potential in the treatment of refractory chronic tendon disorders and will be described in detail. Finally, intervention of bursae and ganglion cysts will be reviewed.

GENERAL PRINCIPLES

The choice of ultrasound probe is critical. High-frequency (7–12 MHz), linear array transducers should be used routinely. To visualize deep structures such as the hip in larger patients, lower frequency curvilinear probes may be required. However, such probes should be avoided when possible because they are prone to anisotropic artifact. Anisotropy is a phenomenon in which the appearance of a structure varies depending on the angle from which it is being examined. Anisotropic artifact is common when imaging acoustically reflective, highly organized structures such as ligaments, tendons, muscles, and nerves. When the insonating sound beam is not perpendicular to the structure of interest, the sound reflects off of the structure and away from the transducer, resulting in a hypoechoic "drop off" (**Fig. 1**).

Regardless of the transducer selected, a complete sonographic examination (including color Doppler) of the area to be punctured is required to define the relationship of adjacent critical structures to be avoided such as nerves and vessels. Only then can a needle trajectory be planned safely. Areas of superficial infection should also be avoided when selecting a needle path to prevent deeper spread. These include areas of cellulitis, septic bursitis, and abscess. In cases of aspiration or biopsy of suspected malignancy, magnetic resonance (MR) imaging should be performed before the procedure, and the proposed needle route should be discussed with an orthopedic oncologic surgeon to avert unnecessary

Sections of Musculoskeletal and Emergency Trauma Radiology, Department of Radiology, Vancouver General Hospital, University of British Columbia, 899 W.12th Ave., Vancouver, BC V5Z 1M9, Canada
E-mail address: luck.louis@vch.ca

Radiol Clin N Am 46 (2008) 515–533
doi:10.1016/j.rcl.2008.02.003

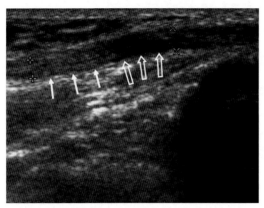

Fig. 1. Anisotropic artifact. Longitudinal sonogram of the ulnar nerve (*solid arrows*) at the level of the wrist using a linear, high-frequency transducer. As the nerve curves toward the transducer face, the insonating sound beams are no longer perpendicular to the nerve. As a result, the nerve appears hypoechoic (*open arrows*), simulating disease. Curvilinear transducers often exacerbate anisotropy because the insonating beams from the ends of the transducer face tend not to be perpendicular to the structure being examined.

transgression of anatomic compartments that may complicate surgical management.[4]

One common localization technique is to perform the puncture without direct ultrasound guidance.[5] In this "safe injection" technique, the lesion is first scanned transversely, and its maximum width is determined. Two dots are marked on the skin surface to either end of the transducer (**Fig. 2**A). The probe is then turned 90°, and the maximum length of the lesion is ascertained. Marks are placed again to either end of the transducer, the depth of the lesion is noted, and the four dots are connected to form a cross hair. The patient's skin is then sterilized, and a needle is inserted through the center of the cross hair at

right angles to the original scan planes and passed to the predetermined depth (**Fig. 2**B). The advantage of this technique is that it is less time consuming because the probe requires no special sterile preparation.

Most musculoskeletal procedures, however, can be performed with a free-hand technique, which allows direct, dynamic visualization of the needle tip. The following is the author's method of choice. After planning a safe route of access, a line parallel to the long axis of the transducer face can be drawn on the skin adjacent to the end of the transducer where the needle will be introduced (**Fig. 3**). Once the patient's skin and transducer are sterilized and draped, the probe can be returned quickly to the same location and orientation by aligning the probe to the skin mark. A 1.5-in (3.8 cm) 25-G needle is then used to infiltrate the subcutaneous tissues with local anesthetic such as lidocaine 1% or 2%. The needle is directed toward the intended target under constant observation with the long axis of the needle parallel and in line with the long axis of the transducer face. The angle at which the freezing needle is advanced should be noted mentally because any other needles introduced afterward will follow an identical path. In many cases, it will be possible to advance the freezing needle into the target directly and use the same needle to perform aspiration or injection. This avoids puncturing the patient multiple times and helps to expedite the case. Glenohumeral joints can be accessed routinely with this single-puncture method as can hip joints and hamstring origins in thinner patients. If one intends to perform a procedure with only one needle, it is prudent to securely screw the needle onto the syringe and then unscrew the needle by an eighth turn. This ensures that the syringe can be removed easily from the needle without disturbing the needle's position once at the target site.

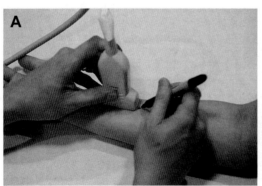
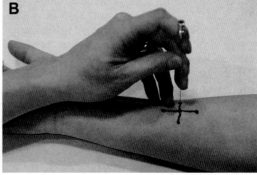

Fig. 2. Safe injection technique. (*A*) Dots are placed on the skin surface to either end of the transducer after determining the maximal length and width of the lesion. (*B*) A cross hair is drawn by connecting the four dots. A needle is then passed through the center of the cross hair to the predetermined depth. (Sterile technique not depicted above.)

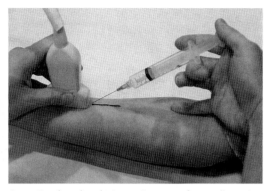

Fig. 3. Freehand technique. Once a safe needle trajectory has been chosen, a line parallel to the transducer face is drawn on the skin at the proposed needle entry site. The needle is introduced to the target along this line under constant ultrasound guidance. (Sterile technique not depicted above.)

It is sometimes difficult to visualize smaller caliber needles, and several strategies are effective in discriminating the needle tip. First, the transducer face should remain as perpendicular to the needle as possible by heel–toe angling and rocking of the probe. When ideally oriented in such a manner, reverberation artifact posterior to the needle is commonly seen, which aids in highlighting the needle (**Fig. 4**). Another approach is to sweep the transducer from side to side while repeatedly moving the needle in and out, which aids in identifying the tip in real time. Injecting a small amount of local anesthetic will disrupt the adjacent soft tissues and also helps to localize the needle tip. At other times, rotating the transducer 90° to examine the needle in short axis may be useful in determining whether the needle has veered off to one side of the intended course.

Sterile skin preparation and aseptic technique vary tremendously between institutions and radiologists. In our department, sterile coupling gel and disposable sterile drapes are always used. Extra-articular structures are routinely punctured after thorough cleansing of the skin and probe only. Disposable plastic probe covers are used, however, for intra-articular work to minimize the risk of septic arthritis. Standoff pads are prone to physically interfere with procedures and are, therefore, never used.

The needle size, length, and type should be selected based on the task at hand. Larger needles (18–20 G) are generally required for aspiration of suspected thick material such as pus, ganglia, or organized hematoma. Smaller needles (22–27 G) suffice for most injections but are inappropriate for aspirations unless the aspirate is thin. Specialized needles with cutting tips such as the Westcott biopsy needle (Becton, Dickinson and Company, Franklin Lakes, New Jersey) or core-biopsy needle sets are often required for soft tissue biopsies.

MEDICATIONS

The most common medications used in musculoskeletal intervention are for local anesthesia. Lidocaine 2% (Xylocaine) is the author's drug of choice and has rapid onset with a duration of action of up to 5 hours.[6] Bupivacaine (Sensorcaine, Marcaine) is an alternate slower-onset anesthetic but one which can last up to 12 hours and is available in 0.25%, 0.5%, and 0.75% concentrations. The duration of action of both drugs is shorter with lower concentration formulations.[6]

Corticosteroids have potent anti-inflammatory properties and are commonly prescribed for injection into soft tissues, bursae, tendon sheaths, and joints. At the author's institution, the two corticosteroids used most routinely are triamcinolone acetonide and methylprednisolone acetate (Depo-Medrol). These are generally mixed 1 part lidocaine 2%, 1 part bupivacaine 0.25%, and 2 parts 40 mg/mL corticosteroid before injection.

Several potential side effects of corticosteroids are relevant to musculoskeletal intervention, which practitioners need to be aware of. First, skin atrophy, fat necrosis, and skin depigmentation may develop from corticosteroids applied topically or injected intralesionally, intradermally, or subcutaneously. Methylprednisolone is less prone to causing skin atrophy than triamcinolone[7–11] and, therefore, is preferred when injecting lesions near the skin surface.

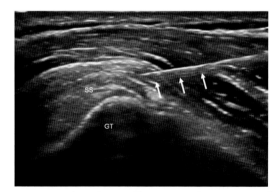

Fig. 4. Reverberation artifact. Coronal sonogram of the distal supraspinatus tendon (SS) upon its insertion onto the greater tuberosity (GT). A 25-G needle introduced for a diagnostic block of the subacromial bursa shows reverberation artifacts (*solid arrows*), which appear as multiple, parallel lines deep to the needle. This artifact, when present, is useful in helping to identify the needle position. Smaller caliber needles tend to produce less, if any, reverberation.

Secondly, animal models have shown that the biomechanical properties of tendons are adversely affected by intratendinous corticosteroid administration.[12,13] Corticosteroids may limit formation of granulation and connective tissue, reduce tendon mass, and decrease the amount of load that a tendon can withstand before mechanical failure. Case reports of tendon rupture after intratendinous corticosteroid injection are common in the literature.[14–16] Although corticosteroids have been used to treat tendon degeneration, or tendinosis, inflammation is not a predominant feature of this condition and, when present, may be important in the healing process.[17] Currently, there is no good evidence to substantiate the use of corticosteroids in treatment of chronic tendon lesions.[18] Even peritendinous injections may predispose to tendon rupture[15,19–21] and, therefore, should be performed with caution.

Corticosteroids have also been implicated in cartilage breakdown when injected into synovial joints, particularly weight-bearing articulations.[22–24] Articular surfaces develop multiple cystic defects, which become filled with necrotic debris. Such lesions appear not to develop in similarly injected non–weight-bearing joints. Reduction in cartilage elasticity has also been shown, which may further accelerate cartilage breakdown as the cushioning effect of cartilage is lost. There has been at least one case report of a Charcot-like arthropathy after intra-articular corticosteroid use.[25]

Currently, there is no consensus and no evidence-based guidelines for the number of safe injections at one site or the appropriate interval between injections.[18] As such, many recommendations for the use of locally injected corticosteroids are anecdotal. **Box 1** summarizes some suggestions for corticosteroid use in soft tissues and joints.

INTRA-ARTICULAR INTERVENTION

Eustace and colleagues[27] found that blind injections for shoulder pain, even in the hands of musculoskeletal specialists, are successful only in the minority of cases. In their series, only 29% of subacromial injections and 42% of glenohumeral joint injections were performed accurately without image guidance. In another recent study that compared ultrasound-guided and blind aspirations of suspected joint effusions, only 32% of cases returned fluid when performed blindly. In contrast, fluid was aspirated in 97% using ultrasound scan.[28] Indeed, ultrasonography has been shown to be effective in guiding difficult joint aspirations throughout the body.[29,30]

Ultrasound-guided joint aspirations may be performed for diagnosis of conditions such as crystal

---

Box 1

Suggestions for corticosteroid injection into soft tissues and joints

- Use methylprednisolone when injecting superficial lesions or superficial joints.
- Mix the corticosteroid with local anesthetic solution to provide immediate but short-term pain relief.
- Avoid intratendinous injections.
- Use caution with peritendinous injections, especially when the adjacent tendon is heavily loaded (such as the patellar and Achilles' tendons) or is torn.
- Avoid intra-articular injections unless there is a specific indication, such as end-stage osteoarthritis.
- Be mindful of injection into structures that communicate with a joint. Examples include the long head of biceps tendon sheath, flexor hallucis longus tendon sheath, and Baker's cysts.
- Advise at least 2 weeks of rest and avoid heavy loading for 6 weeks after peritendinous and intra-articular injections.
- Be careful not to damage the articular cartilage with the needle during injection.
- Allow adequate time between injections to assess its effects, generally a minimum of 6 weeks.
- Be cautious in using more than 3 injections at any one site.
- Do not repeat an injection if at least 4 weeks of symptomatic relief was not achieved after 2 injections.

Data from Speed CA. Fortnightly review: Corticosteroid injections in tendon lesions. BMJ 2001; 323(7309):382–6; and Tehranzadeh J, Booya F, Root J. Cartilage metabolism in osteoarthritis and the influence of viscosupplementation and steroid: a review. Acta Radiol 2005;46(3):288–96.

---

arthropathy and septic arthritis. In the case of an infected joint, aspiration may be therapeutic as well. Septic joint effusions are commonly hypoechoic with low-amplitude internal echoes but fluid may also be hyperechoic or rarely anechoic (**Fig. 5B**).[31,32] In approximately 0.5% of septic joints, the initial ultrasound examination will find no joint effusion.[33] A repeat ultrasound study should be considered if fever and joint pain persist in these cases. Although septic arthritis may be associated with hyperemia, Doppler ultrasound scan is unreliable in differentiating septic from aseptic joints.[34] Finally, intra-articular injection of local anesthetic should be avoided because

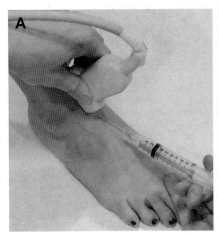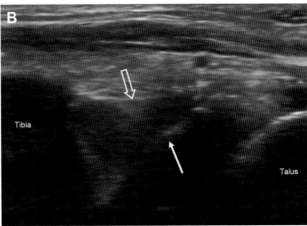

Fig. 5. Ankle joint access from an anterior approach. (A) The transducer is aligned in a sagittal plane at the tibiotalar articulation, and the needle is introduced from an anteroinferior approach. Care should be exercised to avoid puncturing the dorsalis pedis artery and extensor tendons. (B) Sagittal sonogram of the anterior ankle joint in an intravenous drug abuser. A hypoechoic joint effusion containing low-amplitude internal echoes is interposed between the distal tibia and talar dome and displaces the ankle joint capsule anteriorly (open arrow). The needle tip is seen within the joint space (solid arrow). (Sterile technique not depicted above.)

lidocaine is bacteriostatic and may contribute to false-negative results.

Ultrasound-guided joint injections are also commonly performed for diagnosis and therapy. Diagnostic blocks are performed by injecting a small amount of anesthetic into a joint and then clinically assessing whether the procedure has improved the patient's symptoms. Several in vitro and animal-based studies have shown chondrotoxic effects resulting from intraarticular exposure to anesthetic solutions, including lidocaine and bupivicaine.[35–41] Although data are preliminary, these results stress the need to perform all intraarticular interventions with caution and only when there is a reasonable clinical indication. The author uses an equal volume mixture of lidocaine and bupivicaine for this purpose, but the total volume of injected solution will depend on the size of the joint. Most hip and shoulder joints easily receive 10 mL, whereas the small joints of the hands and feet may take less than 1 mL. In all cases, injection should be terminated if the patient complains of excessive discomfort. The procedure is useful in confirming or ruling out the source of pain and, in cases of subsequent surgery, helps to predict postsurgical pain relief. Pain response is graded subjectively on a 10-point scale, and the patient is asked to keep a diary of blockade efficacy over the next 24 hours. Patients should be instructed not to overuse the joint because pain relief, although potentially dramatic, will be short-lived.

Therapeutic intra-articular injection of corticosteroid and viscosupplement are useful in treating osteoarthritis[26] and can be performed under ultrasound guidance. Viscosupplementation is a procedure in which hyaluronic acid, or a derivative, is injected directly into afflicted joints and aims to replace what is believed to be an important factor of joint lubrication. Several formulations are commercially available that vary in their duration of effect and treatment schedules. Although the precise mechanism of action is not entirely understood, numerous clinical trials have shown some improvement in pain and joint function.[42,43]

The following section describes potential routes of access to the most commonly injected joints. As already discussed, every precaution should be taken to prevent septic arthritis. Proper sterile preparation and draping of the patient and of the equipment are essential.

Shoulder Joint

The majority of shoulder joints can be injected while the patient is seated. However, if the patient is known to become faint or is overly anxious, a lateral decubitus position works equally well. Although the glenohumeral joint may be accessed from anteriorly or posteriorly, the preferred approach is the latter. This route is particularly advantageous when performing gadolinium injections before MR imaging because there is less chance of causing interstitial injection of the rotator cuff interval or anterior labrum where misplaced contrast material could simulate disease.

With the patient's hand gently resting on the opposite shoulder, the posterior joint is examined in an axial plane, and the key landmarks of the triangular-shaped posterior labrum, humeral head, and joint capsule are identified (**Fig. 6**).

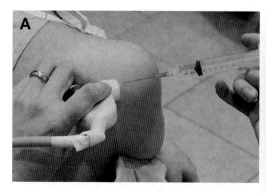
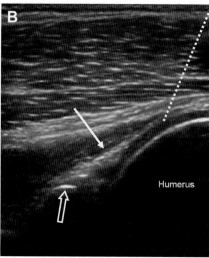

Fig. 6. Shoulder joint access from a posterior approach. (*A*) With the patient seated, the posterior glenohumeral joint is examined in a transverse plane. (*B*) The needle is introduced from a lateral and posterior approach (*dotted line*). Important landmarks include (**1**) the humeral head (Humerus) which is lined by a thin, hypoechoic layer of articular cartilage, (**2**) the bony glenoid rim (*open arrow*), and (**3**) the echogenic, triangular-shaped posterior labrum (*solid arrow*) which arises from the glenoid. (Sterile technique not depicted above.)

The needle is introduced laterally in an axial plane and is advanced medially. The needle target is between the posterior-most aspect of the humeral head and the posterior labrum. Particular care should be taken to not puncture the labrum or articular cartilage, however. Once the needle tip is felt against the humeral head, a small test injection of anesthetic is performed. With correct intra-articular placement, anesthetic will flow easily into the joint. If there is resistance to injection, gently twirling the syringe or withdrawing the needle by 1 to 2 mm while continuing to inject a small amount of anesthetic will often resolve the problem.

In almost all cases, the 1.5-inch 25-G needle used for local anesthesia will suffice in accessing this joint with a single puncture. In larger patients, the use of a longer 22-G spinal needle may be required.

Elbow Joint

The patient is seated or laid supine with the elbow flexed and the arm placed comfortably across the chest (**Fig. 7**A). The ultrasound probe is then positioned along the posterior elbow and is oriented sagittally such that the triceps tendon is visualized

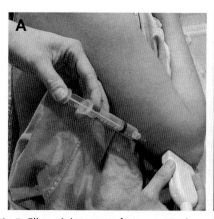
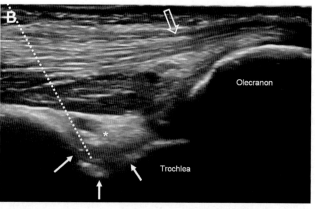

Fig. 7. Elbow joint access from a posterior approach. (*A*) With the patient seated and the affected arm placed across the chest, the posterior joint is examined in a sagittal plane. (*B*) The needle is introduced from a postero-superior approach (*dotted line*), passing adjacent to the triceps tendon (*open arrow*), through the posterior fat pad (*asterisk*) and into the joint. The concave olecranon fossa of the humerus (*solid arrows*) provides a useful landmark. (Sterile technique not depicted above.)

ongitudinally. The probe, which remains parallel to the triceps fibers, is then slid laterally until just out of view of the triceps tendon. Key landmarks are the olecranon fossa of the humerus, the posterior fat pad, and the olecranon (**Fig. 7**B). The needle is introduced from a superior approach, passing beside the triceps tendon and through the posterior fat pad to enter the joint space. This joint is easily accessible with a 1.5-inch long needle.

Hip Joint

There are two common approaches to accessing the hip joint and the choice between the two depends on operator preference, the presence of a joint effusion, and body habitus. In both cases, the patient is laid supine and the joint is punctured anteriorly.

When a joint effusion is present or in larger patients, the best approach is often with the probe aligned along the long axis of the femoral neck. The concave transition between the anterior aspect of the femoral head and neck can be visualized clearly, and the joint capsule is seen immediately superficial (**Fig. 8**). The needle is introduced from an inferior approach and passes through the joint capsule to rest on the subcapital femur. Septic hip arthritis is a frequent clinical concern, particularly in patients with hip arthroplasties. Although a fine needle is useful for joint injections, aspiration for suspected septic arthritis should be performed with an 18-G spinal needle. Not only

will purulent material be easier to aspirate, but a 22-G Westcott biopsy needle can be introduced through the larger needle to obtain synovial biopsies, if required.

In thinner patients, it is often easiest to access the hip joint with the ultrasound probe oriented axially. When positioned correctly, the femoral head and acetabular rim will be in view (**Fig. 9**). The needle is introduced from an anterolateral approach, remaining lateral to the femoral neurovascular bundle. The needle tip is advanced until it rests on the femoral head, adjacent to its most anterior aspect. The hip labrum, which arises from the acetabulum, should be avoided.

Knee Joint

A knee joint distended with effusion is most easily injected or aspirated through the suprapatellar bursa with the patient supine and the knee flexed slightly. A small pillow or sponge placed behind the knee is helpful. The probe is placed in a sagittal plane superior to the patella, whereby the fibers of the distal quadriceps tendon are seen in long axis (**Fig. 10**). The probe is kept parallel to the quadriceps tendon but is slid medially or laterally until the quadriceps fibers disappear from view. A needle is then passed directly into the bursa.

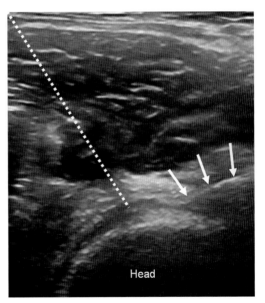

Fig. 9. Hip joint access—short axis technique. With the transducer oriented in a transverse plane, the key landmarks of the femoral head and anterior acetabulum (*solid arrows*) are visualized. The needle is introduced from an anterior and lateral approach (*dotted line*), piercing the anterior joint capsule to rest upon the femoral head. The femoral neurovascular bundle (not shown) is medial to and remote from the needle path.

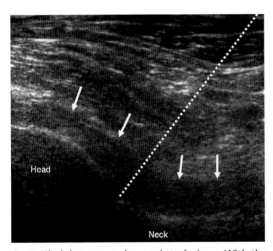

Fig. 8. Hip joint access—long axis technique. With the ultrasound probe aligned along the long axis of the femoral neck, the distinctive concave transition between the femoral head and neck is visualized. In this case, the anterior hip joint capsule (*solid arrows*) is displaced anteriorly by a large joint effusion. The needle is introduced from an inferior and anterior approach (*dotted line*), lateral to the femoral neurovascular bundle (not shown).

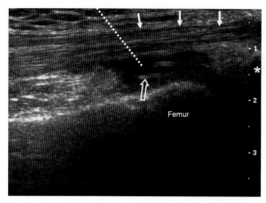

Fig. 10. Knee joint access from anterior approach. Sagittal sonogram of the suprapatellar knee shows the distal quadriceps tendon (*solid arrows*), the distal femur, and the superior patellar pole (*asterisk*). The needle is introduced from an anterior and superior approach (*dotted line*) and is preferably passed to one side of the quadriceps tendon without puncturing it. In this case, synovial plicae (*open arrow*) are present in a mildly distended suprapatellar bursa.

For knee joints with no joint effusion, the medial patellofemoral facet affords an excellent target. After palpating the patella and medial patellofemoral joint line, the probe is placed in an axial plane so that the patella and medial femoral condyle are visible. The probe is then turned 90° and oriented along the joint line. The needle is introduced either from an inferior or superior approach directly into the joint.

Ankle Joint

With the patient supine, the anterior tibiotalar joint is examined in a sagittal plane (see **Fig. 5**A). If there is any doubt of correct probe placement, performing plantar flexion and dorsiflexion maneuvers will readily identify the talus moving across the tibia. The position of the dorsalis pedis artery and extensor tendons should be noted and kept away from during needle placement. A needle then is introduced into the joint in a sagittal plane using an inferior approach (see **Fig. 5**B).

INTRATENDINOUS INTERVENTION

Calcific and noncalcific tendinosis are two potentially symptomatic diseases that are often refractory to conservative management. The ability of ultrasound scan to accurately depict and localize tendon abnormalities makes ultrasound-guided calcium aspiration and prolotherapy invaluable in treating these conditions.

Treatment of Calcific Tendinosis

Rotator cuff **calcific tendinosis** (also commonly referred to as **calcifying tendinitis**), is caused by the deposition of carbonate apatite crystals,[44] most commonly in the critical zone of the supraspinatus tendon roughly 1 cm proximal to its insertion.[45–47] Uhthoff and Loehr[46] described three distinct stages in the disease process, namely the precalcific, calcific, and postcalcific stages. Depending on the phase of disease, the imaging appearance and physical consistency of the calcification differ significantly as do patient symptoms.

The calcific stage consists of three phases. The **formative** and **resting phases** are chronic and may be associated with varying degrees of pain at rest or with movement. Many patients, however, are asymptomatic.[48] These calcifications tend to be well circumscribed and discrete when examined radiographically[49] and often produce significant acoustic shadowing by ultrasound scan (**Fig. 11**).[50] Attempts at aspirating calcifications in these two phases tend to be difficult because the calcifications are quite hard and chalklike.

The **resorptive phase** is the last phase in the calcific stage and is the most symptomatic. Shedding of calcium crystals into the adjacent subacromial bursa may result in severe pain and restricted range of motion.[51] This phase typically lasts for 2 weeks or longer. These calcifications appear ill-defined on radiographs and produce little or no acoustic shadowing by ultrasonography (**Fig. 12**).[50] When aspirated, these calcified deposits typically are soft with a slurrylike consistency.

Calcific tendinosis is usually a self-limiting condition in which the calcification resorbs after a period of worsening pain.[48] However, in some patients, the condition can lead to chronic pain and functional impairment. The resolution of calcification correlates well with clinical improvement of symptoms[52–57] and, therefore, various treatments have been devised to promote their removal. There is no conclusive evidence that intralesional steroid injection,[58] acetic acid iontophoresis,[59,60] or pulsed ultrasound therapy are effective.[48] Extracorporeal shockwave lithotripsy uses acoustic waves to fragment calcium deposits, and substantial or complete clinical improvement has been reported in 66% to 91% of patients.[52,54,61,62] However, access to lithotripter equipment is limited and is less available than ultrasound imaging.

Open or arthroscopic surgery currently provides the greatest long-term relief in terms of substantial or complete clinical improvement with numerous studies reporting between 76.9% and 100% good or excellent results.[49,63–73] However, surgery may be complicated by prolonged post-surgical disability and reflex sympathetic

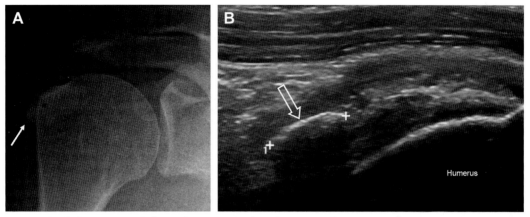

Fig. 11. Hard calcifications in calcific tendinosis. Examples of "hard calcification" that typify the formative phase of calcific tendinosis. (*A*) The anteroposterior radiograph of patient A shows a large, sharply circumscribed calcification within the infraspinatus tendon (*solid arrow*). (*B*) In patient B, the supraspinatus tendon is imaged longitudinally. A large intratendinous calcification (*open arrow*) produces significant posterior acoustic shadowing artifact.

dystrophy.[52,63,74–76] Because conservative measures are successful in up to 90% of patients,[71] surgery is generally indicated only in those who have progressive symptoms, whose symptoms interfere with activities of daily living, and who have not responded to conservative therapy.[77]

Image-guided needle irrigation and aspiration (**barbotage**) of rotator cuff calcifications has been shown to be an effective minimally invasive technique and was first described three decades ago.[78] In a recent study, del Cura and colleagues[56] reported that 91% of patients experienced significant or complete improvement in range of motion, pain, and disability when aspiration was performed under ultrasound guidance. Given the potential risks of surgery, percutaneous calcium aspiration should be considered after failure of

medical therapy.[56,79] Successful aspiration may not be possible in cases in which the calcification appears striated because this is thought to represent calcification of the tendon fibers themselves. Also, clinical outcomes when attempting to remove numerous, diffuse, small (<5 mm) calcifications are only fair to poor, even when treated surgically.[80]

Image-guided barbotage techniques vary greatly, and there is no accepted standardized methodology. Needle sizes have ranged from 15 G[81] to 25 G,[58] and some investigators have advocated a two-needle irrigation system,[76,82,83] whereas others have used only one.[56,57,76] In some published results, as many as 15 passes were made through the same calcification,[78,83,84] whereas other researchers opted to limit potential

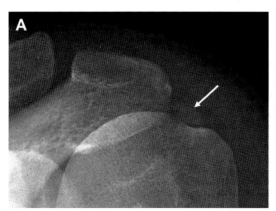
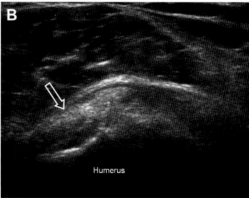

Fig. 12. Soft calcification in calcific tendinosis. Examples of "soft calcification" that characterize the resorptive phase of calcific tendinosis. (*A*) Faint, ill-defined calcification (*solid arrow*) is seen on the anteroposterior radiograph of patient A who suffers from excruciating shoulder pain. (*B*) In patient B, a vague, hyperechoic area is seen anteriorly within the supraspinatus tendon, which is scanned in short axis (*open arrow*).

iatrogenic cuff damage by performing a single lesional puncture only.[56,57]

At our institution, we routinely perform a full-shoulder ultrasound examination before any intervention. This is done to ensure that there are no co-existing disorders such as rotator cuff tears. We also ensure a recent set of radiographs has been performed to characterize the calcifications more fully and to act as a baseline for follow-up. The patient is placed into the lateral decubitus position opposite the affected side. Although the procedure can be done sitting, patients have been documented to become syncopal during aspiration.[56] Depending on the location of the calcification in the cuff, the arm is positioned appropriately. In the case of the supraspinatus tendon, a "hand in back pocket" position is used. The calcification is then targeted under ultrasound scan before sterile preparation of the skin and equipment. A 20-G needle connected to a syringe filled with 2% lidocaine is advanced into the subacromial bursa where a small amount of anesthetic is injected before the needle continues into the calcification. Importantly, lidocaine is injected into the calcification without first aspirating to prevent the needle tip from becoming obstructed. Several short injections, each followed by release of pressure on the plunger, are performed. If successful, lidocaine and calcium fragments will evacuate into the syringe. The syringe should be held below horizontal to prevent re-injection of aspirated material. Also, new lidocaine-filled syringes can be exchanged for when required. Barbotage should be continued until no more calcification can be aspirated. However, it may not be possible to aspirate very hard calcifications, in which case the calcification can be ground gently with the needle tip by rotating the syringe (**Fig. 13**). This mechanical perturbation of the deposit is hypothesized to stimulate cell-mediated resorption.[57,76,78,85] There is collaborative evidence in the surgical literature that suggests that calcific deposits need not be removed completely to achieve successful outcomes.[72,78] The needle is then withdrawn into the subacromial bursa where a combination of 1 mL 2% lidocaine and 1 mL of 40 mg/mL triamcinolone is injected to mitigate the risk of post-procedural bursitis (**Fig. 14**).

Patients are instructed to rest the shoulder for up to a week and are advised to take nonsteroidal anti-inflammatory medication, as needed, to manage discomfort. A follow-up appointment is made for 6 weeks after barbotage and includes repeat ultrasound and plain film studies.

Treatment of Noncalcific Tendinosis

Tendon degeneration, often referred to as "tendinopathy" or "tendinosis," is not characterized by an inflammatory response but rather infiltration of fibroblasts and vessels.[86] Tendinosis is generally considered to be caused by repetitive microtrauma with an ensuing chronic cycle of tendon degeneration and repair resulting in a weakened tendon. These changes have been shown to appear as hypoechoic areas on sonography (**Fig. 15**).[87] Several techniques have been described to treat tendinosis. Autologous blood, which contains fibroblast growth factors, has been used successfully in treatment of refractory medial and lateral epicondylitis of the

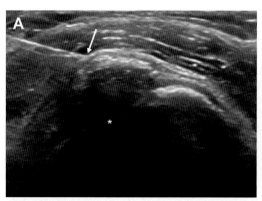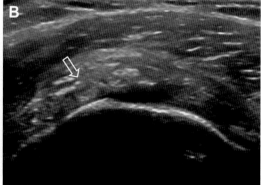

Fig. 13. Incomplete aspiration of supraspinatus calcification. (*A*) Sonogram of the supraspinatus tendon in short axis shows placement of a needle (*solid arrow*) at the edge of a "hard" calcified deposit. There is marked posterior acoustic shadowing that obscures the humeral cortical surface (*asterisk*). Only a small amount of calcification could be aspirated. The calcification instead was gently ground with the needle tip. (*B*) Follow-up sonogram 6 weeks later shows marked change in the appearance of the calcification with loss of the acoustic shadowing seen previously (*open arrow*). The patient's symptoms improved significantly between the two examinations.

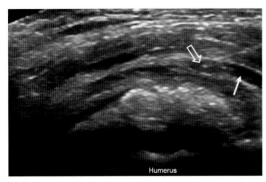

Fig. 14. Subacromial bursal injection. An oblique short-axis sonogram of the supraspinatus tendon shows placement of a needle (*open arrow*) within the subacromial bursa (*solid arrow*). The bursa has been distended partially with injected lidocaine and corticosteroid at the end of a barbotage procedure.

elbow.[86,88–90] Ohberg and Alfredson reported significant improvement in chronic achillodynia after obliteration of neovessels using polidocanol as a sclerosing agent.[91]

Prolotherapy is another treatment option that has shown promising results. It is a technique in which injection of an irritant solution (the proliferant) into a ligament or tendon incites a local inflammatory response, which, in turn, induces fibroblast proliferation and collagen synthesis.[92–94] One popular proliferant solution that has been studied is hyperosmolar dextrose, which has an excellent safety profile and is inexpensive.[95] As little as 0.6% extracellular D-glucose (dextrose) has been shown experimentally to stimulate human cells in producing growth factors within minutes to hours[96] and dextrose concentrations greater than 10% result in a brief inflammatory reaction.[93] In a recent review of the prolotherapy literature, Rabago and colleagues[97] reported positive results compared with controls in both nonrandomized

and randomized, controlled studies. Good results have been reported previously after treatment of tendons such as the thigh adductor origins and suprapubic abdominal insertions without image guidance.[98] Intra-articular dextrose administration has also been experimentally used in treatment of osteoarthritis and ACL laxity.[99–101]

Maxwell and colleagues[95] significantly advanced this technique by using ultrasonography to treat chronic Achilles tendinosis. Focal areas of tendinosis and partial tearing were precisely targeted and then injected with 25% dextrose monohydrate solution (**Fig. 16**). In their study, patients showed a significant reduction in tendon pain at rest (88%), with normal activity (84%), and after exercise (78%). The number of intrasubstance tears decreased by 78% and areas of neovascularity diminished by up to 55%. At 1-year follow-up, 67% of patients continued to be asymptomatic, 30% had mild symptoms, and only 3% had moderate symptoms.

As with all interventional procedures, a formal ultrasound examination of the entire area is performed first to characterize the extent and nature of the disease and to exclude other pathology. A 25% dextrose solution is produced by mixing 1 mL of 50% dextrose monohydrate and 1 mL of 2% lidocaine. Once the needle route is planned, and sterile preparation has been performed, a 25-G needle and lidocaine solution are used for local anesthesia. The needle then is advanced directly into the tendon at the site of tendinosis or tearing (**Fig. 17**). Areas of neovascularity are not targeted specifically, but neovessels frequently will coexist in areas of tendinosis and often will decrease with treatment (**Fig. 18**). As advocated by Maxwell and colleagues[95] usually 0.5 mL or less solution is injected into any one lesion. However, several lesions may be injected during a single treatment session.

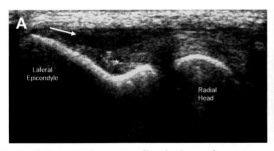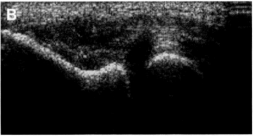

Fig. 15. Common extensor tendinosis. Coronal sonograms of the common extensor tendon origin of the elbow in a patient with lateral epicondylitis clinically. (*A*) A large, hypoechoic area (*solid arrow*) is seen along the superficial aspect of the tendon, characteristic of tendinosis. Normal tendon is seen immediately deep to the lesion (*asterisk*). (*B*) The corresponding color Doppler examination of the same area shows marked hypervascularity, which is a common, albeit nonspecific, finding in tendinosis.

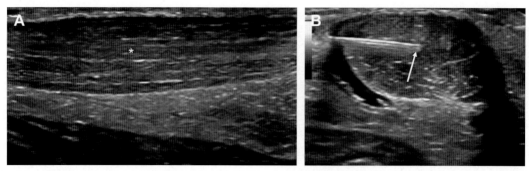

Fig. 16. Achilles tendinosis and prolotherapy. (A) On the initial longitudinal sonogram of the Achilles tendon, marked fusiform swelling of the tendon is present (*asterisk*) in its midportion. There are diffuse echopoor areas within the tendon, and the normal fibrillar echotexture is disrupted, particularly along its superficial aspect. (B) Short axis sonogram of the tendon at the maximal site of swelling shows needle placement (*solid arrow*) before injection of hyperosmolar dextrose. The patient's symptoms nearly completely resolved after five treatments.

Postprocedure instructions include avoidance of any heavy tendon loading for 2 weeks. Also, nonsteroidal anti-inflammatory medications should not be used for pain relief because they may inhibit the dextrose-stimulated inflammatory reaction. Patients are re-assessed at 6-week intervals, and repeat injections are performed until the patient is asymptomatic or no longer derives any benefit from the treatment. It is worthwhile noting that the tendons in some patients who report

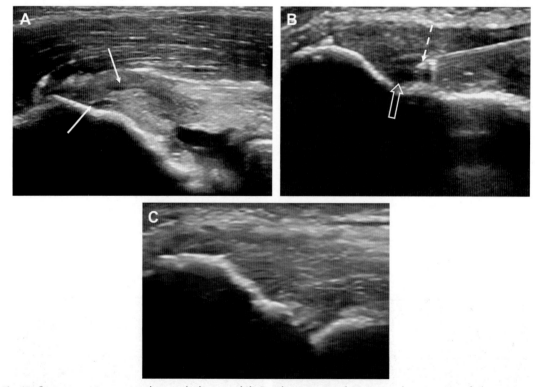

Fig. 17. Common extensor tendon prolotherapy. (A) On the preprocedure coronal sonogram of the common extensor tendon of the elbow, two prominent partial tears are present (*solid arrows*). (B) A needle is seen within the deeper of the two tears (*dashed arrow*), which has been distended with a small amount of injected dextrose solution (*open arrow*). (C) After 10 months (6 injections), the partial tears are no longer seen, and the patient's symptoms had improved subjectively by 90%. However, the tendon continues to be diffusely echopoor and slightly thickened. In the author's experience, even successfully treated tendons often continue to appear quite heterogeneous.

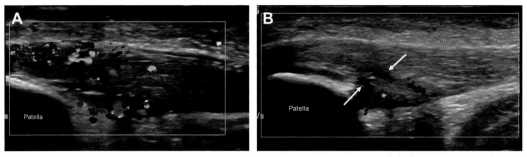

Fig. 18. Jumper's knee and prolotherapy. (*A*) Sagittal sonogram of the patellar tendon origin in a world-class water skier shows a marked amount of hypervascularity and tendon thickening. (*B*) Repeat sonogram after several prolotherapy injections shows significant reduction in the number of vessels present. However, small partial tears are evident along the deep surface of the tendon (*solid arrows*).

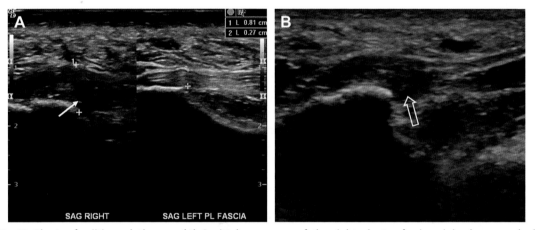

Fig. 19. Plantar fasciitis prolotherapy. (*A*) Sagittal sonogram of the right plantar fascia origin shows marked thickening and a large partial tear (*solid arrow*) when compared with the asymptomatic left side. (*B*) After several dextrose injections, the partial tear had decreased substantially in size (*open arrow*), and the patient's symptoms had completely resolved. Despite this, the tendon remains thickened and heterogeneous.

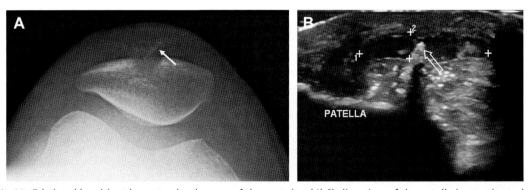

Fig. 20. Frictional bursitis at bone-tendon-bone graft harvest site. (*A*) Skyline view of the patella in a patient who previously underwent ACL repair. The patellar graft harvest site is surrounded by osseous fragments (*solid arrow*). (*B*) Sagittal sonogram of the patella shows a fluid collection (indicated by the calipers) centered over one such fragment (*open arrow*). Progressive swelling and pain with knee flexion and extension had developed over several weeks after surgery.

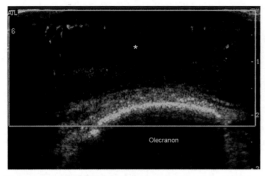

Fig. 21. Septic olecranon bursitis. Short axis sonogram of the olecranon bursa. The synovial-lined bursal walls are markedly thickened and hyperemic, and there is a small amount of anechoic fluid present centrally (*asterisk*). The appearances are nonspecific, and differentiation between septic and aseptic bursitides by ultrasound scan is unreliable.

complete cessation of symptoms continue to appear thickened and hypoechoic and show hypervascularity (**Fig. 19**). In our series of unpublished results, the majority of patients who derive some benefit from prolotherapy only do so after four or five injections. Prospective patients are made aware of this fact before beginning treatment to circumvent any unrealistic expectations.

INTERVENTION OF GANGLION CYSTS AND BURSAE

Ultrasonography is the ideal modality for image-guided aspiration and injection of most cysts and bursae in the musculoskeletal system. The ability of ultrasound imaging to target even very small collections while avoiding adjacent critical structures in real time is essential in treating these lesions successfully.

Treatment of Bursitis

Bursae are fluid-filled sacs that serve to decrease friction between adjacent structures and may or may not be lined with synovium.[102] Inflammation of a bursa may be caused by repetitive use, infection, systemic inflammatory conditions, and trauma. In treating bursitis, it is important to establish the likely cause. Corticosteroids, which are used commonly to treat bursitis resulting from overuse (**Fig. 20**), would be contraindicated in septic bursitis (**Fig. 21**). Caution should also be exercised when injecting corticosteroids into bursae that communicate with a joint to prevent potential steroid-mediated cartilage damage. Therefore, when treating subacromial-subdeltoid bursitis, rotator cuff tearing should be excluded before injection.

In the case of bursae that are distended with a large amount of fluid, immediate and dramatic improvement in symptoms can be achieved by thorough aspiration (**Fig. 22**). However, if performing a corticosteroid injection into a very small collection, incomplete aspiration of the bursa is sometimes advantageous and will help ensure that the potential space is not collapsed entirely before the medication can be injected intrabursally (**Fig. 23**).

Treatment of Ganglion Cysts

Ganglion cysts are the most common cause of a soft tissue mass in the distal upper extremity.[103] The etiology of ganglia is controversial. One widely held view is that cyst formation occurs as a result of trauma or tissue irritation, whereby mucin is produced by modified synovial cells lining the synovial–capsular interface.[104] The mucin eventually pools behind valvelike structures formed by capsular ducts, resulting in ganglion formation.

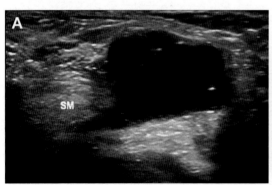
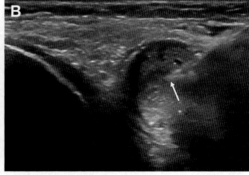

Fig. 22. Semimembranosus bursitis. (*A*) Transverse sonogram of the posteromedial knee. An irregular fluid collection is seen along the medial aspect of the semimembranosus tendon (SM), typical of semimembranosus bursitis. (*B*) A needle (*solid arrow*) has been introduced into the bursa, which has been nearly completely aspirated. The patient experienced immediate relief in his symptoms.

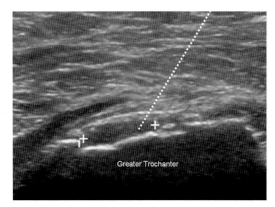

Fig. 23. Greater trochanteric bursitis. Sagittal sonogram of the hip shows a small amount of fluid (indicated by the calipers) adjacent to the greater trochanter. With the patient in a lateral decubitus position, a fine needle can be placed easily into the collection (*dotted line*).

Many lesions are asymptomatic and require no treatment. In fact, 40% to 60% of ganglia have been reported to resolve spontaneously.[105,106] However, in other cases, symptoms related to mass effect may mandate intervention (**Fig. 24**). Patients may complain of restricted range of motion, aching, paresthesias, or weakness. Furthermore, cysts that drain externally are at risk of a deep soft tissue or joint infection.

Although surgery has been stated to have success rates of 99%,[107] complications such as joint instability, postoperative stiffness, decreased range of motion, and neurovascular injury make minimally invasive techniques a viable alternative in symptomatic patients. Success rates for blind, percutaneous aspiration vary tremendously from 33%[108] to 85%.[109] In one of the largest published series of wrist ganglia undergoing nonoperative management, 85 patients were randomly assigned to two groups: aspiration alone or aspiration followed by injection of 40 mg of methylprednisolone.[108] The investigators found no difference in the success rate between these two groups. Interestingly, 96% of those ganglia that did not subsequently recur were treated successfully after only one attempt. Of those lesions requiring a second or third aspiration, only 4% eventually resolved. In this series, multiple aspirations were of little benefit. The major limitation of this study was that all punctures were performed without image guidance.

Breidahl and Adler[110] were the first to describe the use of ultrasound guidance in treatment of ganglia. In their small study population, nine of ten patients derived significant or complete relief after aspiration with a 20-G needle and injection of 40 to 80 mg of triamcinolone. However, the use of corticosteroids in treating ganglia remains controversial.

Ganglia appear as cystic masses by ultrasonography and typically are oval or lobulated in shape (**Fig. 25**).[103,111,112] Internally, a ganglion may be anechoic or contain low-amplitude echoes and septae. An 18-G needle is recommended for

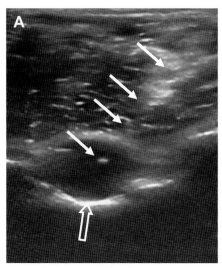
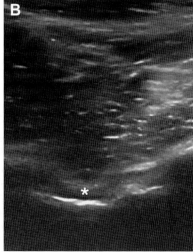

Fig. 24. Spinoglenoid notch ganglion cyst aspiration. (*A*) Transverse sonogram of the spinoglenoid notch (*open arrow*) depicts a small ganglion cyst, presumably impinging upon the suprascapular nerve. An 18-G needle was advanced into the cyst but is only partially visualized along its course (*solid arrows*). (*B*) Transverse sonogram of the spinoglenoid notch after aspirating 2 mL of gelatinous material. The cyst cavity has completely collapsed (*asterisk*). The chronic, dull aching in the posterior shoulder experienced by the patient for months had improved dramatically by the end of the examination.

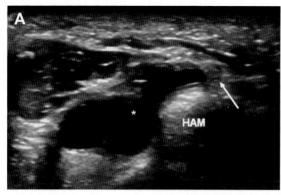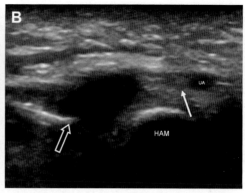

Fig. 25. Aspiration of ganglion cyst causing ulnar nerve palsy. Transverse sonograms of the palmar ulnar wrist. (*A*) A lobulated ganglion cyst (*asterisk*) is seen extending superficial to the hamate (HAM) to abut the ulnar nerve (*solid arrow*). (*B*) A needle (*open arrow*) has partially decompressed the ganglion, which has receded from the ulnar nerve (*solid arrow*) and ulnar artery (UA). The patient's symptoms resolved slowly over the course of several weeks after aspiration.

aspiration of all suspected ganglion cysts because cyst contents are invariably thick and gelatinous.

SUMMARY

Ultrasound-guided intervention is probably underutilized currently in North America. However, the dynamic, multiplanar capability of ultrasonography makes it an attractive alternative to procedures that might otherwise be performed under fluoroscopic or computed tomography guidance. Indeed, the majority of joints, cysts, and bursae can be accessed routinely under sonographic control. In the cases of barbotage and prolotherapy, ultrasonography has given fresh breath to old concepts and has afforded radiologists new options to treat difficult and chronic tendon problems. It is hoped that this review has served as a springboard for the reader to further investigate the important and diverse role ultrasound imaging is able to play in musculoskeletal intervention.

ACKNOWLEDGEMENTS

This article would not have been possible without the outstanding contributions of the medical sonography team at UBC Hospital. In particular, the author wishes to thank Anne Hope, Maureen Kennedy, and Pam Grossman for their unwavering enthusiasm and support. The author also wishes to recognize Paulina Louis for her invaluable help in preparing the manuscript.

REFERENCES

1. Cardinal E, Beauregard CG, Chhem RK. Interventional musculoskeletal ultrasound. Semin Musculoskelet Radiol 1997;1(2):311–8.

2. Dodd GD 3rd, Esola CC, Memel DS, et al. Sonography: the undiscovered jewel of interventional radiology. Radiographics 1996;16(6):1271–88.

3. Rubens DJ, Fultz PJ, Gottlieb RH, et al. Effective ultrasonographically guided intervention for diagnosis of musculoskeletal lesions. J Ultrasound Med 1997; 16(12):831–42.

4. Liu PT, Valadez SD, Chivers FS, et al. Anatomically based guidelines for core needle biopsy of bone tumors: implications for limb-sparing surgery. Radiographics 2007;27(1):189–205 [discussion: 206].

5. van Holsbeeck MT, Introcaso JH. Interventional musculoskeletal ultrasound. 2nd edition. St. Louis (MO): Mosby, Inc.; 2001.

6. Repchinsky C, editor. Compendium of pharmaceuticals and specialties. Ottawa (ON): Canadian Pharmacists Association; 2007.

7. Beardwell A. Subcutaneous atrophy after local corticosteroid injection. Br Med J 1967;3:1.

8. Cassidy JT, Bole GG. Cutaneous atrophy secondary to intra-articular corticosteroid administration. Ann Intern Med 1966;65(5):1008–18.

9. Fisherman EW, Feinberg AR, Feinberg SM. Local subcutaneous atrophy. JAMA 1962;179:971–2.

10. Schetman D, Hambrick GW Jr, Wilson CE. Cutaneous changes following local injection of triamcinolone. Arch Dermatol 1963;88:820–8.

11. Goldman L. Reactions following intralesional and sublesional injections of corticosteroids. JAMA 1962;182:613–6.

12. Kapetanos G. The effect of the local corticosteroids on the healing and biomechanical properties of the partially injured tendon. Clin Orthop Relat Res 1982;(163):170–9.

13. Ketchum LD. Effects of triamcinolone on tendon healing and function. A laboratory study. Plast Reconstr Surg 1971;47(5):471–82.

14. Clark SC, Jones MW, Choudhury RR, et al. Bilateral patellar tendon rupture secondary to repeated local steroid injections. J Accid Emerg Med 1995; 12(4):300–1.

15. Ford LT, DeBender J. Tendon rupture after local steroid injection. South Med J 1979;72(7):827–30.

16. Kleinman M, Gross AE. Achilles tendon rupture following steroid injection. Report of three cases. J Bone Joint Surg Am 1983;65(9):1345–7.

17. Wong ME, Hollinger JO, Pinero GJ. Integrated processes responsible for soft tissue healing. Oral Surg Oral Med Oral Pathol Oral Radiol Endod 1996;82(5):475–92.

18. Speed CA. Fortnightly review: corticosteroid injections in tendon lesions. BMJ 2001;323(7309):382–6.

19. Bickel KD. Flexor pollicis longus tendon rupture after corticosteroid injection. J Hand Surg [Am] 1996;21(1):152–3.

20. Gottlieb NL, Riskin WG. Complications of local corticosteroid injections. JAMA 1980;243(15): 1547–8.

21. Unverferth LJ, Olix ML. The effect of local steroid injections on tendon. J Sports Med 1973;1(4):31–7.

22. MacLean CH, Knight K, Paulus H, et al. Costs attributable to osteoarthritis. J Rheumatol 1998; 25(11):2213–8.

23. McDonough AL. Effects of corticosteroids on articular cartilage: a review of the literature. Phys Ther 1982;62(6):835–9.

24. Moskowitz RW, Davis W, Sammarco J, et al. Experimentally induced corticosteroid arthropathy. Arthritis Rheum 1970;13(3):236–43.

25. Hagen R. [Charcot-like arthropathy following intra-articular injections of corticosteroids]. Nord Med 1971;85(12):381 [in Norwegian].

26. Tehranzadeh J, Booya F, Root J. Cartilage metabolism in osteoarthritis and the influence of viscosupplementation and steroid: a review. Acta Radiol 2005;46(3):288–96.

27. Eustace JA, Brophy DP, Gibney RP, et al. Comparison of the accuracy of steroid placement with clinical outcome in patients with shoulder symptoms. Ann Rheum Dis 1997;56(1):59–63.

28. Balint PV, Kane D, Hunter J, et al. Ultrasound guided versus conventional joint and soft tissue fluid aspiration in rheumatology practice: a pilot study. J Rheumatol 2002;29(10):2209–13.

29. van Holsbeeck MT, Introcaso JH. Musculoskeletal ultrasonography. Radiol Clin North Am 1992; 30(5):907–25.

30. Chhem RK, Kaplan PA, Dussault RG. Ultrasonography of the musculoskeletal system. Radiol Clin North Am 1994;32(2):275–89.

31. Fessell DP, Jacobson JA, Craig J, et al. Using sonography to reveal and aspirate joint effusions. AJR Am J Roentgenol 2000;174(5): 1353–62.

32. Shiv VK, Jain AK, Taneja K, et al. Sonography of hip joint in infective arthritis. Can Assoc Radiol J 1990; 41(2):76–8.

33. van Holsbeeck MT, Introcaso JH. Sonography of large synovial joints. 2nd edition. St. Louis (MO): Mosby, Inc.; 2001.

34. Strouse PJ, DiPietro MA, Adler RS. Pediatric hip effusions: evaluation with power Doppler sonography. Radiology 1998;206(3):731–5.

35. Chu CR, Izzo NJ, Papas NE, et al. In vitro exposure to 0.5% bupivacaine is cytotoxic to bovine articular chondrocytes. Arthroscopy 2006;22:693–9.

36. Dogan N, Erdem AF, Erman Z, et al. The effects of bupivacaine and neostigmine on articular cartilage and synovium in the rabbit knee joint. J Int Med Res 2004;32:513–9.

37. Gomoll AH, Kang RW, Williams JM, et al. Chondrolysis after continuous intra-articular bupivacaine infusion: an experimental model investigating chondrotoxicity in the rabbit shoulder. Arthroscopy 2006;22:813–9.

38. Nole R, Munson NM, Fulkerson JP. Bupivacaine and saline effects on articular cartilage. Arthroscopy 1985;1:123–7.

39. Petty DH, Jazrawi LM, Estrada LS, et al. Glenohumeral chondrolysis after shoulder arthroscopy: case reports and review of the literature. Am J Sports Med 2004;32:509–15.

40. Piper SL, Kim HT. Comparison of ropivacaine and bupivacaine toxicity in human articular chondrocytes. J Bone Joint Surg Am 2008;90:986–91.

41. Karpie JC, Chu CR. Lidocaine exhibits dose- and time-dependent cytotoxic effects on bovine articular chondrocytes in vitro. Am J Sports Med 2007; 35:1621–7.

42. van den Bekerom MP, Lamme B, Sermon A, et al. What is the evidence for viscosupplementation in the treatment of patients with hip osteoarthritis? Systematic review of the literature. Arch Orthop Trauma Surg 2007; [epub ahead of print].

43. Waddell DD. Viscosupplementation with hyaluronans for osteoarthritis of the knee: clinical efficacy and economic implications. Drugs Aging 2007; 24(8):629–42.

44. Hamada J, Ono W, Tamai K, et al. Analysis of calcium deposits in calcific periarthritis. J Rheumatol 2001;28(4):809–13.

45. Bradley M, Bhamra MS, Robson MJ. Ultrasound guided aspiration of symptomatic supraspinatus calcific deposits. Br J Radiol 1995;68(811):716–9.

46. Uhthoff HK, Loehr JW. Calcific tendinopathy of the rotator cuff: pathogenesis, diagnosis, and management. J Am Acad Orthop Surg 1997;5(4):183–91.

47. Rothman RH, Parke WW. The vascular anatomy of the rotator cuff. Clin Orthop Relat Res 1965;41:176–86.

48. Speed CA, Hazleman BL. Calcific tendinitis of the shoulder. N Engl J Med 1999;340(20):1582–4.

49. Depalma AF, Kruper JS. Long-term study of shoulder joints afflicted with and treated for calcific tendinitis. Clin Orthop 1961;20:61–72.

50. Farin PU. Consistency of rotator-cuff calcifications. Observations on plain radiography, sonography, computed tomography, and at needle treatment. Invest Radiol 1996;31(5):300–4.

51. Neer CS II. Less frequent procedures. Philadelphia: WB Saunders; 1990.

52. Rompe JD, Zoellner J, Nafe B. Shock wave therapy versus conventional surgery in the treatment of calcifying tendinitis of the shoulder. Clin Orthop Relat Res 2001;(387):72–82.

53. Wang CJ, Ko JY, Chen HS. Treatment of calcifying tendinitis of the shoulder with shock wave therapy. Clin Orthop Relat Res 2001;(387):83–9.

54. Wang CJ, Yang KD, Wang FS, et al. Shock wave therapy for calcific tendinitis of the shoulder: a prospective clinical study with two-year follow-up. Am J Sports Med 2003;31(3):425–30.

55. Loew M, Daecke W, Kusnierczak D, et al. Shock-wave therapy is effective for chronic calcifying tendinitis of the shoulder. J Bone Joint Surg Br 1999;81(5):863–7.

56. del Cura JL, Torre I, Zabala R, et al. Sonographically guided percutaneous needle lavage in calcific tendinitis of the shoulder: short- and long-term results. AJR Am J Roentgenol 2007;189(3): W128–34.

57. Aina R, Cardinal E, Bureau NJ, et al. Calcific shoulder tendinitis: treatment with modified US-guided fine-needle technique. Radiology 2001;221(2):455–61.

58. Uhthoff HK, Sarkar K. The shoulder, vol. 2. Philadelphia: WB Saunders; 1990.

59. Leduc BE, Caya J, Tremblay S, et al. Treatment of calcifying tendinitis of the shoulder by acetic acid iontophoresis: a double-blind randomized controlled trial. Arch Phys Med Rehabil 2003; 84(10):1523–7.

60. Perron M, Malouin F. Acetic acid iontophoresis and ultrasound for the treatment of calcifying tendinitis of the shoulder: a randomized control trial. Arch Phys Med Rehabil 1997;78(4):379–84.

61. Daecke W, Kusnierczak D, Loew M. Long-term effects of extracorporeal shockwave therapy in chronic calcific tendinitis of the shoulder. J Shoulder Elbow Surg 2002;11(5):476–80.

62. Maier M, Stabler A, Lienemann A, et al. Shockwave application in calcifying tendinitis of the shoulder–prediction of outcome by imaging. Arch Orthop Trauma Surg 2000;120(9):493–8.

63. Ark JW, Flock TJ, Flatow EL, et al. Arthroscopic treatment of calcific tendinitis of the shoulder. Arthroscopy 1992;8(2):183–8.

64. Ellman H, Kay SP. Arthroscopic subacromial decompression for chronic impingement. Two- to five-year results. J Bone Joint Surg Br 1991;73(3):395–8.

65. Gschwend N, Patte D, Zippel J. [Therapy of calcific tendinitis of the shoulder]. Arch Orthop Unfallchir 1972;73(2):120–35 [in German].

66. Rubenthaler F, Wittenberg RH. [Intermediate-term follow-up of surgically managed tendinosis calcarea (calcifying subacromion syndrome–SAS) of the shoulder joint]. Z Orthop Ihre Grenzgeb 1997; 135(4):354–9 [in German].

67. Tillander BM, Norlin RO. Change of calcifications after arthroscopic subacromial decompression. J Shoulder Elbow Surg 1998;7(3):213–7.

68. Hedtmann A, Fett H. Die sogenannte Periarthropathia humeroscapularis. Z Orthop Ihre Grenzgeb 1989;127:643–9.

69. Huber H. Ist bei der Tendinitis calcarea die operative Kalkentfernung gerechtfertigt. Orthop Praxis 1992;3:179–83.

70. McLaughlin HL. The selection of calcium deposits for operation; the technique and results of operation. Surg Clin North Am 1963;43:1501–4.

71. Rochwerger A, Franceschi JP, Viton JM, et al. Surgical management of calcific tendinitis of the shoulder: an analysis of 26 cases. Clin Rheumatol 1999;18(4):313–6.

72. Seil R, Litzenburger H, Kohn D, et al. Arthroscopic treatment of chronically painful calcifying tendinitis of the supraspinatus tendon. Arthroscopy 2006; 22(5):521–7.

73. Hurt G, Baker CL Jr. Calcific tendinitis of the shoulder. Orthop Clin North Am 2003;34(4):567–75.

74. Wittenberg RH, Rubenthaler F, Wolk T, et al. Surgical or conservative treatment for chronic rotator cuff calcifying tendinitis–a matched-pair analysis of 100 patients. Arch Orthop Trauma Surg 2001; 121(1–2):56–9.

75. Rubenthaler F, Ludwig J, Wiese M, et al. Prospective randomized surgical treatments for calcifying tendinopathy. Clin Orthop Relat Res 2003;(410): 278–84.

76. Parlier-Cuau C, Champsaur P, Nizard R, et al. Percutaneous treatments of painful shoulder. Radiol Clin North Am 1998;36(3):589–96.

77. Gschwend N, Scherer M, Lohr J. Die tendinitis calcarea des schultergelenks (T. c.). Orthopade 1981;10:196–205.

78. Comfort TH, Arafiles RP. Barbotage of the shoulder with image-intensified fluoroscopic control of needle placement for calcific tendinitis. Clin Orthop Relat Res 1978;(135):171–8.

79. Normandin C, Seban E, Laredo JD. Aspiration of tendinous calcific deposits. New York: Springer-Verlag; 1988.

80. Resch KL, Povacz P, Seykora P. Excision of calcium deposit and acromioplasty? Paris: Elsevier; 1997.

81. Lam F, Bhatia D, van Rooyen K, et al. Modern management of calcifying tendinitis of the shoulder. Current Orthopaedics 2006;20:446–52.

82. Farin PU, Jaroma H, Soimakallio S. Rotator cuff calcifications: treatment with US-guided technique. Radiology 1995;195(3):841–3.

83. Farin PU, Rasanen H, Jaroma H, et al. Rotator cuff calcifications: treatment with ultrasound-guided percutaneous needle aspiration and lavage. Skeletal Radiol 1996;25(6):551–4.

84. Pfister J, Gerber H. Chronic calcifying tendinitis of the shoulder-therapy by percutaneous needle aspiration and lavage: a prospective open study of 62 shoulders. Clin Rheumatol 1997;16(3):269–74.

85. Laredo JD, Bellaiche L, Hamze B, et al. Current status of musculoskeletal interventional radiology. Radiol Clin North Am 1994;32(2):377–98.

86. Connell DA, Ali KE, Ahmad M, et al. Ultrasound-guided autologous blood injection for tennis elbow. Skeletal Radiol 2006;35(6):371–7.

87. Movin T, Kristoffersen-Wiberg M, Shalabi A, et al. Intratendinous alterations as imaged by ultrasound and contrast medium-enhanced magnetic resonance in chronic achillodynia. Foot Ankle Int 1998;19(5):311–7.

88. Edwards SG, Calandruccio JH. Autologous blood injections for refractory lateral epicondylitis. J Hand Surg [Am] 2003;28(2):272–8.

89. Suresh SP, Ali KE, Jones H, et al. Medial epicondylitis: is ultrasound guided autologous blood injection an effective treatment? Br J Sports Med 2006;40(11):935–9 [discussion: 939].

90. Iwasaki M, Nakahara H, Nakata K, et al. Regulation of proliferation and osteochondrogenic differentiation of periosteum-derived cells by transforming growth factor-beta and basic fibroblast growth factor. J Bone Joint Surg Am 1995;77(4):543–54.

91. Ohberg L, Alfredson H. Ultrasound guided sclerosis of neovessels in painful chronic Achilles tendinosis: pilot study of a new treatment. Br J Sports Med 2002;36(3):173–5 [discussion 176–7].

92. Banks AR. A rationale for prolotherapy. J Orthop Med 1991;13:54–9.

93. Reeves KD. Prolotherapy: basic science, clinical studies, and technique. 2nd edition. Philadelphia: Hanley & Belfus; 2000.

94. Liu YK, Tipton CM, Matthes RD, et al. An in situ study of the influence of a sclerosing solution in rabbit medial collateral ligaments and its junction strength. Connect Tissue Res 1983;11(2–3):95–102.

95. Maxwell NJ, Ryan MB, Taunton JE, et al. Sonographically guided intratendinous injection of hyperosmolar dextrose to treat chronic tendinosis of the Achilles tendon: a pilot study. AJR Am J Roentgenol 2007;189(4):W215–20.

96. Oh JH, Ha H, Yu MR, et al. Sequential effects of high glucose on mesangial cell transforming growth factor-beta 1 and fibronectin synthesis. Kidney Int 1998;54(6):1872–8.

97. Rabago D, Best TM, Beamsley M, et al. A systematic review of prolotherapy for chronic musculoskeletal pain. Clin J Sport Med 2005;15(5):376–80.

98. Topol GA, Reeves KD, Hassanein KM. Efficacy of dextrose prolotherapy in elite male kicking-sport athletes with chronic groin pain. Arch Phys Med Rehabil 2005;86(4):697–702.

99. Reeves KD, Hassanein K. Randomized, prospective, placebo-controlled double-blind study of dextrose prolotherapy for osteoarthritic thumb and finger (DIP, PIP, and trapeziometacarpal) joints: evidence of clinical efficacy. J Altern Complement Med 2000;6(4):311–20.

100. Reeves KD, Hassanein K. Randomized prospective double-blind placebo-controlled study of dextrose prolotherapy for knee osteoarthritis with or without ACL laxity. Altern Ther Health Med 2000;6(2):68–74, 77–80.

101. Reeves KD, Hassanein KM. Long-term effects of dextrose prolotherapy for anterior cruciate ligament laxity. Altern Ther Health Med 2003;9(3):58–62.

102. O'Connor PJ, Grainger AJ. Ultrasound imaging of joint disease. In: McNally EG, editor. Practical musculoskeletal ultrasound. Philadelphia: Churchill Livingstone; 2005. p. 245–62.

103. Miller TT, Potter HG, McCormack RR Jr. Benign soft tissue masses of the wrist and hand: MRI appearances. Skeletal Radiol 1994;23(5):327–32.

104. Angelides AC. Ganglions of the hand and wrist. 4th edition. Philadelphia: Churchill Livingstone; 1999.

105. McEvedy B. The simple ganglion: a review of modes of treatment and an explanation of the frequent failures of surgery. Lancet 1954; 266(6803):135–6.

106. Hvid-Hansen O. On the treatment of ganglia. Acta Chir Scand 1970;136(6):471–6.

107. Angelides AC, Wallace PF. The dorsal ganglion of the wrist: its pathogenesis, gross and microscopic anatomy, and surgical treatment. J Hand Surg [Am] 1976;1(3):228–35.

108. Varley GW, Needoff M, Davis TR, et al. Conservative management of wrist ganglia. Aspiration versus steroid infiltration. J Hand Surg [Br] 1997; 22(5):636–7.

109. Zubowicz VN, Ishii CH. Management of ganglion cysts of the hand by simple aspiration. J Hand Surg [Am] 1987;12(4):618–20.

110. Breidahl WH, Adler RS. Ultrasound-guided injection of ganglia with corticosteroids. Skeletal Radiol 1996;25(7):635–8.

111. Cardinal E, Buckwalter KA, Braunstein EM, et al. Occult dorsal carpal ganglion: comparison of US and MR imaging. Radiology 1994;193(1):259–62.

112. Bianchi S, Abdelwahab IF, Zwass A, et al. Ultrasonographic evaluation of wrist ganglia. Skeletal Radiol 1994;23(3):201–3.

Embolization of Musculoskeletal Tumors

Richard J.T. Owen, MB BCh, MRCP, FRCR*

KEYWORDS

• Transarterial embolization • Bone tumors • Metastases

Transarterial embolization (TAE) has been widely practiced for many years. Initial reports involved embolization of organ-based tumors[1] closely followed by the preoperative embolization of metastatic tumors using Gelfoam (Pharmacia and Upjohn, Mississauga, Ontario, Canada)[2] Since those early days indications have widened to include both benign and malignant bone tumors. There are now many options of embolic agent, techniques, and end points but all aim to devascularize the tumor either as a primary treatment or as an adjunct to surgery. The addition of chemotherapy and sclerosants has also gained favor in some areas. A role for direct lesion embolization may also be present in some types of tumor where the TAE route is not feasible.

The term "musculoskeletal tumor" includes primary and metastatic tumors of benign or malignant etiology occurring within the skeleton, joint structures, and muscles. This article is confined to those occurring in the skeleton. A wide spectrum of tumors can be encountered and many are rare entities. Literature-based evidence is at best level II and the bulk of the evidence level III, with many case reports and case series from individual centers. There are no randomized controlled trials.

PRESENTATION

The presence of tumor within bone presents in several ways. Where destruction of normal adjacent bone, infiltration of the periosteum, and expansion occur, pain is a common presenting feature. When adjacent structures, such as joints, neural structures, and soft tissues, are infiltrated or compressed loss of function and pain may occur. Where the structural integrity of the bone is threatened microtrabecular fractures or complete fractures may occur; both are commonly accompanied by pain. The presence of a bone tumor may also be noted as an incidental finding or in the course of investigations to establish the extent of disease.

TECHNIQUE

The aim of embolization is to devascularize the tumor as a palliative procedure to alleviate symptoms, as a preoperative measure to reduce perioperative blood loss to allow more definitive surgery, or in some cases as a curative option. In all cases TAE aims to occlude as much of the tumor supply as possible avoiding nontarget embolization. The outcome ranges from complete tumor necrosis to degrees of ischemia and hypovascularity. Preprocedure planning with MR imaging, CT, and ultrasound is generally advisable allowing identification of arterial blood supply, venous drainage, extent into adjacent tissues, and proximity of vital structures sharing potential blood supply. CT angiography is particularly useful in complex lesions with multiple possible routes of arterial supply.

Following preprocedure planning, catheter-based angiography performed at the time of TAE confirms imaging findings and ultimately determines the safety of embolization. For example, before embolization of spinal lesions identification of arterial supply to the spinal cord determines whether TAE is feasible with acceptable safety parameters.

Parameters pertaining to safe angiography including coagulation times, International Normalized Ratio prothrombin time or partial thromboplastin time in patients on heparin, platelet count,

Radiology and Diagnostic Imaging, University of Alberta, Edmonton, AB, Canada
* Walter Mackenzie Health Sciences, 8440 112 Street, Edmonton, AB T6G 2B7, Canada.
E-mail address: drrichardowen@tbwifi.ca

Radiol Clin N Am 46 (2008) 535–543
doi:10.1016/j.rcl.2008.02.002

and blood count need correction if abnormal. Many of the particulate embolic agents, embolization coils, and injectable thrombogenic agents require a functioning intrinsic clotting system, and a normal coagulation profile assists in their effectiveness.

Once the diagnostic angiogram has been performed the various feeding vessels can be identified and cannulated either with the initial 4 or 5 French diagnostic catheter or with a microcatheter. Microcatheters offer several advantages. The embolic agent can be delivered further from the parent vessel and potentially reduce the chance of nontarget embolization. The feeding vessels to these tumors are often hypertrophied unnamed vessels and cannulation with the larger catheters may be more difficult. Arterial spasm with larger-caliber catheters may lead to false end points for embolization and reduce efficacy of these procedures.

Figures demonstrate a case of renal cell carcinoma metastases embolized before intramedullary nail placement (**Figs. 1–6**).

CHOICE OF EMBOLIC MATERIAL

There are many factors that determine the best choice of embolic material, the most important of which is operator experience. In a life-threatening situation or in preoperative embolizations of metastatic tumors many operators may opt for a combination of particulate emboli (polyvinyl alcohol particles [PVA]) and stainless steel or platinum coils. There is very little published on comparative results from embolic material. In one study looking at operative blood loss after embolization, no clinically significant difference was observed between trisacryl gelatin microspheres and PVA in this

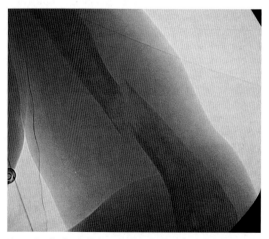

Fig. 1. Pathologic fracture through a renal cell metastases in left humoral diaphysis.

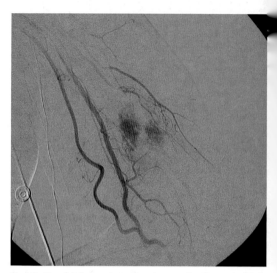

Fig. 2. Brachial angiogram demonstrating multiple arterial feeders from brachial and profunda brachii.

setting.[3] Particulate agents may offer some potential advantages because there is a decreased incidence of nontarget embolization.[4]

POLYVINYL ALCOHOL PARTICLES

PVA is ground from blocks of foam and then separated into different size groupings. Available sizes range from 50 to 1000 μm; the commonest size used is in the 300 to 500 μm range. PVA has a number of desirable characteristics. It is a particulate material capable of penetrating the tumor blood supply and occluding it, it is relatively inexpensive, and it is easy to deliver. Most interventional radiologists have extensive experience in its use and both animal studies and the published experience in patients suggest that it is safe without any known long-term side effects. The traditional preparation (Contour, Boston Scientific Corp., Mississauga, Ontario, Canada) characteristically has a very irregular outline and as a result occludes vessels larger than itself because of particle aggregation.[5] Some of the newer preparations have a smoother outline. Contour SE Microspheres (Boston Scientific Corp.) are engineered PVA particles with more uniform size and because of their microporous nature are compressible with some delivery benefits through small catheters.

EMBOSPHERE MICROSPHERES

Embosphere Microspheres (Biosphere Medical, Rockland, Maryland) are clear acrylic copolymer (trisacryl) microspheres that were previously used as a microcarrier for cell culture, which helped confirm their biocompatibility. Similar to PVA, they are available in sizes from 40 to 1200 μm.

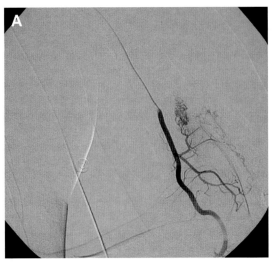
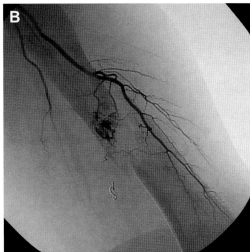

Fig. 3. Selective catheterization and angiographic imaging of multiple arterial feeding vessels.

There are some attractive characteristics of this material, which is widely used in the treatment of uterine fibroids. The spheres are compressible, allowing easy passage through a microcatheter with a luminal diameter smaller than that of the spheres; the spheres are more uniform in size than PVA; and particle size does not changed in liquids. They have little tendency to clump after injection, and animal studies indicate that they have less tissue reaction than is typically seen with PVA.

GELATIN SPONGE

Gelatin sponge (Gelfoam) is a dissolvable sponge-like material that has been used for many years in surgery. It comes in small flat rectangular blocks that can be cut with scissors into elongated rectangles and rolled into pledgets, which can then be injected by diagnostic catheters or microcatheters. Alternatively, the material can be cut into small cubes and mixed vigorously in a syringe (two syringes connected by a stopcock works best to form a slurry). Gelfoam is considered a temporary occluding agent,[6] with the occluded vessel recannalizing in 2 to 4 weeks, although the evidence for this exact time frame is limited.

Once stasis or near stasis has been achieved many operators use coil embolization for final and complete vessel occlusion. As many branches

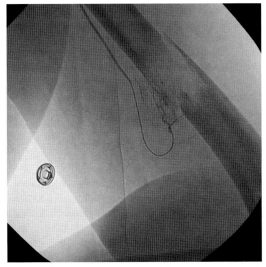

Fig. 4. Distal catheterization of feeding vessel with particulate embolization.

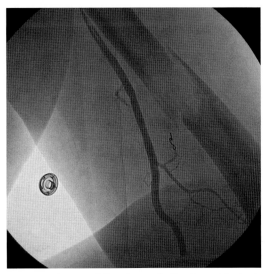

Fig. 5. Angiogram following embolization with single embolization coil in proximal feeding vessel.

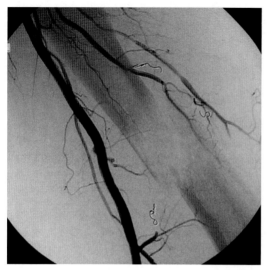

Fig. 6. Completion angiogram demonstrating effective devascularization; patient proceeded to intramedullary nail placement without incident and minimal blood loss.

as can be safely embolized are treated avoiding occluding vessels supplying vital structures. Care should be taken in the femoral region to avoid embolizing supply to the sciatic nerve, in the humoral area to avoid circumflex femoral nerve, and the lateral cutaneous nerve of the thigh. In general, thought should be given to the location and vascular supply of at-risk vital structures.

LIQUID AGENTS

Liquid embolic agents include N-butyl cyanoacrylate; absolute alcohol; Ethibloc (Ethicon, Norderstedt, Germany); sodium tetradecyl sulfate; and Onyx (Microtherapeutics, Irvine, California). Published results involving the use of these agents in embolization of bone tumors is limited. In a non–end organ, such as bone, with multiple arterial feeders liquid agents may increase the potential for nontarget embolization. Ethibloc, cyanoacrylates, and Onyx have been used for tumor embolization, however, and in a potential cure situation may have a role to play. In general, where the goal is to devascularize the tumor there is little advantage over particulate emboli.

EMBOLIZATION COILS

Stainless steel fibered coils and platinum coils have been used for many years for vascular occlusion. Usually reserved for larger vessel occlusion, they do have a role in tumor embolization. Prior to particulate or liquid embolization, coils may be placed to protect the distal vasculature from these

agents. This situation may occur when the vessel is giving off several small vessels to the tumor and continuing on to supply a distal structure that cannot be sacrificed. The use of embolization coils in this instance may reduce nontarget embolization. Following particulate embolization, coils may be used to permanently occlude the vessel and in the emergency situation where either the expertise or time is lacking for other forms of embolization.

CONTRAINDICATIONS

The usual contraindications to intravascular procedures apply with attention to the presence of coagulopathy, thrombocytopenia, or anemia.

PREOPERATIVE EMBOLIZATION

Tumor within bone may present as pain, as an incidental finding, as loss of function, or as a pathologic fracture. In many cases surgery to debulk the tumor, completely resect, or augment the affected bone is planned. In the case of pathologic fracture the fractures do not heal and tumor deposits often lead to fractures if untreated. Many metastatic lesions, notably renal cell carcinoma and primary bone tumors, are highly vascular with excessive bleeding reported at surgery, and one of the earliest reports of selective TAE was in 1975 when the technique was used to reduce perioperative blood loss.[7] There is now a broad range of indications for TAE of primary or metastatic bone tumors: to reduce operative and postoperative hemorrhagic risks, to simplify surgery, pain palliation, fever, bleeding, and hypercalcemic and other rheologic indications. Embolization may also increase tumor sensitivity to chemotherapy or radiation therapy.

Preoperative tumor embolization has been found to be useful in a number of etiologies[8]; avoids major blood loss during surgery[9,10]; and the resultant smaller tumor volume enables complete resection that is safer, easier, and more complete.[10] In addition, preoperative TAE reduces the size of inoperable metastases before other therapies, such as radioiodine therapy, and as a purely palliative measure for pain. A retrospective review of 21 patients who underwent embolization of painful renal cell carcinoma metastases published in 2007 demonstrated effective palliation in this group where therapeutic options are limited. Thirty procedures were performed to treat 39 lesions (18 pelvic, 8 lower extremity, 3 upper extremity, 5 rib-chest wall, and 5 vertebral lesions). Clinical response was achieved at 36 of 39 sites with a mean duration of treatment response of 5.5 months.[11] When the procedure is followed by surgery, it is recommended that the surgery be performed within 3 days to avoid revascularization. In one study blood loss was increased in patients operated on 3 or more days following the embolization procedure.[12]

METASTASES

Renal cell and thyroid carcinoma metastases are hypervascular and treated the most frequently. Aims of treatment are directed at quality of life outcomes; in the case of metastatic thyroid cancer there is some evidence that patients experience a rapid reduction in pain levels and a reduction in neurologic symptoms.[13] Reduction in pain is thought related to decompression of the periosteum. In renal cell carcinoma spinal neurologic symptoms have been treated in this manner.[14–16] In 16 cases of renal cell carcinoma expected bleeding was significantly reduced when tumor enhancement was reduced by more than 70%.[15] One study looking at the effectiveness of TAE for renal cell carcinoma metastases reviewed the case histories of 21 patients with painful metastatic lesions. Thirty embolization procedures to treat 39 metastatic lesions were performed (18 pelvic, 8 lower extremity, 3 upper extremity, 5 rib-chest wall, and 5 vertebral lesions). PVA was used in all cases with additional embolic material in 16 procedures. A clinical response was seen in 36 of 39 sites with the mean duration of response 5.5 months.[11]

TAE has been used in the treatment of metastatic lesions in patients with hepatocellular carcinoma. In one series of 33 patients, 39 metastatic bone lesions from hepatocellular carcinomawere treated with TAE.[17] Each lesion underwent TAE alone (N = 11); TAE in conjunction with radiotherapy (N = 17); or radiotherapy alone (N = 11). Based on the results TAE was found to be effective in relieving pain immediately and improving quality of life but a combination of TAE and radiotherapy was recommended for permanent pain relief. A further series of seven patients underwent TAE for osseous metastases; in the five that had successful embolization all became symptom free within 1 week.[18]

METASTATIC SPINAL TUMORS

Hypervascular spinal and pelvic metastases represent a difficult surgical group. In a series of 32 patients treated with TAE before anterior resection of spinal metastases (N = 21) or pelvic metastases (N = 11) there was a significant difference in blood loss and transfusion requirements in both groups compared with a nonembolized control group. Operating time was also shorter, and no neurologic deficits attributable to the embolization procedure occurred.[19] A further study of 24 patients undergoing preoperative embolization concluded that radical tumor resection was facilitated and that the procedure could be performed without permanent neurologic deficit or skin or muscle deficit. PVA was the embolic material used; in two cases partial embolization was performed because of the proximity of the artery of Adamkiewicz.[14] Direct injection of these hypervascular spinal metastases preoperatively is an alternative route and in one series direct intralesional injection of N-butyl cyanoacrylate mixed with lipiodol was used in conjunction with TAE; there were no neurologic deficits and subsequent surgery was thought to have been facilitated.[20]

GIANT CELL TUMORS

Giant cell tumors of the sacrum can be very difficult to manage with significant complications of surgery and radiotherapy and a local recurrence rate of 33%.[21] Sacrectomy has been described but often requires sacrifice of the sacral nerve roots with potentially severe morbidity.[22,23] Blood loss at surgery is typically high. Serial arterial embolization has been reported to be a useful primary treatment modality for sacral giant cell tumors. A series of nine cases treated with repeated TAE (mean 4.8 treatments per patient) demonstrated a substantial improvement in pain scores, and no tumor progression was seen in seven of nine cases with mean follow-up of 8.96 years; minimal progression was seen in two cases over the study period. Various embolic techniques were used over the study period (1984–2006) but with a similar aim: to reduce tumor vascularity. Embolization was continued until no further tumor supply could be seen.[24]

A series of 18 patients aged 17 to 59 years with sacral giant cell tumors were managed with selective intra-arterial embolization over a 26-year period. Results indicate a durable response in 50% of patients with local recurrence rates of 31% at 10 years and 43% at 15 and 20 years.[25] A total of 50% of the patients receive adjunctive cisplatin therapy. Embolization technique involved Gelfoam or PVA. Typically embolizations were performed at 2- to 4-month intervals until there was no longer a hypervascular mass or the patient's condition was improved (mean number of treatments, 4.4). In this study embolization involved the middle sacral, superior and inferior lateral sacral, lumbar segmental, internal iliac, iliolumbar, and superior and inferior and rectal arteries. Embolization was continued to stasis. One patient died 1 day after embolization (cause of death was not specified but was considered treatment related); three patients experienced neurologic complications; two cases of unilateral weakness of ankle dorsiflexion and one case of transient numbness involving the great toe all were associated with embolization of the lateral sacral artery. Transient pain and fever occurred in nearly all patients. No patients had compromise of bowel or bladder function as a result of embolization. Of 18 patients, 14 (78%) demonstrated an objective, favorable radiographic response characterized by a decrease in vascularity and increase in ossification on CT and plain films rather than a percentage reduction in size. Other studies support this favorable response to embolization.[26–28]

Giant cell tumor may also occur in the remaining areas of the spine, and again TAE has been shown to be useful in these circumstances, particularly in newly diagnosed cases.[29] In a further case a rare giant cell tumor of the atlas was treated with a combined surgical and preoperative embolization of the right vertebral artery.[30] Where tumors are located in the cervical spine, angiography is important in identifying the vertebral arteries and in the lower thoracic spine to identify the artery of Adamkiewicz. Where vertebral artery sacrifice is to be considered a vertebral test balloon occlusion may be required. Spinal embolization, however, has significant risks, particularly relating to long-term neurologic function; in one case although a patient was disease free following TAE he had permanent lower limb paralysis.[31]

Overall, these results are encouraging and embolization should be considered in the treatment algorithm of patients with sacral or spinal giant cell tumor where surgical treatment and radiation are associated with high morbidity and high recurrence rates. TAE may be used alone or in conjunction with other therapies.

ANEURYSMAL BONE CYSTS

Curettage and resection are the treatments of choice for aneurismal bone cysts; however, other treatments, such as radiation, cryotherapy, and embolization, have been used for inaccessible or recurrent lesions.[32] TAE has also been used in combination with surgery to reduce operative blood loss,[33,34] and excessive blood loss during surgery without prior embolization has been reported.[35] In one case,[36] a sacral aneurismal bone cyst confirmed with cytology was embolized with PVA 500 to 700 μm in diameter following catheterization of the main feeding artery arising from the left inferior epigastric. The embolization procedure was followed by curettage and bone grafting with no evidence of recurrence at 6-month follow-up.

A further paper describes embolization of aneurismal bone cysts in the thoracic spine and long bones.[33] Peripheral aneurismal bone cyst may also be treated with embolization. Four aneurismal bone cysts embolized with PVA were presented by Boruban and colleagues.[37] In three cases embolization was followed by surgery, in one case of a distal femur lesion this was considered cured by embolization at 2 years.

VERTEBRAL HEMANGIOMA

Vertebroplasty for vertebral hemangioma remains one option for treating these highly vascular lesions and is generally reserved for lesions without neurologic deficit. Traditionally, where presentation has involved spinal pain or cord compression with neurologic deficit radiation or decompression surgery has been the treatment of choice. Surgery is, however, often associated with massive hemorrhage from these highly vascular lesions[38,39] and preoperative TAE has been found to be a useful adjunctive step reducing perioperative blood loss.[40] Results support the role of TAE in this context as an adjunctive to surgery.[41] Although TAE has been advocated by some as a stand-alone treatment,[42] long-term data are lacking.

In one case the patient with multicentric intraosseous hemangiomas presented with intractable retromolar hemorrhage. The bleeding was effectively controlled with transoral direct lesion puncture and injection of N-butyl cyanoacrylate.[43] Direct lesional injection with ethanol has also been described.[44]

OSTEOSARCOMA

Chemoembolization in combination with limb salvage surgery had encouraging results when data were presented by Chu and colleagues[45] in 2007. Transarterial chemoembolization was used in 32 patients before limb salvage surgery. An intra-arterial three-drug regimen was given: methotrexate (1–2 g); pharmorubicin (30–50 mg); and cisplatin (60–100 mg). Vascular isolation of the treated limb was performed using ligation for a period of 15 minutes in each case. Following the infusion of the chemotherapeutic agent the vessels were embolized with a variety of embolic agents: adriblastine gelatin microspheres, anhydrous alcohol, gelatin sponge particles, and common bletilla tuber. Results confirmed tumor necrosis and the addition of a chemotherapeutic agent does seem to increase tumor necrosis and may result in less local recurrence. Convincing survival benefits, however, have yet to be demonstrated. TAE without chemotherapy has also been shown to be effective as an adjunct to surgery.[46–48]

ARTERIOVENOUS MALFORMATION OF BONE

There are a number of references to TAE or transvenous embolization of arteriovenous malformations involving the bone[49,50] and in one case by direct lesional puncture following failure of TAE to control hemorrhage.[51] TAE seems to be a valuable primary or adjunctive treatment in these rare cases.

CERVICAL SPINE OSTEOBLASTOMAS

Three cases of TAE are reported in the literature with favorable adjunctive results with surgery, where the procedure was thought to reduce intraoperative bleeding, increase the chance of complete resection, and reduce postoperative complications with the potential to improve patient outcomes.[52] These results were supported by a further small study.[53] PVA was used as the embolic agent (150–250 μm) in these cases, and there were no reported complications.

OTHER BONE TUMORS

Isolated reports involving other pathologies have been reported, preoperative embolizations in hemangiopericytoma have been described,[54,55] and postoperative embolization in a case of angiosarcoma.[56]

SUMMARY

TAE should be considered in the treatment algorithm of primary or secondary bone tumors. Specific benefit is present where there is a high risk of bleeding at surgery, where there is spinal involvement and neural encroachment, where active bleeding is present, or in awkward surgical locations where prolonged surgery is anticipated.

REFERENCES

1. Bucheler E, Hupe W, Hertel EU, et al. Catheter embolization of renal tumours. Rofo 1976;124(2):134–8.
2. Carpenter PR, Ewing JW, Cook AJ, et al. Angiographic assessment and control of potential operative hemorrhage with pathologic fractures secondary to metastasis. Clin Orthop Relat Res 1977;123:6–8.
3. Basile A, Rand T, Lomoschitz F, et al. Trisacryl gelatin microspheres versus polyvinyl alcohol particles in the preoperative embolization of bone neoplasms. Cardiovasc Intervent Radiol 2004;27(5):495–502.
4. Munk PL, Legiehn GM. Musculoskeletal interventional radiology: applications to oncology. Semin Roentgenol 2007;42(3):164–74.
5. Yamamoto A, Shigeki I, Makito K, et al. Evaluation of tris-acryl gelatin microsphere embolization with monochromatic x rays: comparison with polyvinyl alcohol particles. J Vasc Interv Radiol 2006;17:1797–802.
6. Vlahos L, Benakis V, Dimakakos P, et al. A comparative study of the degree of arterial recanalization in kidneys of dogs following transcatheter embolization with eight different materials. Eur Urol 1980;6(3):180–5.
7. Feldman F, Caserella WJ, Dick HM, et al. Selective intraarterial embolization of bone tumors: a useful adjunct in the management of selected lesions. Am J Roentgenol Radium Ther Nucl Med 1975;123:130–9.
8. Fenoy AJ, Greenlee JD, Menezes AH, et al. Primary bone tumors of the spine in children. J Neurosurg 2006;105:252–60.
9. Reuter M, Heller M, Heise U, et al. Transcatheter embolization of tumors of the muscular and skeletal systems. Rofo 1992;156(2):182–8.
10. Gellad TE, Sadato N, Numaguchi Y, et al. Vascular metastatic lesions of the spine: preoperative embolization. Radiology 1990;176:683–6.
11. Forauer AR, Kent E, Cwikiel W, et al. Selective palliative transcatheter embolization of bony metastases from renal cell carcinoma. Acta Oncol 2007;46(7):1012–8.
12. Barton PP, Waneck RE, Kamel FJ, et al. Embolization of bone metastases. J Vasc Interv Radiol 1996;7:81–8.
13. Van Tol KM, Hew JM, Jager PL, et al. Embolization in combination with radio-iodine therapy for bone metastases from differentiated thyroid carcinoma. Clin Endocrinol 2000;52:653–9.
14. Guzman R, Dubach-Schwizer S, Heini P, et al. Preoperative transarterial embolization of vertebral metastases. Eur Spine J 2005;14(3):263–8.
15. Sun S, Lang EV. Bone metastases from renal cell carcinoma: preoperative embolization. J Vasc Interv Radiol 1998;9:263–9.
16. Chatziioannou AN, Johnson ME, Pneumaticos SG, et al. Preoperative embolization of bone metastases from renal cell carcinoma. Eur Radiol 2000;10:593–6.
17. Uemura A, Fujimoto H, Yasuda S, et al. Transcatheter arterial embolization for bone metastases from hepatocellular carcinoma. Eur Radiol 2001;11(8):1457–62.
18. Nagata Y, Nakano Y, Abe M, et al. Osseous metastases from hepatocellular carcinoma: embolization for pain control. Cardiovasc Intervent Radiol 1989;12(3):149–53.
19. Wirbel RJ, Roth R, Schulte M, et al. Preoperative embolization in spinal and pelvic metastases. J Orthop Sci 2005;10(3):253–7.
20. Schirmer CM, Malek AM, Kwan ES, et al. Preoperative embolization of hypervascular spinal

metastases using percutaneous direct injection with N-butyl cyanoacrylate: technical case report. Neurosurgery 2006;59(2):431–2.

21. Turcotte RE, Sim FH, Unni KK. Giant cell tumor of the sacrum. Clin Orthop Relat Res 1993;291:215–21.

22. Simpson AH, Porter A, Davis A, et al. Cephalad sacral resection with a combined extended ilioinguinal and posterior approach. J Bone Joint Surg Am 1995;77:405–11.

23. Gokaslan ZL, Romsdahl MM, Kroll SS, et al. Total sacrectomy and Galveston L-rod reconstruction for malignant neoplasms. [technical note]. J Neurosurg 1997;87:781–7.

24. Hosalkar HS, Jones KJ, King JJ, et al. Serial arterial embolization for large sacral giant-cell tumors: mid- to long-term results. Spine 2007;32(10):1107–15.

25. Lin PP, Guzel VB, Moura MF, et al. Long-term follow-up of patients with giant cell tumor of the sacrum treated with selective arterial embolization. Cancer 2002;95(6):1317–25.

26. Wallace S, Granmayah M, DeSantos LA, et al. Arterial occlusion of pelvic bone tumours. Cancer 1979; 15:1223–7.

27. Chuang VP, Soo CS, Wallace S, et al. Arterial occlusion: management of giant cell tumor and aneurismal bone tumor and aneurismal bone cyst. AJR Am J Roentgenol 1981;136:1127–30.

28. Eftekhari F, Wallace S, Chuang VP, et al. Intraarterial management of giant-cell tumors of the spine in children. Pediatr Radiol 1982;12:289–93.

29. Luther N, Bilsky MH, Hartl R. Giant cell tumor of the spine. Neurosurg Clin N Am 2008;19(1):49–55.

30. Tsuchiya H, Kokubo Y, Sakurada K, et al. A case of giant cell tumor in atlas. No Shinkei Geka 2005; 33(8):817–23.

31. Finstein JL, Chin KR, Alvandi F, et al. Postembolization paralysis in a man with a thoracolumbar giant cell tumor. Clin Orthop Relat Res 2006;453:335–40.

32. Guzey FK, Emel E, Aycan A, et al. Pediatric vertebral and spinal epidural tumors: a retrospective review of twelve cases. Pediatr Neurosurg 2008;44(1):14–21.

33. Fraser RK, Coates CJ, Cole WG. An angiostatic agent in treatment of a recurrent aneurismal bone cyst. J Pediatr Orthop 1993;13:668–71.

34. Konya A, Szendroi M. Aneurysmal bone cysts treated by superselective embolization. Skeletal Radiol 1992;21:167–72.

35. Han X, Dong Y, Sun K, et al. A huge occipital osteoblastoma accompanied with aneurismal bone cyst in the posterior cranial fossa. Clin Neurol Neurosurg 2008;110(3):282–5.

36. Yildirim E, Ersozlu S, Kirbas I, et al. Treatment of pelvic aneurismal bone cysts in two children: selective arterial embolization as an adjunct to curettage and bone grafting. Diagn Interv Radiol 2007;13:49–52.

37. Boruban S, Sancak T, Yildiz Y, et al. Embolization of benign and malignant bone and soft tissue tumors

of the extremities. Diagn Interv Radiol 2007;13: 164–71.

38. Pastushyn AI, Slin'ko EI, Mirzoyeva GM. Vertebral hemangiomas: diagnosis, management, natural history and clinicopathological correlates in 86 patients. Surg Neurol 1998;50:535–47.

39. Fox MW, Onofrio BM. The natural history and management of symptomatic and asymptomatic vertebral hemangiomas. J Neurosurg 1993;78:36–45.

40. Bandiera S, Gasbarrini A, De lure F, et al. Symptomatic vertebral hemangioma: the treatment of 23 cases and a review of the literature. Chir Organi Mov 2002;87:1–15.

41. Acosta FL Jr, Dowd CF, Chin C, et al. Current treatment strategies and outcomes in the management of symptomatic vertebral hemangiomas. Neurosurgery 2006;58(2):287–95.

42. Jayakumar PN, Vasudev MK, Srikanth SG. Symptomatic vertebral haemangiona: endovascular treatment of 12 cases. Spinal Cord 1997;35:624–8.

43. Syal R, Tyagi I, Goyal A, et al. Multiple intraosseous hemangiomas-investigation and role of N-butylcyanoacrylate in management. Head Neck 2007;29(5): 512–7.

44. Doppman JL, Oldfield EH, Heiss JD. Symptomatic vertebral hemangiomas: treatment by means of direct intralesional injection of ethanol. Radiology 2000;214(2):341–8.

45. Chu JP, Chen W, Li JP, et al. Clinicopathologic features and results of transcatheter arterial chemoembolization for osteosarcoma. Cardiovasc Intervent Radiol 2007;30(2):201–6.

46. Crews KR, Liu T, Rodriguez-Galindo C, et al. High dose methotrexate pharmacokinetics and outcome of children and young adults with osteosarcoma. Cancer 2004;100:1724–33.

47. Philip T, Iiescu C, Demaille M-C, et al. High dose methotrexate and HELP [holoxan (isofamide), eldesine (vindesine), platinum] doxorubicin in non-metastatic osteosarcoma of the extremity: a French multicentre pilot study. Ann Oncol 1999;10:1065–71.

48. Wang MQ, Dake MD, Wang ZP, et al. Isolated lower extremity chemotherapeutic infusion for treatment of osteogenic sarcoma: experimental study and preliminary clinical report. J Vasc Interv Radiol 2001; 12:731–7.

49. Katzen BT, Said S. Arteriovenous malformation of bone: an experience with therapeutic embolization. AJR Am J Roentgenol 1981;136:427–9.

50. Beek FJ, Ten Broek FW, Van Schaik JP, et al. Transvenous embolization of an arteriovenous malformation of the mandible via a femoral approach. Pediatr Radiol 1997;27(11):855–7.

51. Resnick SA, Russell EJ, Hanson DH, et al. Embolization of a life threatening vascular malformation by direct percutaneous transmandibular puncture. Head Neck 1992;14(5):372–9.

52. Trubenbach J, Nagele T, Bauer T, et al. Preoperative embolization of cervical spine osteoblastomas: report of three cases. AJNR Am J Neuroradiol 2006; 27(9):1910–2.

53. Denaro V, Denaro L, Papalia R, et al. Surgical management of cervical spine osteoblastomas. Clin Orthop Relat Res 2007;455:190–5.

54. Findik S, Akan H, Baris S, et al. Preoperative embolization in surgical treatment of a hemangiopericytoma of the rib: a case report. J Korean Med Sci 2005;20(2): 316–8.

55. Deneuve S, Lezy JP, Cyna-Gorse F, et al. Mandibular hemangiopericytoma, a malignant vascular tumor. Rev Stomatol Chir Maxillofac 2007;108(2):146–9.

56. Sanchez-Mejia RO, Ojemann SG, Simko J, et al. Sacral epitheliod angiosarcoma associated with a bleeding diathesis and spinal epidural hematoma: case report. J Neurosurg Spine 2006;4(3):246–50.

Venous Malformations: Classification, Development, Diagnosis, and Interventional Radiologic Management

Gerald M. Legiehn, MD, FRCPC[a],*, Manraj K.S. Heran, MD, FRCPC[b,c]

KEYWORDS
- Classification • Vascular malformation
- Venous malformation • Sclerotherapy • Embolization
- Radiology • Hemangioma

Venous malformations (VMs) are a commonly encountered entity in clinical practice, with an estimated incidence of 1 to 2 in 10,000[1] births and a prevalence of 1%.[2,3] VMs are also responsible for more than 50% of referrals to vascular anomaly centers.[4–6] Despite this, the collective experience of this group of patients before final referral has often included unacceptably high rates of misdiagnosis, resulting in incorrect, ineffective, and often overly invasive therapy.[7,8] Delays in arriving at the appropriate diagnosis and management in VM patients, if viewed within the context of the broader family of vascular anomalies, are understandable and predictable in light of several historical and clinical factors. Foremost, the power of a name has greatly influenced understanding and progress within the realm of vascular anomalies. For several centuries, a myriad of cutaneous or visceral masses, pigmentations, or spaces that resulted in a predominantly disturbed vascular morphologic pattern were named and categorized according to appearance, location, fluid content, and often inconsistent or unpredictable clinical behavior.[9] Until only recently, this purely descriptive nomenclature resulted in a severely bloated lexicon that was redundant, difficult to understand or conceptualize, and predisposed to frequent misdiagnosis and incorrect management.[10] Further understanding of etiology, disease process relationships, and the development and testing of novel therapies was also impeded because these earlier categorization schemes were not founded on the currently accepted belief that a much smaller group of vascular defects or entities are responsible for the protean clinical appearances and manifestations of most vascular anomalies. Furthermore, although the prevalence of congenital vascular malformations may be higher than that of other inborn errors,[2,3,11] there is a persistent and pervasive lack of diagnostic familiarity with and accessibility to appropriate therapy for vascular malformations, resulting in the all too often default and erroneous diagnosis of "hemangioma."[12,13] Over time, experienced

[a] Division of Interventional Radiology, Department of Radiology, Vancouver General Hospital, University of British Columbia, 899 West 12th Avenue, Vancouver, BC V5Z 1M9, Canada
[b] Division of Neuroradiology, Department of Radiology, Vancouver General Hospital, University of British Columbia, 899 West 12th Avenue, Vancouver, BC V5Z 1M9, Canada
[c] Division of Pediatric Interventional Radiology, Children's and Women's Health Center of British Columbia, University of British Columbia, 4500 Oak Street, Vancouver, BC V6H 3N1, Canada
* Corresponding author.
E-mail address: gerald@telus.net (G.M. Legiehn).

Radiol Clin N Am 46 (2008) 545–597
doi:10.1016/j.rcl.2008.02.008

multidisciplinary vascular anomaly teams have evolved that allow the establishment of clear lines of communication and the use of the most current clinical, pathologic, and image-based standards available. Only through such a clinical body can one reasonably expect accurately to diagnose, appropriately treat, and follow the patient presenting with a vascular malformation.[12–14]

The correct clinical, pathologic, and imaging diagnosis of VMs requires discrimination between various overlapping characteristics found in other vascular anomalies and syndromes, which can often mimic the appearance of a VM. The diagnostic and interventional radiologist serving on the multidisciplinary team must possess a working understanding of the comparative anatomy of these entities and the position of VMs within current classification schemes if they are to direct an appropriate imaging work-up and arrive at an accurate diagnosis before therapy. If the diagnosis of VM is made, the interventional radiologist must be aware of the natural history of the lesion, and indications for percutaneous sclerotherapy based on firmly established clinical criteria. If appropriate, he or she must then address morphologic issues specific to VMs and their effect on choice of sclerosant, technique, complication rate, and efficacy of sclerotherapy so as to allow both the patient and responsible caregivers to make the most informed choices. This article addresses these issues and further provides a detailed description of the rationale, patient preparation and follow-up, and technique of percutaneous image-guided sclerotherapy with respect to VMs.

MODERN CLASSIFICATION SCHEMA OF VASCULAR ANOMALIES
Historical Background

Because most vascular anomalies involve the skin to variable degrees,[10] they tend to be visible and have consequently received colorful appellations since ancient times. As recently as the nineteenth century, causative factors implicating the mother resulted in names such as naevus maternus or "mother's mark."[15] Other systems used food descriptors, such as strawberry, port-wine, or cherry, terms that unfortunately still persist in common medical parlance today.[10,16] Virchow and Wegner developed histologic-based classification schemes for vascular anomalies in the later nineteenth century. Vascular lesions were considered to be vascular tumors and were further subdivided into angioma simplex (later known as the "capillary" or "strawberry" hemangioma); angioma cavernosum (later used to describe both the infantile hemangioma or the VM); and the angioma

racemosum (used to describe a cirsoid aneurysm or arteriovenous hemangioma).[10,15–18] This classification hypothesized an underlying cause of abnormal vascular cellular proliferation or dilatation at work, but did little to address the biologic behavior of these lesions.[16] As early as 1932, De Takats[19] proposed that these angiomas represented persistent rests of embryonic angioblastic tissue that failed to resorb fully or differentiate because of aberrations in vasculogenesis occurring in specific stages of embryonic development. The concept of these lesions being tumors persisted in the literature,[20] however, fostering the ubiquitous use of the term "hemangioma" that was often accompanied by host of prefixes. This practice continued throughout the remainder of the twentieth century, perpetuating the disconnect between misleading nomenclature and the true biologic nature of the lesion its name was meant to describe.

Historical Development of the Modern International Society for the Study of Vascular Anomalies Classification

By 1971, there was general agreement by attendees of the International Symposia on Angiological Nosology in Florence that a new vascular anomaly classification scheme "was absolutely necessary for didactic and practical purposes" that was to be "in so far as possible, schematic and simplified."[21] As a result, based on the concepts proposed by Malan[22] and described by Degni and coworkers,[23,24] congenital vascular defects were simply categorized as predominantly arterial, venous, arteriovenous, lymphatic, or mixed. In 1976, further to address ongoing nosologic and research concerns, Mulliken and Young founded the International Workshop for the Study of Vascular Anomalies, later becoming the International Society for the Study of Vascular Anomalies (ISSVA) in Budapest in 1992. Meeting biennially since its inception, this Society served in the vanguard for developments within this rapidly evolving multidisciplinary field dedicated to the accurate classification, diagnosis, and management of all vascular anomalies.

In 1982, in a landmark publication, Mulliken and Glowacki[15] proposed what would become the foundation of modern vascular anomaly classification. Based on the lesion's biologic and pathologic differences, all vascular anomalies were assigned to one of two broad categories: hemangiomas and vascular malformations (**Table 1**). Hemangiomas were described as those exhibiting rapid neonatal growth and hypercellularity during a proliferating phase, followed by an involutive phase characterized by diminished cellularity and

Table 1
Classification of vascular lesions in infants and children

Hemangiomas	Malformations
Proliferating phase	Capillary
Involuting phase	Venous
	Arterial
	Lymphatic
	Fistulae

Data from Mulliken JB, Glowacki J. Hemangiomas and vascular malformations in infants and children: a classification based on endothelial characteristics. Plast Reconstr Surg 1982;69:412–20.

fibrosis. This former category was later expanded to include vascular tumors. The suffix "-oma" was only to be reserved for those lesions exhibiting increased cellular turnover, the classic example within this category being the infantile hemangioma. The term "vascular malformation" was applied to those lesions present at birth growing commensurately or pari passu with the child. The vascular malformations were composed of normal "mature" flat endothelial-lined vascular spaces with normal rates of cell turnover and were further subdivided into capillary malformation; VM; arterial (arteriovenous malformation [AVM]); lymphatic malformation (LM); and fistulae initially. In 1983, Burrows and coworkers[25] incorporated angiographic differentiation and flow characteristics into the classification.

To incorporate the hypothesized level of embryologic defect responsible for each type of anomaly described earlier by Malan and Degni, Belov[21,26,27] went on subdivide each of these anomaly categories into two distinct anatomic-pathologic subtypes: truncular and extratruncular. The often more severe truncular form arose as a consequence of a relatively late embryonic error of maturation within a differentiated vascular trunk leading to the development of regional vascular aplasia, obstruction, or dilatation. The usually less severe extratruncular form was caused by a relatively early embryonal dysplasia within the primitive undifferentiated capillary network and presented in either a diffuse-infiltrating or limited-localized pattern. In 1988, at the 7th Meeting of the ISSVA in Hamburg, the work of Malan, Degni, and Belov formed the "Hamburg Classification" of vascular defects (**Table 2**).

In 1993, Jackson and coworkers[28] later identified the need for further augmentation of Mulliken's classification to "answer the (therapeutic) questions of 'what to do' and 'when to do it'." He elegantly simplified flow patterns within vascular malformations as either low flow (VMs) or high flow (AVMs), keeping separate categories for LMs and hemangiomas, with the purpose of creating a "system directly related to investigation and treatment" (**Box 1**). LMs have since been subdivided into macrocystic, microcystic, and mixed varieties based on lesion cavity size. For simplicity, many now consider LMs to reside in Jackson's low-flow category.

In 1992 at the ISSVA meeting in Colorado, a final nosologic consensus clarified the umbrella term of "vascular anomaly" to describe all vascular tumors and malformations and the use of the

Table 2
Anatomopathologic classification of vascular defects (Hamburg classification)

Type	Forms	
	Truncular	Extratruncular
Predominantly arterial defects	Aplasia or obstructive	Infiltrating
	Dilatation	Limited
Predominantly venous defects	Aplasia or obstructive	Infiltrating
	Dilatation	Limited
Predominantly lymphatic defects	Aplasia or obstructive	Infiltrating
	Dilatation	Limited
Predominantly AV shunting defects	Deep	Infiltrating
	Superficial	Limited
Combined/mixed vascular defects	Arterial and venous	Infiltrating hemolymphatic
	Hemolymphatic	Limited hemolymphatic

Based on 7th Meeting of the International Workshop on Vascular Malformations, Hamburg, Germany, 1988.
Abbreviation: AV, arteriovenous.
Data from Ref. 21,26,27.

Box 1
Classification of vascular anomalies by vascular dynamics

I. Hemangioma
II. Vascular malformations
    a. Low-flow (VM)
    b. High-flow (AVM)
III. LM

suffix "-oma" to refer only to lesions demonstrating cellular hyperplasia.[29] The final modern classification of vascular anomalies after Mulliken based on histology, clinical behavior, and flow characteristics was adopted at the ISSVA in Rome 1996,[29] with the most recent and complete version appearing in 2007 (**Table 3**).[30]

COMPARATIVE VENOUS MALFORMATION ANATOMY
Gross Inspection

VMs are composed of abnormal collections of veins that have a variable luminal size and wall thickness and geographically can appear superficial, deep, diffuse, localized, and not uncommonly multiple.[31] The lesions are often less well circumscribed than vascular tumors, such as infantile hemangiomas[31], and can be interspersed with adipose tissue or within variably atrophic or degenerative muscle.[13,32]

Conventional Microscopy

As with all vascular malformations, conventional hematoxylin-eosin staining techniques for VMs reveal irregular variably dilated or thickened dysplastic-appearing vascular channels lined with flat mature endothelial cells in contrast to hypercellularity seen in vascular tumors.[15,16,31,32] These vascular spaces are usually filled with an abundance of erythrocytes (**Fig. 1**). Capillaries and venules may reside within the VM substance. In addition to the absence of internal elastic lamina, there is a relative paucity or intermittent absence of smooth muscle within the VM channel wall[13,31] with occasional locules of disorganized smooth muscle identified emanating from the vascular wall into the surrounding stroma (**Fig. 2**).[31] Localized intravascular coagulopathy is frequently present within VMs[33] and as a result, luminal thrombi can develop and become calcified and form phleboliths. During the process of recanalization of thrombosed segments, the local endothelium can undergo a papillary endothelial hyperplasia known as "Masson's vegetant intravascular hemangioendothelioma" or more aptly "papillary endothelial hyperplasia" that can lead to further vascular restriction.[13,31,34] This phenomenon can evolve into a mass-like lesion within the malformation containing cores of hyalinized tissue lined by endothelial tissue in a sinusoidal or papillary pattern.

VMs are contrasted with LMs, because the latter are predominantly filled with lymphatic fluid or much fewer erythrocytes than VMs. The frequent LM findings of surrounding lymphocytic infiltrates containing lymphoid follicles set in a loose connective tissue stroma are not usually identified in pure VMs[31] but may be identified in mixed lesions and in syndromes containing VMs. Aside from having obviously different clinical presentations, VMs can be histologically discriminated from AVMs, because the latter demonstrates heterogeneous architecture, dilated arterial structures, and thick-walled veins (**Fig. 3**).

Table 3
International society for the study of vascular anomalies classification of vascular anomalies

| Tumors | Vascular Malformations | |
	Simple	Combined
Infantile hemangioma	Capillary (C)	Arteriovenous fistula
Congenital hemangioma	Lymphatic (L)	Arteriovenous malformation (AVM)
Tufted angioma	Venous (V)	CVM
Kaposiform hemangioendothelioma		CLVM
Hemangiopericytoma		LVM
Pyogenic granuloma		CAVM
Spindle-cell hemangioendothelioma		CLAVM

Based on Scientific Committee of the 11th Meeting of the International Society for the Study of Vascular Anomalies, Rome, Italy, 1996.
Data from Enjolras O. Classification and management of the various superficial vascular anomalies: hemangioma and vascular malformation. J Dermatol 1997;24:701–10; and Garzon MC, Huang JT, Enjolras O, et al. Vascular malformations: Part I. J Am Acad Dermatol 2007;56:353–70 [quiz: 371–4].

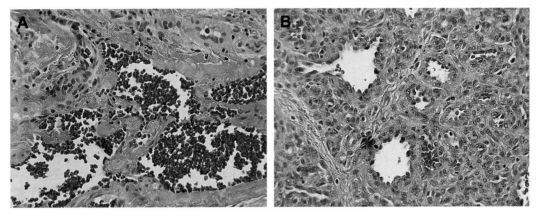

Fig. 1. Comparative histology of VMs and infantile hemangioma. (*A*) Conventional hematoxylin-eosin staining of a VM under 400× magnification revealing typical enlarged erythrocyte-filled vascular spaces lined with flattened mature nonhypercellular endothelium. (*B*) Hematoxylin-eosin staining of an infantile hemangioma under 400× magnification revealing diffuse hypercellularity with vascular spaces lined with nonmature-appearing endothelium. (*Courtesy of* C. Senger, MD, Vancouver, BC.)

Immunohistochemical Staining

Although the vascular channels in VMs are surrounded by a normal reticulin network,[15] anti-smooth muscle α-actin stains reveal an absent or patchy mural smooth muscle distribution in clumps, which is thought to be the major causative factor in the histologically observed vascular ectasia that results in the mass-like appearance of VMs.[5,35–37]

VMs share many histologic characteristics with LMs and AVMs, and to a much lesser extent, vascular tumors. In those cases of mixed or ambiguous histology, the addition of immunohistochemical staining to a detailed clinical and imaging work-up may be required to arrive at the correct diagnosis. All vascular malformations are negative for glucose transporter-1 that is expressed exclusively by infantile hemangiomas (**Fig. 4**).[38] Conversely, nerve tissue avid S-100 immunostain has recently identified nerve bundles to be consistently present within vascular malformations and consistently absent in hemangiomas.[39] D2-40, a monoclonal antibody to oncofetal antigen M2A, is highly avid for normal lymphatic endothelium and interestingly also within kaposiform hemangioendotheliomas.[40–43] This allows discrimination between VMs and frequently similar appearing LMs (particularly microcystic varieties) with the former staining negative for this antibody and the latter staining positive.[42]

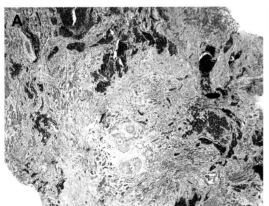
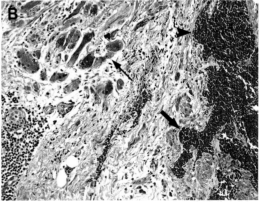

Fig. 2. VM architecture. (*A*) Masson trichrome staining of an intramuscular VM under 40× magnification demonstrates multiple vascular channels interspersed between regions of striated muscle. (*B*) Further magnification to 200× reveals regions of vascular channels associated with disorganized clumps of smooth muscle (*thick arrow*) and regions where vascular spaces have little or no surrounding smooth muscle (*arrowhead*). The lesion is interwoven between striated muscle (*thin arrow*) and inflammatory lymphocytic infiltrate (*lower left margin*). (*Courtesy of* C. Senger, MD, Vancouver, BC.)

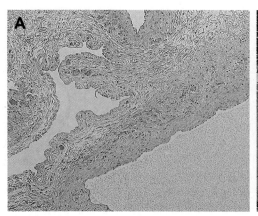 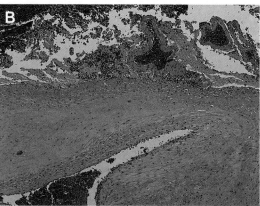

Fig. 3. Comparative histology between VMs and other vascular malformations. (*A*) Typical appearance of a LM with hematoxylin-eosin staining under x40 maginification demonstrating enlarged lymphatic spaces lined by bland endothelial cells not contiguous with normal lymphatic channels (*From* Legiehn GM, Heran MK. Classification, diagnosis, and interventional radiologic management of vascular malformations. Orthop Clin North Am 2006;37:435–74; with permission). (*B*) Hematoxylin-eosin staining of an AVM under x40 magnification revealing variably enlarged hypertrophic arterial and venous spaces. (*Courtesy of* C. Senger, MD, Vancouver, BC.)

DEVELOPMENTAL ETIOLOGY OF VENOUS MALFORMATIONS

Because many vascular malformations are not clinically obvious in early life, it is not generally appreciated that all vascular malformations are present at birth.[31] For that reason, it has long been held that a localized defect or defects within vascular morphogenesis is responsible for all vascular malformations whether caused by hereditable or sporadic mutation, altered gene expression, or environmental factors. To comprehend the

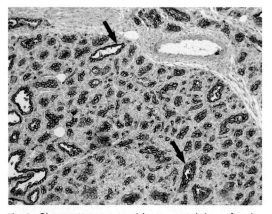

Fig. 4. Glucose transporter-1 immunostaining of an infantile hemangioma. Innumerable irregular hypercellular vascular channels (*arrows*) stain positively for glucose transporter-1 within an infantile hemangioma. VMs do not stain positively by this method, serving as an important means of differentiating between these two entities. (*Courtesy of* C. Senger, MD, Vancouver, BC.)

hypothesized mechanisms leading to the development of a VM, one must first possess an understanding of normal vascular morphogenesis.

Embryology: Vascular Morphogenesis

The cardiovascular system is the first functional system to form in the embryo[44] and begins development at approximately 13 to 15 days gestation with the urgent embryonic need for increased nourishment and oxygenation. Vascular morphogenesis is divided into two phases. The first phase, termed "vasculogenesis," begins in the extraembryonic mesoderm of the yolk sac.[45] Mesodermal hemangioblasts congregate into clusters of blood islands that cavitate centrally. Outer layers differentiate into endothelial progenitors called angioblasts,[46] whereas the inner layers form primitive plasma and blood cells.[45] These "shells" organize to form a lattice of short tubes or canaliculi that constitute the primary capillary plexus. The second phase, angiogenesis, occurs as a result of four distinct processes.[6,47,48] Sprouting results in additional capillaries "budding" from existing capillaries. Nonsprouting occurs as a result of extracellular matrix transcapillary pillars or posts cleaving or fusing existing vessels. These first two processes occur simultaneously on the primary capillary plexus to create a juvenile vascular network. Further deletions are made in the juvenile network through the third process of pruning. The fourth and final process, termed "maturation," occurs as a result of an interaction between the primitive endothelium and the surrounding mesenchyme to form fully differentiated smooth muscle cells and pericytes-adventitia surrounding mature endothelium. This gives rise to a fully differentiated multilayered vascular structure within a mature circulatory system (**Fig. 5**).

Molecular Genetics: Endothelial-Pericyte Interactions

Given the histologic abnormalities of the smooth muscle–pericyte component within vascular channel walls of VMs, it is not surprising that a hypothesized defect in this interaction has garnered a great deal of attention by molecular biologists as a potential cause of many VMs.[6] In a recent study of 1685 patients, 98.8% of VMs occurred sporadically in a noninherited fashion.[49] The few inherited varieties often appear as multifocal lesions clinically.[4,6,50] Some entities are thought to be the result of mosaicism.[51] The molecular biologic study of these inherited lesions allows a more complete understanding of the genes coding for endothelial cell–mesenchymal pericyte interaction and those genes and proteins that are responsible for the observed malformation phenotypes.[1,4–6,36,44,52–55]

The study of a rare autosomal-dominant inherited condition named "familial cutaneomucosal VM," characterized by the appearance of multiple cutaneous and mucosal VMs within two separate families, reveals a genetic linkage to a locus on the short arm of chromosome 9.[4,50] Identical R849W mutations occurred in the region coding for the tyrosine kinase or TIE-2 receptor.[36,56] In addition to this location, later studies have found another Y897S mutation within the TIE-2 gene.[57] Located on the surface of the endothelial cell, TIE-2 is critical to maintaining this multilayer vascular stability between endothelial cells and smooth muscle cells during angiogenesis through activation-inactivation by the angiopoietin (Ang) family of ligands.[44,58–61] Late in angiogenesis (or in nonhypoxic states), Ang-1 produced by the surrounding smooth muscle cell stimulates the TIE-2 receptor on the endothelial cell promoting smooth muscle cell–pericyte proliferation and adherence to the endothelial cells (assembly). Early in angiogenesis (or hypoxemic states) vascular endothelial growth factor leads to the endothelial cell production of Ang-2, which antagonizes the Ang-1 signal on the TIE-2 receptor, leading to loss of endothelial cell perivascular cell adherence (disassembly), which allows for more sprouting.[44,52,62] In animal models of underexpression of Ang-1, overexpression of Ang-2, or absence of the TIE-2 receptor, vasculogenesis proceeds normally; however, disrupted angiogenesis results in disordered vascular assembly.[59,61,62]

During angiogenesis, freshly sprouted endothelial cells induce the surrounding mesenchyme to express platelet-derived growth factor receptor-β. The new endothelial cells secrete platelet-derived growth factor B, which interacts with the mesenchymal receptor leading to smooth muscle proliferation and adherence.[63] The interaction between pericyte and endothelium is also mediated by transforming growth factor-β1 signaling, which is critical for smooth muscle differentiation.

Glomuvenous malformation is an autosomal-dominant inherited subtype of VM resulting in multiple raised purple subcutaneous nodular VMs surrounded by "glomus cells" within the extremities that are painful on palpation.[1,5,44,53] The entity accounts for 5.1% of all VMs and is inherited in 63.8% of cases.[49] A mutation at chromosome 1p21-22 coding for previously unknown protein

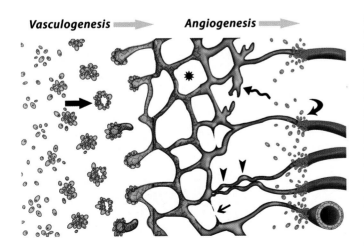

Vasculogenesis ➡ **Angiogenesis** ➡

Fig. 5. Vascular morphogenesis. Vascular morphogenesis is divided into two sequential phases: vasculogenesis followed by angiogenesis. During vasculogenesis mesodermal hemangioblasts form blood islands (*thick arrow*) that cavitate centrally. The outer layer angioblasts form short tubes that coalesce to form the primary capillary plexus (*star*). During angiogenesis, sprouting results in additional capillaries budding from existing capillaries (*spiral arrow*). Nonsprouting occurs as transcapillary pillars cleave or fuse existing vessels (*arrowheads*). Pruning results in the deletion of some vessels of the juvenile network (*thin arrow*). Through maturation, the surrounding mesenchymal cells interact with vascular endothelium to form fully differentiated smooth muscle cells that encapsulate the vessel resulting in a mature multilayered vascular structure (*curved arrow*).

glomulin is thought to be responsible.[64] Based on anti–smooth muscle α-actin staining and electron microscopy, glomus cells are thought to be deranged smooth muscle cells.[65–67] Glomulin is normally thought to control differentiation of smooth muscle cells by competitively inhibiting inhibitors of the transforming growth factor-β1 pathway.[53,68] In the mutated state, this effect is lost, leading to the glomuvenous malformation phenotype.

Klippel-Trénaunay syndrome has recently revealed three chromosomal abnormalities resulting in "increased" angiogenesis.[55,69] Genetic analyses of many other VM-containing syndromes are ongoing.

CLINICAL PRESENTATION AND DIAGNOSIS
The Classic Venous Malformation

The diagnosis of VM and differentiation from other malformations can usually be made purely by clinical history and physical examination. Although all VMs are present at birth,[31] they may not be identified until later in childhood or young adulthood. Usually, the period of greatest enlargement of the lesion occurs from infancy to puberty.[30] Occasionally, the VM may be of insufficient size during the childhood phase of pari passu or commensurate lesional growth and may escape detection. With the end of somatic growth in later adolescence, however, continued linear growth within the malformation often results in clinical manifestations later in life and is typically the case in deeper lesions.[70] Adults presenting with the erroneous label of "acquired" VM on closer questioning often give a history of the formative lesion or related symptoms being present for years to decades earlier.[9] Some have reported accelerated growth because of trauma, hemorrhage, partial resection, or the hormonal influences of pregnancy.[37,71]

Those patients with visible VMs are, as expected, the most common referrals to vascular anomaly centers.[13] These lesions are typically soft, compressible variably blue-tinged masses that can enlarge with dependant positioning and Valsalva.[72] The blue tinge is considered pathognomonic and is caused by the known dilated venous channels within the dermis.[30] The lesions may also possess associated superficial ecchymoses, telangiectasias, or varicosities. Unlike AVMs, there is no hyperemia, increased temperature, pulsatility, or palpable local thrill (Fig. 6).

Forty percent of VMs occur in the head and neck region[37,71] and may involve mucosal surfaces of the tongue, palate and orbital, mandibular, or neck region. Mandibular lesions typically present as a painless slow-growing masses that infiltrate bony structures, dentition, and affect speech and lead to dysphagia. Local infiltration can cause orbital or ocular issues or airway obstruction.[30,73]

VMs occurring in the extremities and trunk make up the remaining 40% and 20% of lesions, respectively,[37] and are usually localized or segmental. Although superficial manifestations may be present, VMs in the extremities often violate surrounding fascial planes and can infiltrate subcutaneous tissue, muscle, bone, joints, neurovascular structures, and even viscera. As such, patients commonly experience symptoms as a result of five related mechanisms. (1) Venous engorgement secondary to dependant positioning, exercise, and after prolonged stasis, such as after morning awakening, frequently results in significant swelling and pain.[37,71] (2) Mass effect may cause local compression or distention of local nerve, fascial, or capsular structures, leading to pain. (3) Local infiltration or mass effect may cause muscular contracture or restricted range of motion of an adjacent joint. (4) Local hemorrhage, or even

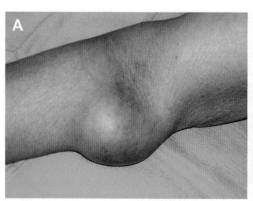
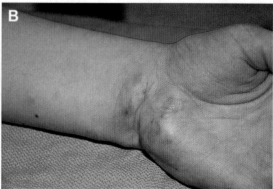

Fig. 6. Clinical appearance of venous malformations. (A) Protuberant subcutaneous VM near the elbow resulting in a mild "blue tinge" on examination. (B) Superficially visible component of a much deeper and diffusely infiltrative VM involving the entire elbow, forearm, and wrist.

hemarthrosis can cause significant pain and impairment. (5) Local stasis on a background of a chronic low-grade localized intravascular coagulopathy thrombophilic state within the lesion[33,74] frequently results in local thrombosis and thrombophlebitis. Interestingly, there is little or no literature concerning the incidence of pulmonary embolism in the setting of untreated nonsyndromic VMs.

Glomuvenous malformations differ slightly in clinical presentation from most VMs in that they are usually more superficial, plaque-like, and demonstrate a rough nodular, papular, or cobblestone appearance sometimes associated with hyperkeratosis. These lesions are less compressible than most VMs, painful with sustained compression, and are less likely to involve deeper structures.[30,49,73]

Syndromes of Containing Venous Malformations

First described in 1900,[75] Klippel-Trénaunay syndrome is currently defined by ISSVA as a combined capillary VM or a combined capillary lymphovenous malformation with associated soft tissue or bony hypertrophy of the affected limb. The entity is only rarely bilateral and involves more than one limb unilaterally in only 10% to 15% of cases. The capillary malformation presents as either a localized well-defined geographic or more diffuse nongeographic cutaneous stain (**Fig. 7**). Geographic stains are usually obvious at birth and may indicate a more significant LM involvement and greater complication rates.[76] They may bleed and may appear vesicular because of LM components. Lymphedema and macrocystic LMs can coexist.[73] Nongeographic stains are less intense colored and predict a slower progression of disease. Venous varicosities develop with age and usually involve the entire limb. Multiple anomalies within the deep venous system including atresias, valvular incompetence, dilatations, and persistent embryonic dorsal veins have been identified.[77–81] Klippel-Trénaunay is complicated by venous stasis phenomena of dermatitis, ulceration, thrombophlebitis, deep venous thrombosis, and pulmonary embolus. LM complications can lead to lymphedema, cellulitis, and skin breakdown and sepsis.

Blue rubber bleb nevus syndrome (or Bean syndrome) is comprised of multiple variably blue-tinged cutaneous VMs that have been likened to a "rubber nipple" in combination with multiple predominantly small bowel VMs. The cutaneous lesions are usually present at birth and increase in number and size throughout childhood and are typically painful to compression. The

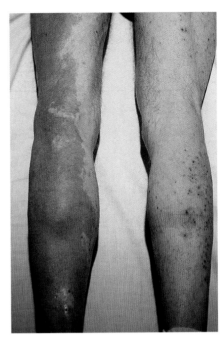

Fig. 7. Clinical appearance of Klippel-Trénaunay syndrome. Posterior view of a large cutaneous stain produced by a capillary malformation involving the left leg in a patient with Klippel-Trénaunay syndrome.

gastrointestinal lesions can bleed and lead to chronic anemia.[82,83]

Several other syndromes are comprised of VMs in whole or in combination with other malformations and are included in table form (**Table 4**).

COMPARATIVE IMAGING DIAGNOSIS OF VENOUS MALFORMATIONS

Although the diagnosis of most cutaneously visible or palpable VMs can be made largely on the basis of clinical history and physical examination, diagnostic imaging is often required for the evaluation of deeper lesions or in the setting of an atypical history to allow differentiation from other malformations or nonmalformation lesions. Imaging may also be performed for confirmation or to alleviate persisting concerns regarding the possibility of malignancy.

Conventional Radiography

Because of limited soft tissue contrast resolution, there is little to be offered by conventional radiography for the evaluation and diagnostic work-up of VMs. Conventional radiography can reveal varying degrees of dystrophic calcification that can commonly occur within VMs and more rarely in LMs.[9] The pathognomonic finding within VMs is the phlebolith caused by thrombosis and calcification

Table 4
Syndromes containing venous malformations

Syndrome	Components				ISSVA Nomenclature	Associations/Comments
	C	V	L	AVM		
Klippel-Trénaunay	●	●	●		CVM, CLVM	Low-flow combined lesion–port-wine stain (capillary malformation), VMs with phleboliths, soft tissue or osseous hypertrophy/limb overgrowth, with possible associated lymphedema or LM
Blue-rubber bleb nevus		●				Multiple VMs of skin and gastrointestinal tract associated with hemorrhage
Familial cutaneomucosal venous malformation		●			VMCM?	Autosomal-dominant inherited TIE-2 mutation resulting in multiple venous malformations in skin and mucosal (but not gastrointestinal) membranes
Maffucci's		●	●			Multiple enchondromas, exostoses, and venous and LMs in association with spindle cell hemangioendotheliomas
Proteus	●	●	●			Cutaneous and subcutaneous nevi, lipomas, hyperpigmentation, and mixed vascular malformations
Gorham-Stout	●	●	●			Focal areas of bone loss and replacement with fibrous tissue (disappearing bone disease) associated with vascular malformations (more lymphatic than venous), usually self limited
Bockenheimer		●				Congenital progressive diffuse phlebectasia of upper more commonly than lower extremities

Abbreviations: AV, arteriovenous; AVM, arteriovenous malformation; C, capillary; ISSVA, International Society for the Study of Vascular Anomalies; L, lymphatic; LM, lymphatic malformation; V, venous; VM, venous malformation.

(**Fig. 8**).[9,13,25,31,37,71,84] When a VM is of sufficient size, mass effect or adjacent bony distortion can be identified. In an early study, 34% of vascular malformations demonstrated some form of bony change.[25] VMs within or near bone can cause hypoplasia, cortical thinning, demineralization, and even osteolysis (the latter being a more common finding in high-flow lesions).[25,71,85] Other than those effects caused by frequent direct mechanical forces on adjacent bone, it has been suggested that bony distortion may be caused by either local environmental changes in oxygen tension and blood flow or by the intrinsic nature of the regional dysmorphogenic process acting on the bone (**Fig. 9**).[85] It is known that venous hypertension and stasis can lead to bony hypertrophy,[86,87] and in the authors' experience cortical thickening

by way of an organized periosteal reaction is the most common finding within soft tissue or juxtaosteal VMs (**Fig. 10**).[9] Overall, bony distortion, hypertrophy, and hypoplasia have been described with VMs and other low-flow lesions with a predilection for lymphatic lesions to cause greater hypertrophy than venous lesions (ie, as in Klippel-Trénaunay syndrome).[25,85,88]

Other ancillary radiographic findings can be identified within VM-containing syndromes. In addition to hemihypertrophy, subtle discrepant phalangeal lengths can be detected and syndactyly, polydactyly, and congenital hip dislocation have been described in Klippel-Trénaunay syndrome.[89]

Plain-film findings of Maffucci's syndrome include the sine qua non finding of multiple enchondromas with associated VMs predisposed to

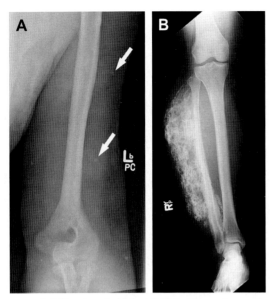

Fig. 8. Calcifications in VMs. (*A*) Plain film radiographs reveal multiple phleboliths (*arrows*) identified within an extensive infiltrative VM of the entire left arm. (*B*) Diffuse dystrophic calcifications and associated fibular bony changes caused by the presence of a large VM within the anterior compartment of the right calf.

phlebolith formation. Dysmorphic bone, shortened long bones, and pathologic fractures can be seen.[90] Because a high percentage of enchondromas can undergo malignant degeneration to chondrosarcoma, clinical and radiographic vigilance is a must (**Fig. 11**).

Gorham-Stout syndrome,[91,92] or disappearing bone disease, is a rare skeletal disorder that is associated with diffuse VMs. The disease is characterized of progressive relentless osteolysis usually within the skull, shoulder, or pelvis that may be preceded by trauma. Intramedullary and subcortical lucent foci coalesce to diminish the diaphyses resulting in tapered ends of the long bone creating a cone-like or "sucked candy" appearance. Bone

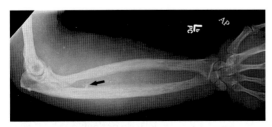

Fig. 9. Dysmorphic bony changes in the presence of VMs. Bowing, thickening, and diffuse alteration in bony texture is identified within a diffuse infiltrative VM. Note is made of multiple phleboliths, some of which are lamellated (*arrow*).

loss can be complete, does not respect joints, and does not regenerate even in the setting of spontaneous remission.[93–95]

Ultrasonography

Ultrasound is usually the first modality used in the imaging work-up of a suspected vascular malformation because it is widely available, low cost, noninvasive, and does not use ionizing radiation. This latter point is particularly important given the relatively young vascular anomaly population.[84,96] Ultrasound is also the modality of choice for image-guided biopsy or intervention of these vascular lesions if clinically indicated. Ultrasound does, however, have the disadvantages of low spatial resolution; a narrow field of view that often does not encompass the entire lesion; and the inability to evaluate deep, osseous, or periosseous pathology.[3] For optimal imaging, a high-frequency linear array transducer of 5 to 10 MHz[37] or even 15 MHz should be used.

It is important to realize that the diagnostic usefulness or goals of ultrasound for vascular malformations is a function of clinical presentation. In the work-up of the typical high-clinical probability for malformation presentation, the focus or goal of the ultrasound examination is to differentiate between a high-flow (AVM) and low-flow lesion, and if the latter, then to decide if the lesion is a VM or a macrocystic or microcystic LM. In the case of the atypical presentation where the clinical probability of malformations is much lower, one must take into account that there is significant overlap of imaging features between vascular malformations and other benign, aggressive, or malignant entities. As a result, one must possess a very low threshold to proceed with additional imaging or biopsy if there are insufficiently specific or equivocal historical or imaging findings confidently to diagnose a malformation.[96,97] The same can be stated for any imaging modality at any point in the work-up of a suspected vascular anomaly.

On gray-scale imaging, VMs nearly always appear heterogeneous (98%). Relative to adjacent tissue, the lesions are usually hypoechoic (82%), but can be hyperechoic (10%) or isoechoic (8%).[98] Tubular anechoic structures representing vascular channels are seen in a minority of cases (4%–50%).[37,98] The pathognomonic phlebolith, as expected, appears as a hyperechoic focus with acoustic shadowing; however, unfortunately this is only detected in 16% of cases.[98] If near the skin surface, the lesions are compressible. On occasion the only sonographic finding is isoechoic skin thickening without discernible mass or vascular channels (**Fig. 12**).[96]

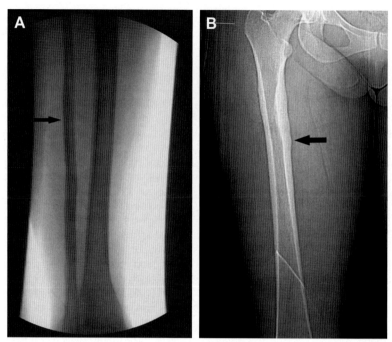

Fig. 10. Alteration in bony cortex in the presence of VMs. (*A*) Diffuse VM in the anterior tibial compartment leading to periosteal/cortical thickening of the fibula (*arrow*). (*B*) Multiple juxtaosteal VMs associated with focal cortical thickening within the medial proximal femur (*arrow*).

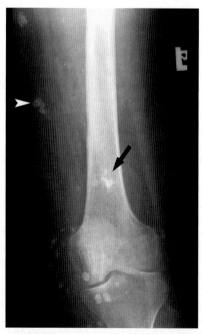

Fig. 11. Maffucci's syndrome. Focal enchondroma (*arrow*) within the distal femur associated with multiple phleboliths (*arrowhead*) in the setting of soft tissue VMs. (*Courtesy of* P. L. Munk, MD, FRCPC, Vancouver, BC.)

Color and pulsed Doppler analysis of the VMs reveal flow in 84% of lesions, with monophasic and biphasic flow seen in 78% and 6%, respectively. Only 16% reveal no discernible flow, which has been proposed may indicate lesion thrombosis or flow below detectible limits (**Fig. 13**).[98]

In the typical suspected malformation presentation, high-flow AVMs can easily be differentiated from VMs, because the former possess enlarged vascular channels with a relative absence of a well-defined soft tissue mass. Color Doppler and spectral analysis identify high vessel density, high systolic flow, and AV shunting.[71] If the diagnosis of VM cannot be confirmed by the presence of phleboliths, they can usually easily be differentiated from macrocystic LMs because the latter typically reveal enlarged anechoic cystic spaces that are separated by thin septa, and may contain dependant debris. The cystic spaces do not reveal Doppler flow; however, the septa or surrounding stroma may possess limited arterial or venous flow (**Fig. 14**).[71,96,98,99] Microcystic LMs can be confused with VMs; however, microcystic lesions tend to be more echogenic because of the high density of reflective interfaces of their many small cystic spaces and usually do not exhibit significant Doppler flow.[71,99]

Klippel-Trénaunay patients demonstrate the expected finding of diffuse lymphovenous malformations affecting the involved extremity. Despite the

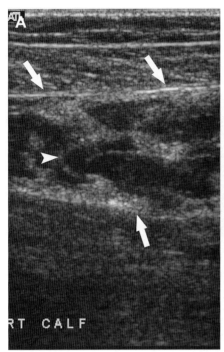

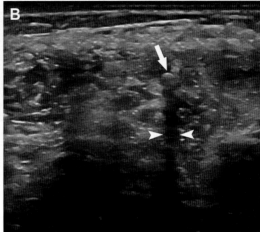

Fig. 12. Ultrasound of VMs. (*A*) Gray scale imaging of a VM reveals its extent (*arrows*) and typical heterogeneous echotexture containing hypoechoic vascular spaces (*arrowhead*). (*B*) Highly reflective phlebolith (*arrow*) within a diffuse VM resulting in acoustic shadowing (*arrowheads*).

theoretic high incidence of deep venous obstructions and atresias, however, ultrasound can demonstrate the presence of a patent deep venous system in many patients (**Fig. 15**).[78,89,100]

Computed Tomography

CT is of limited use in the work-up of most focal VMs because of several factors. CT, even with contrast enhancement, usually provides poor lesion conspicuity relative to adjacent potentially critical structures and does not usually provide

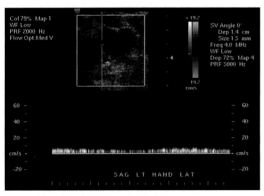

Fig. 13. Doppler ultrasound of VMs. Doppler evaluation of a VM reveals a typical monophasic venous waveform.

assessment of internal malformation vascular architecture, two variables that have significant impact on therapeutic decisions. On noncontrast CT, VMs are usually of low attenuation and appear homogeneous or, as is commonly the case, heterogeneous if infiltrated with adipose tissue.[37] Contrast administration results in a similar pattern of gradual peripheral to central enhancement as is seen in hepatic VMs; however, contrast CT can still underestimate lesion extent.[37,71] CT scan can identify dystrophic calcifications and phleboliths when present, and can be extremely helpful in providing detailed anatomic information regarding adjacent bony pathology if required (**Fig. 16**).[9]

With the introduction of multidetector CT technology, the ability rapidly to perform thinly collimated contrast-enhanced scans over large body segments with subsequent multiplanar reconstructions has provided the opportunity to evaluate very large vascular malformations. Klippel-Trénaunay patients are particularly well suited to this technology given that their lesions are large and the venous structures to be evaluated are of a largely macroscopic "truncular" nature, and consequently are easily resolved when contrast enhanced. Recently described techniques of multidetector CT venography for this subgroup of patients have allowed detection of abnormalities of the superficial and deep venous systems,

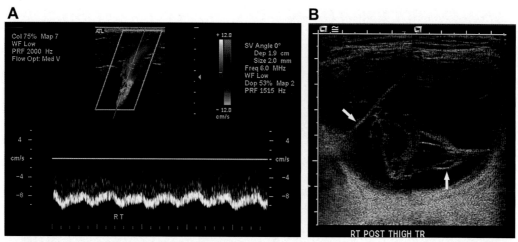

Fig. 14. Comparative ultrasound findings within other vascular malformations. (*A*) Doppler evaluation of an AVM reveals the expected high-flow findings of high amplitude arterial waveform and spectral broadening. (*B*) Typical ultrasound appearance of a macrocystic LM demonstrating large anechoic spaces separated by thin-walled septa (*arrows*).

presence or absence of aberrant lateral or sciatic veins, course of major venous drainage, and the presence or absence of pelvic or abdominal extension of the lesion.[84,100] In addition to being noninvasive, this technique allows for the syndrome's accompanying capillary malformation and limb hypertrophy findings to be evaluated simultaneously in a "one-stop shop" manner. In a recent series of 10 patients, no patient required additional sonography or conventional venography for vascular mapping before planned intervention (**Fig. 17**).[100]

MR Imaging

The introduction of MR imaging has allowed a giant leap forward in the noninvasive assessment of vascular anomalies by providing superior lesion and soft tissue discrimination to CT, semiquantitative flow assessment, and three-dimensional reconstruction, all without subjecting the patient to ionizing radiation.[9,84,101] As a result, MR imaging has become the imaging modality of choice for these lesions.[84,102] Not only can MR imaging influence therapeutic decision making by defining the internal architecture of a malformation and its relationship to adjacent critical structures, but it can also serve an objective method quantitatively to assess therapeutic outcomes through serial MR imaging monitoring of treated lesion size and signal characteristics.[9,37,84,101,102] Recent advances now even use MR imaging for image guidance during percutaneous therapy of vascular malformations.[103–105] The disadvantages of MR imaging are not unique to malformations, because imaging requires a cooperative, nonclaustrophobic patient

and sometimes long scan duration for larger lesions.

The usual basic MR imaging protocol used in the evaluation of a suspected VM should ideally start with an spin-echo or fast spin-echo T1-weighted evaluation of the lesion morphology allowing maximal definition of tissue planes and relationship to critical osseous or neurovascular structures. This should be followed by fat-saturated T2-weighted and T2-weighted short tau inversion recovery sequences, which allow one to define maximal extent of the lesion. T1- and T2-weighted sequences should be performed in at least two planes. The identification of hemosiderin, dystrophic calcification, or phleboliths can be achieved through the use of gradient echo T2*-weighted sequences that can also aid in evaluation of high versus low flow. The study should be completed with pre–gadolinium- and post–gadolinium-enhanced fat-saturated T1-weighted imaging.[9,37,102]

VMs classically appear as either isointense or hypointense[9,13,37,71,102,106,107] on T1-weighted sequences. They may appear more hyperintense,[108] however, particularly if the lesion contains fat.[107] The lesion can appear focal or diffuse, or demonstrate lobulated margins.[102] A more heterogenous appearance can be identified in the setting of hemorrhage or thrombosis, and often dilated or serpiginous vascular structures can be identified compatible with abnormal veins.[37,71] Lower signal areas or signal voids may represent dystrophic calcification or phleboliths on all imaging sequences.[37,101,102,107] T2-weighed or short tau inversion recovery imaging of VMs consistently demonstrate high signal intensity[9,13,37,71,102,106–110]

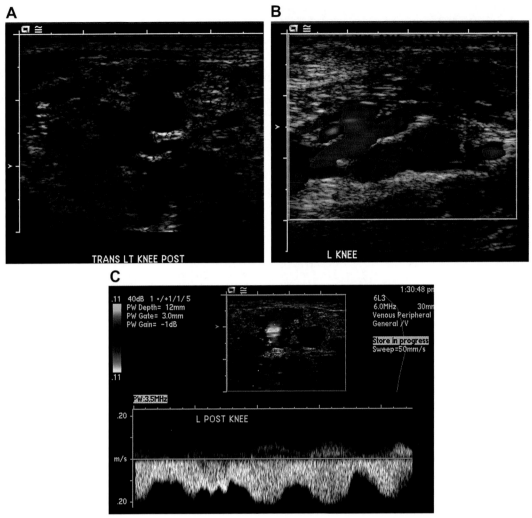

Fig. 15. Ultrasound findings in Klippel-Trénaunay syndrome. (*A*) Multiple dilated anechoic venous collaterals are demonstrated within superficial to deep layers. (*B*) Color Doppler evaluation reveals flow within enlarged vascular spaces. (*C*) Doppler evaluation reveals variable venous flow.

and reveal the fullest extent or infiltration at the margins of the lesion, often more so than that defined on T1-weighted imaging. In addition to calcifications or phleboliths, lower signal areas on T2 can be caused by either vascular channels or fibrofatty septa.[37,107] Gradient echo imaging can demonstrate areas of low signal corresponding to calcification or hemosiderin.[37] Gadolinium administration results in homogenous or heterogenous enhancement within the substance of a VM.[102,109] Gadolinium-enhanced fat-saturated sequences demonstrate the level of vascularity within the lesion and allow clear separation of the lesion from commonly inspissated or perilesional fat (**Figs. 18–20**).[9,37] MR imaging can be used to monitor clinical outcomes after sclerotherapy with successful treatment resulting in reduction

of lesion size.[9,37] Treated portions demonstrate increased heterogeneity, decreased T1 and T2 signal intensity, and decreased enhancement, and if necessary, allows for targeting of specific untreated regions for future therapy (**Fig. 21**).[9,37]

VMs are usually easily differentiated from other vascular malformations based on several criteria. VMs are differentiated from high-flow malformations because the latter have low T1 and T2 signal and signal void among tangles of hypertrophied arteries, turbulent shunts, and engorged venous spaces that are focally higher signal on gradient echo.[71,101,102,108] Very importantly, AVMs characteristically lack a definable mass or soft tissue component quite unlike VMs (**Fig. 22**).[102,111] Only rarely can an AVM demonstrate a pseudomass because of edema, fatty hypertrophy, diffuse

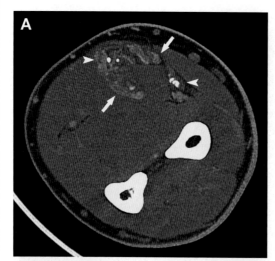

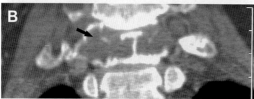

Fig. 16. CT findings in VMs. (*A*) Contrast-enhanced CT scan defines the mass effect and extent (*arrows*) of a VM containing several foci of phleboliths (*arrowheads*). (*B*) CT coronal reconstruction revealing bony infiltration and lysis of C7 (*arrow*) in a patient with Gorham's disease. ([*B*] *Courtesy of* P. L. Munk, MD, FRCPC, Vancouver, BC.)

atrophy, or confinement to a fascial compartment.[9,112] VMs are readily differentiated from macrocystic LMs because the latter reveal large cystic septated spaces that do not enhance with gadolinium.[71,102,108,109,113] Occasionally, the septal walls may enhance causing "rings or arcs" or cyst walls may enhance when inflamed, such as with infection or after sclerotherapy.[102,109] Differentiating VMs from microcystic LMs can prove difficult. Because microcystic lesions consist of innumerable small spaces beyond the resolution of MR imaging, a more homogenous VM-like appearance is seen that may minimally enhance or may not enhance at all (**Fig. 23**).[102,109] Because conventional MR imaging is exquisitely sensitive but not specific for the detection and characterization of vascular malformations,[114] all diagnoses have to be made in the context of clinical history and physical examination. As with any other noninvasive imaging, if MR imaging findings are atypical or suspicious or merely nonspecific, one should consider proceeding to diagnostic phlebography or angiography, or biopsy.[9,37]

Because MR imaging can so exquisitely demonstrate intralesional and extralesional morphologic characteristics relevant to intervention, a number of different classifications schemes of VM morphologies based on different imaging modalities have been proposed (**Table 5**). These MR imaging classification schemes provide a framework for correlation and stratification of lesion morphology of VMs with optimal therapy and outcome. One described strategy[110] categorizes MR imaging grade 1 lesions being less than 5 cm in maximal diameter and demonstrating well-defined margins. MR imaging grade 2 lesions are either greater than 5 cm or have ill-defined margins. MR imaging grade 3 lesions are both greater than 5 cm in diameter and are ill defined (**Fig. 24**). Using this framework, lower-grade lesions correlated with better outcomes to sclerotherapy.

Conventional time-of-flight and phase-contrast techniques of MR imaging angiography faced unique challenges in the evaluation of vascular malformations, particularly with the common VM situation of large deep lesions with very slow flow.[102] These techniques have gradually been supplanted by dynamic contrast-enhanced MR angiographic and venographic techniques that are not flow dependent and result in relatively high temporal and spatial resolution.[102,115,116] These techniques require optimization of bolus administration[102] but allow differentiation of high- and low-flow lesions and can provide information on draining venous anatomy.[114,115,117,118] Whereas conventional MR imaging has 100% sensitivity and 24% to 33% specificity in discriminating venous from non-VMs, adding dynamic contrast MR angiography increases specificity to 95%.[114] Techniques, such as parallel imaging and time-resolved or four-dimensional MR angiograph,[119] have obviated the need for test doses and, together with post–contrast-enhanced conventional imaging, have allowed the acquisition of both morphologic and kinetic information within a malformation.[115] This allows highly sensitive and specific discrimination between high-flow and low-flow malformations and offers a technique of semiquantitatively monitoring outcomes of embolosclerotherapeutic procedures (**Fig. 25**).

Direct Percutaneous Phlebography

Direct percutaneous phlebography, as the name implies, involves direct fine-needle puncture of the lesion and contrast injection under fluoroscopy and is currently used in several distinct scenarios. The study provides the diagnostic gold standard for specificity in situations requiring confirmation of a VM that may be equivocal on previous imaging modalities, or for treatment planning, or to exclude the possibility of neoplasm in cases where biopsy

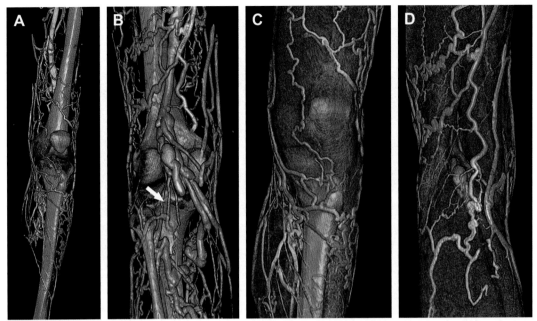

Fig. 17. CT venographic findings in Klippel-Trénaunay syndrome. (*A*) Anterior view revealing diffuse superficial venous collateralization and dilatation in a patient with Klippel-Trénaunay syndrome. (*B*) Posterior magnified view of the popliteal region reveals aplasia or obstruction of the popliteal vein (*arrow*). (*C*) Anterior and (*D*) posterior soft tissue renderings in the same patent demonstrating venous anatomy relative to muscular and other soft tissue planes.

is being contemplated. The technique can also be used in the evaluation of LMs. More commonly, direct percutaneous phlebography is performed as the initial diagnostic evaluation of venous (or lymphatic) malformation morphology and flow characteristics within the sclerotherapy procedure.[9,37] Further discussions of the technique, findings, and therapeutic implications can be found under the section "Image Guided Sclerotherapy of Venous Malformations."

Diagnostic Angiography

In current practice, there is no role for diagnostic angiography in the diagnostic work-up or management of purely low-flow vascular malformations if one follows a prescribed algorithm.[9,120] Unfortunately, patients are still not uncommonly referred to vascular anomaly centers under the erroneous outside diagnosis of "hemangiomas" that have been dutifully evaluated with arteriography and even, on rare occasion, have been previously treated by transarterial embolization. Arteriography may have a role in the specialized work-up of mixed lesions that may have a high-flow component. Historically, arteriography of VMs reveals either no findings, or a delayed mass-associated venous or capillary blush with variable stasis, pooling, or puddling (**Fig. 26**).[9,102] Feeding vessels are

either normal or slightly enlarged and draining veins may be dilated (**Fig. 27**).[25]

Nuclear Medicine

Tc-99m–tagged red blood cell whole-body blood pool scintigraphy is a rarely described technique that uses scintigraphic quantification of systemically administered radiotracer activity within venous or AVMs to evaluate baseline lesion size and change with therapy. Whole-body blood pool scintigraphy can also allow differentiation of venous from LMs.[14,121,122]

Summary: Diagnostic Imaging Algorithm of Vascular Malformations

Because of significant overlap of clinical and imaging findings, entities both within and outside of the domain of vascular malformations, such as sarcomas or inflammatory masses, could masquerade as a VM in the adult. A diagnostic algorithm for the work-up of venous and vascular malformations must allow for these subtle discriminations so as to avoid delayed diagnosis or misdiagnosis. All diagnoses have to be made in the context of clinical history and physical examination. As with any other noninvasive imaging, if imaging findings are atypical, suspicious, or merely nonspecific, one

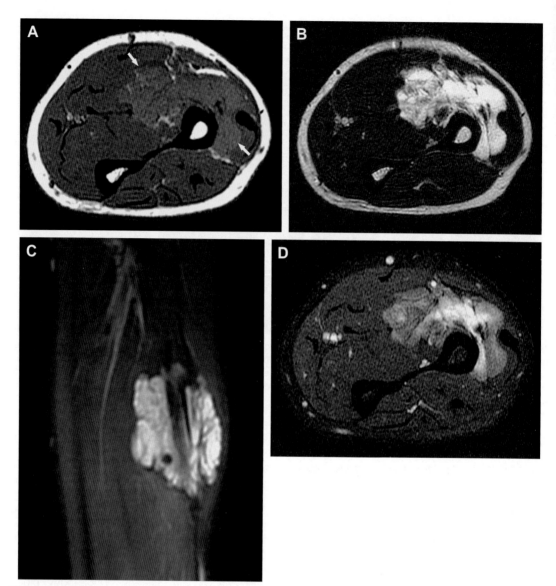

Fig. 18. Typical MR imaging findings in VMs. (*A*) T1-weighted image revealing an isointense VM with the lesion extent (*arrows*) appearing inconspicuous relative to adjacent muscular tissue. (*B*) T2-weighted fast spin echo imaging reveals hyperintense signal within the VM with excellent definition of lesion extent. (*C*) Coronal fast short tau inversion recovery sequence (FSTIR) demonstrates similar lesion characteristic to T2-weighted imaging. (*D*) Gadolinium-enhanced fat-saturated T1-weighted sequence reveals variable heterogenous enhancement of the VM.

should consider proceeding to diagnostic phlebography, angiography, or biopsy (**Fig. 28**).

GENERAL CONCEPTS OF THERAPY FOR VENOUS MALFORMATIONS
The Multidisciplinary Approach

Given the relative rarity, complexity, diagnostic overlap, and variable presentation, prognosis, and evolving treatment within this divergent group of diseases, the patient facing the possible diagnosis of a vascular anomaly requires the attention and input of state-of-the-art services and knowledge that are impossible to achieve and maintain in any one given specialty. This mandate can only be fulfilled by the assembly of an experienced multidisciplinary team of specialists possessing a comfortable working knowledge in the latest diagnostic and therapeutic techniques and controversies within the field of vascular anomalies.[9,12–14,71,101,121,123–125] Based on the patient populations specific to each institution (eg, pediatric, adult, and so forth), the core constituents of this team vary. The team most commonly includes

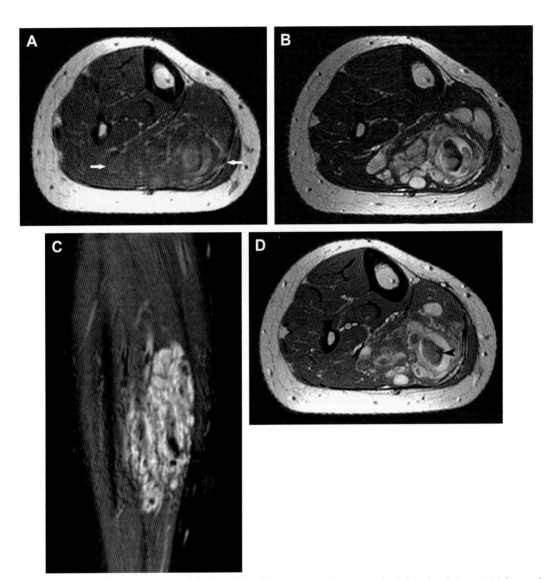

Fig. 19. MR imaging findings in VMs. (*A*) T1-weighted image revealing a poorly defined isointense VM (*arrows*). (*B*) T2-weighted fast spin echo image revealing the full extent and complexity of the lesion's internal architecture. (*C*) FSTIR imaging further defines extent of lesion. (*D*) Gadolinium-enhanced fat-saturated T1-weighted sequence results in luminal enhancement and further definition of an area of organizing thrombus (*arrowhead*) within a larger venous space.

a general, plastic, orthopedic, or head and neck surgeon; dermatologist; internist or pediatrician; radiologist or interventional radiologist; physiotherapist; medical photographer; nurse practitioner; and patient care coordinator.[12,121] Because these patients require multiple investigations and doctor visits, collegiality, speed, and ease of communication and ideas between members is critical to the proper functioning and rapid assessment and triaging of patients.[12] Because outside referrals, although well intentioned, are frequently maldirected, some suggest patient referrals initially be directed to a care coordinator who can more efficiently triage the referral to its appropriate starting point. The care coordinator can also centralize all necessary patient follow-up and provide a common pathway for patients to make direct contact with the system.[12] Because expectations, impressions, and memory can change with time, diligent use of medical photography is essential in maintaining objective assessment on follow-up and is beneficial to both caregivers and the patient and families, particularly within the pediatric group. As with any quaternary medical association, meticulous record keeping, frequent academic interdisciplinary rounds, and

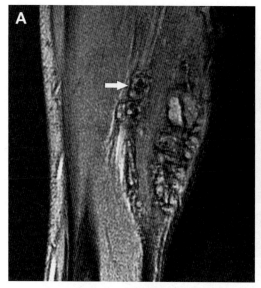
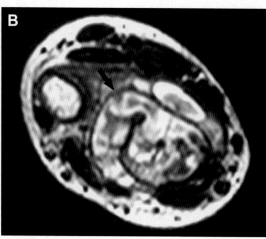

Fig. 20. Other MR imaging findings in VMs. (*A*) Sagittal multiplanar gradient recalled acquisition performed in same patient as in Fig.16A revealing low signal regions corresponding to phleboliths (*arrow*). (*B*) T1-weighted imaged of the distal forearm revealing massive inflammatory infiltration and near complete destruction of the distal radius (*arrow*) in a patient with Gorham's disease. (*Part B courtesy of* P. L. Munk, MD, FRCPC, Vancouver, BC.)

regularly scheduled internal review and assessment by morbidity and mortality rounds are essential for the sustained health of the organization.

Conservative Management of Venous Malformations

The decision to intervene versus conservatively treat the VM patient can be complicated by the fact that they are simultaneously counseled by several medical specialties on a very chronic non–life-threatening medical condition whose symptoms are often temporally highly variable. This underscores the importance of having a unified team that clearly establishes the patient's level, duration, and frequency of symptoms before offering management decisions. Often in the patient with only mild intermittent pain or mass effect, the only significant complaint is that of anxiety regarding the diagnosis, prognosis, and natural history. This can be successfully resolved by reassuring the patient of the lesion's indolent non-neoplastic nature and that intervention can be considered at such time that symptoms warrant.

Patients whose symptoms do not meet the threshold for intervention (see next) or do not wish intervention can be managed with elevation of the involved area during sleep and avoidance of those activities that maximally bring about symptoms. Because some lesions may be hormonally sensitive, cessation of oral contraceptives may provide relief.[126,127] Most (88%) patients have localized intravascular coagulopathy, have low

fibrinogen levels and platelet count, and elevated fibrin degradation products,[33,70] and as a result some advocate all large VM patients undergo a full coagulation profile.[84] Chronic low-grade localized intravascular coagulopathy leads to thrombosis and paroxysmal pain that has been successfully managed with aspirin therapy.[13,37,126] In larger lesions, the thrombophilic profile also predisposes these patients to deep venous thrombosis and even pulmonary embolism; some have advocated prophylactic treatment with low-molecular-weight heparin during high-risk states, such as pregnancy, prolonged bedrest, surgery, and sclerotherapy.[33,70]

Pressure garments or stockings alone or in conjunction with other more active interventions are critical to the successful reduction of symptoms and potentiation of concomitant therapies and should be implemented early and continuously in the patient's course.[13,37,70,128] Elastic garments, when properly fitted, not only slow the progression of venous distention, deformity, ulceration, and pain, but also have been shown to reduce the chronic localized intravascular coagulopathy state.[70] In one series of successfully treated VMs at a major center,[13] 8% had no treatment and 24% had aspirin and compression garments.

Indications for Intervention in Venous Malformations

The decision to treat a VM nonconservatively should only be the result of a consensus within

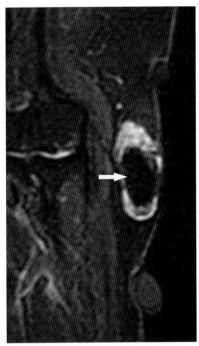

Fig. 21. Changes in VM signal characteristic after sclerotherapy. FSTIR sequence of a VM after two sessions of sclerotherapy reveals marked diminished size and signal intensity within the central treated portions of the lesion (*arrow*).

the multidisciplinary team. One must take into consideration the natural history and expected level of risk related to the VM's size, location, depth, and proximity to other structures relative to the patient's level of morbidity in deciding not only if to

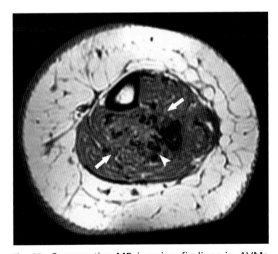

Fig. 22. Comparative MR imaging findings in AVMs. Axial T1-weighted image of a deep calf trifurcation AVM that demonstrates the typical absence of definable mass within the region (*arrows*) and the presence of enlarged high-flow vascular spaces seen as flow voids (*arrowhead*).

treat, but whether treatment should be radiologic, surgical, or both.[14,129] Treatment is generally indicated if the lesion causes pain; functional impairment; or aesthetic problems, as in craniofacial lesions.[37] Because signs and symptoms of VMs may be difficult to quantify objectively, various criteria providing absolute and relative indications for therapy have evolved further to direct management (**Table 6**).[121,123,124] Irrespective of indication, patient status and level of satisfaction must be continuously revisited before each round of intervention is contemplated.

Surgery Versus Interventional Radiology

Lesion morphology, availability of expertise, and patient preference determine whether surgical, interventional radiologic, or combined techniques are used in the treatment of a VM.[9] It should also be noted that there is a distinct subset of VMs that may benefit from laser therapy; however, that discussion is not within the scope of this article. In the initial surgical literature, because sclerotherapy was not considered curative, surgical resection was considered preferable if the lesion could be completely removed so as to avoid recurrence. This includes patients with focal well-defined VMs that are thrombosed, confined to a single or specialized muscle group, or causing a neurologic or compression syndrome, and patients where there is good possibility of anatomic and function restoration.[13,84] Many lesions are infiltrative, however, and involve multiple muscle groups or fascial planes where surgical excision results in an unacceptably high functional and cosmetic deficit.[14,84,126] Sclerotherapy has been increasingly incorporated into surgical regimens and literature and now has been described as either an indispensable adjunct to surgery or the stand-alone therapy of choice for most VMs.[3,30,37,121,123,124] A number of algorithms dictating therapy have evolved.[3,14,28,130–132]

The Hamburg Classification most elegantly provides a framework through which current trends can be observed. Truncular VMs are often geographically more extensive and involve large venous structures with associated venous aneurysms and anomalous veins that require vascular resection and reconstruction to correct hemodynamic factors, and are best treated surgically with or without adjunctive sclerotherapy. Extratruncular, diffuse infiltrating VMs are best treated with sclerotherapy with or without adjunctive surgery. Extratruncular localized VMs are predominantly treated by sclerotherapy; however, they can be treated by either modality based on lesion-specific characteristics.[14,121,123,124,130,133]

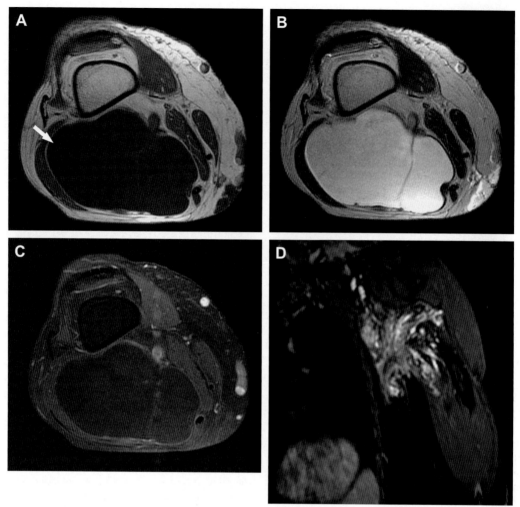

Fig. 23. Comparative MR imaging findings in LMs. (*A*) T1-weighted image of a macrocystic LM demonstrates a large well-defined low-signal cystic space in the popliteal fossa (*arrow*). (*B*) T2-weighted fast spin echo sequence reveals high-signal fluid with septations within the same lesion. (*C*) Gadolinium-enhanced fat-saturated T1-weighted sequence in the same patient reveals characteristic lack of enhancement within the mass but possible enhancement within the cyst wall. (*D*) Coronal FSTIR imaging in a different patient reveals an ill-defined high-signal mass composed of a range of small to imperceptible spaces in a microcystic LM. These findings can be easily confused with the MR imaging appearance of a VM.

IMAGE-GUIDED SCLEROTHERAPY OF VENOUS MALFORMATIONS
Rationale

Within a VM, as in any vascular space, the endothelial cell serves as the "center of operations" controlling the local "milieu" of vascular channel growth and function and maintaining and restoring patency through processes of clearance and recanalization.[134] The continued disordered growth controlled at the endothelial cell level is the factor most responsible for VM symptoms bringing patients to medical attention. It stands to reason that, short of resection, only therapy directed at the endothelial cell level is effective.[134,135] Because

no corrective pharmacologic or genetic endothelial interventions have yet been conceived, only an endothelial-cidal approach can offer the potential to reduce, retard, or eradicate the disease process. The technique of sclerotherapy induces this local endothelial damage by the selective intraluminal delivery of an endothelial-cidal agent or sclerosant into a chosen abnormal intravascular space that then exerts its injurious effect on the endothelial cell by direct contact in a dose-dependant manner.[13,134] Apart from the choice of agent, the therapeutic effect of sclerotherapy on a given endothelial surface is dependant on two major variables: the in vivo sclerosant concentration, and the

Table 5
Image-based classifications and treatment implications based on venous malformation morphology

Author	Image Modality	Category	Anatomic Definition	Implications for Sclerotherapy Alone
Goyal[110]	MR imaging	Grade 1	Well defined ≤5 cm diameter	71% excellent result 29% good result 0% poor result
		Grade 2A	Well defined >5 cm diameter	22% excellent result 44% good result 33% poor result
		Grade 2B	Ill defined ≤5 cm diameter	26% excellent result 15% good result 60% poor result
		Grade 3	Ill defined >5 cm diameter	0% good result 43% good result 57% poor result
Fayad[a],[106]	MR imaging	Extent	Focal Multifocal Diffuse	Require multifocal and additional treatments
		Tissue layer involvement	Skin Subcutaneous Muscle Tendon Bony cortex Marrow	Establishes risk regarding skin or nerve injury Muscular involvement: risk of contracture Bone or marrow involvement: risk of fracture
		Connection	Deep venous system	Increased risk of deep venous thrombosis
Dubois[37]	Phlebography	Cavitary	Cavities with late venous drainage without evidence of abnormal veins	Better results
		Spongy	Small "honeycomb" cavities and late venous drainage	Difficult to treat, especially when intramuscular
		Dysmorphic	Rapid opacification of dysmorphic veins	Better results, prone to recurrence
Dubois[b],[171] Puig[3],[131]	Phlebography	Type I	Isolated, well circumscribed without visible venous drainage	Highest rate of cure or satisfactory result,[171] 92.3% complication-free predictive value[131]
		Type II	Malformation/venous lakes draining into normal veins	High rate of cure or satisfactory result,[171] 93.8% complication-free predictive value[131]
		Type III	Malformation draining into ectatic dysplastic veins	50% exclusion rate, higher risk of complications[3],[131]
		Type IV[c]	Venous ectasia	60% exclusion rate, higher risk of complications[3],[131]

a Modified from Fayad,[106] only data pertaining to venous malformations selected.
b Original data from Dubois[171] classified and enumerated venous malformations as Types 1, 2, and 3. Data herein modified to correspond to Puig.[3],[131]
c Present only in Puig.[3],[131] not Dubois.[171]

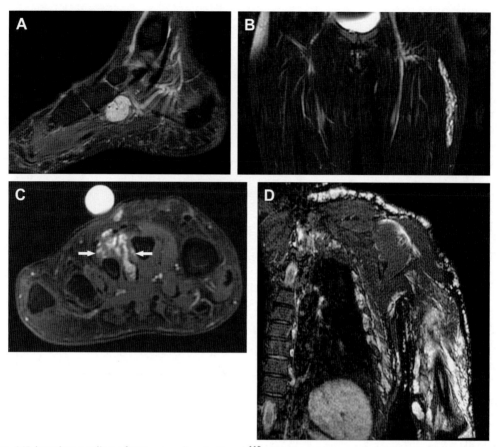

Fig. 24. MR imaging grading of VMs according to Goyal.[110] (*A*) MR imaging grade 1 VM of the foot demonstrating well-defined margins and measuring less than 5 cm diameter. (*B*) MR imaging grade 2A lesion appearing well defined but greater than 5 cm diameter. (*C*) MR imaging grade 2B VM less than 5 cm diameter but exhibiting ill-defined margins (*arrows*) particularly medially. (*D*) MR imaging grade 3 ill-defined lesions extensively involving the upper thorax and arm.

length of time of sclerosant contact with the endothelial layer or "dwell-time."[9,120,136] In vivo concentration is proportional to in vitro concentration, injection rate, and length of time of agent administration and is inversely proportional to volume of distribution within the lesion. Lesion flow rate has an inverse proportional relationship with in vivo concentration and dwell time. The flow rate is fortunately low or negligible within VMs, as seen on Doppler[98]; this variable is of only nominal concern. All of these variables can be manipulated to varying degrees to optimize the therapeutic effect on the vascular endothelium of the lesion while minimizing nontarget trauma to nonmalformation structures within and adjacent to the lesion.

Major Sclerosing Agents

A number of sclerosing agents have been or are currently being used in the treatment of VMs that vary in degree of relative toxicity, viscosity, and complication profile. There are no known retrospective or prospective trials analyzing the therapeutic efficacy or complication rates of the various sclerosants within true VMs.[137] At present, familiarity and availability of the agent and lesion morphology influence the choice of sclerosant for a given patient or lesion.[9]

Ethanol is probably the most widely used sclerosant because it is user-friendly, relatively inexpensive, readily available, and has a long shelf-life.[138,139] As with all sclerosants, ethanol acts through direct contact with the vascular wall causing dehydration of endothelial cells, precipitation of the cytoplasm, followed by sloughing or denuding of this monolayer. The vascular wall fractures to the level of the internal elastic lamina and blood proteins precipitate.[134,140] Given the role of the endothelial cell in angiogenesis and directing removal of thrombus and debris, the elimination of the endothelial cell and its accompanying changes are thought to be responsible, at least by indirect

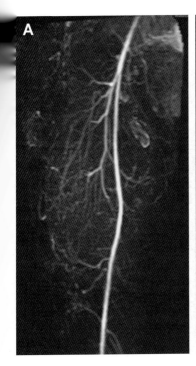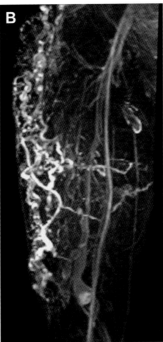

Fig. 25. MR angiography and venography. (*A*) Arteriographic phase in a patient with a VM of the right thigh and buttock reveals no obvious abnormality. (*B*) Venographic phase demonstrating an extensive grade 3 VM with associated deep venous abnormalities.

evidence, for the relative permanence of occlusion and lack of recanalization seen after sclerotherapy with ethanol.[134,140] Although ethanol is clearly a highly if not the single most effective agent in achieving vascular closure, it is also very toxic, with a low therapeutic index or ratio, and must be used with extreme caution.[141] The agent must be given with superselective positioning beyond any reasonable doubt as to the possibility of normal tissue between delivery point and target. Nontarget embolization can occur whereby inflow into interstitial tissue leads to rapid penetration of vascular walls and devitalization of normal tissue.[136,140] As a result, one of the most common major ethanol-related complications is juxtalesional necrosis, particularly skin necrosis, thought to be the result of reflux into superficial venous channels or capillaries during the sclerotherapy procedure.[131] In addition to skin necrosis, other commonly encountered complications encountered during the treatment of venous or vascular malformations with ethanol include nerve impairment or palsy and hemoglobinuria.[135–137,142,143] Administration of intravascular ethanol has been noted to cause precapillary pulmonary arterial vasospasm with increased right heart pressures and right heart failure in rare cases.[140] Sustained pulmonary hypertension has been noted in 30% of patients per ethanol treatment session, but does not seem to have a lasting effect, and does not seem to be correlated with total dose administered. There does not seem to be a tendency for

increased pulmonary reactivity with multistage ethanol therapy.[138] Other rare complications reported are intoxication,[142] bronchospasm,[144] hyperthermia,[145] pulmonary embolus,[135] cardiopulmonary collapse,[146] and death.[147] To reduce the incidence of local and systemic complications, it has been recommended that the administration of ethanol for any given sclerotherapy procedure not exceed 1 mL/kg.[134] In addition to this complication profile, the administration of ethanol is invariably very painful and usually mandates general anesthesia during the procedure.

Sodium tetradecyl sulfate (STS) is an anionic surfactant that appears as a white waxy solid; however, in injectable form, has a soapy consistency and contains 2% benzyl alcohol.[134] STS is much less toxic than ethanol and acts by causing sludging of erythrocytes; thrombosis of the vessel; and obliteration of the vessel by intimal necrosis, adventitial fibrosis, and luminal collapse.[148] This agent has historically been used extensively in the treatment of esophageal varices and varicose veins; however, after reports of nonvariceal use beginning in the 1980s,[149–153] STS has very gradually appeared in the literature for the treatment for VMs.[13,120,137,141,148] STS clearly results in lower rates of skin necrosis, nerve impairment, and systemic complications.[120,148] In higher doses, however, urticaria, anaphylaxis, and hematuria have been reported.[137] This agent has been found to be less effective at permanent closure of vascular structures within high-flow lesions.[134] Similarly,

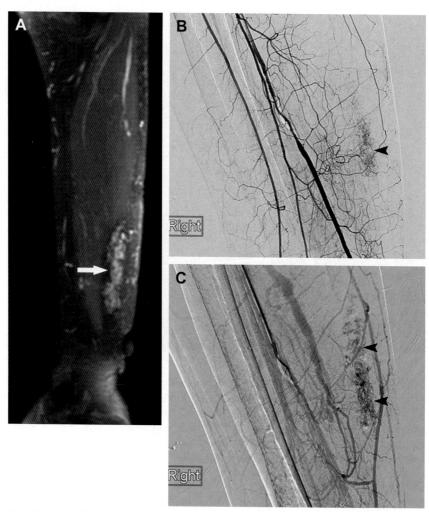

Fig. 26. Typical angiographic findings in VMs. (*A*) Coronal MR image revealing a longitudinally oriented VM of the lower lateral calf (*arrow*). (*B*) Selective tibial digital subtraction angiogram in mid-arterial phase within the same patient reveals a "blush" and contrast pooling and puddling in the lesion (*arrowhead*). (*C*) Angiogram in capillary venous phase reveals further pooling and puddling within the VM (*arrowheads*) and demonstrates some abnormal venous drainage.

within VMs, a lower rate of permanent closure is observed,[13,141] with larger versus smaller venous cavities demonstrating recurrence.[120] Despite these findings, some authors believe that the lower reported complications of STS compared with ethanol make it a more attractive initial option for sclerotherapy of VMs,[120,141] saving ethanol for more resistant lesions.[148]

Polidocanol is an increasingly popular nonionic surfactant that was initially developed as a topical anesthetic in 1936 but was later found to have a vascular sclerosing effect that made it unsuitable for parenteral use.[154,155] Being an anesthetic agent, its intravascular use is virtually painless; however, 1% lidocaine can be added to the agent to ensure minimal pain.[156] Polidocanol consists of

95% hydroxypolyethoxydodecane and 5% ethanol as a preservative, and is available in concentrations ranging from 0.25% to 4%.[154,157,158] This detergent agent acts by causing rapid overhydration of endothelial cells, with consequent vascular injury and closure, and has direct effects on the intrinsic pathway of coagulation.[159] It does not incite as much endothelial damage as ethanol, STS, or ethanolamine oleate.[160] As such, there has been a relatively low rate of reported local complications, such as skin necrosis or nerve impairment; however, they can occur.[154,161] Systemic complications of hemolysis and hemoglobinuria and elevation of D dimers and thrombin-antithrombin III are relatively common[162]; however, more significant events, such as reversible cardiac arrest,

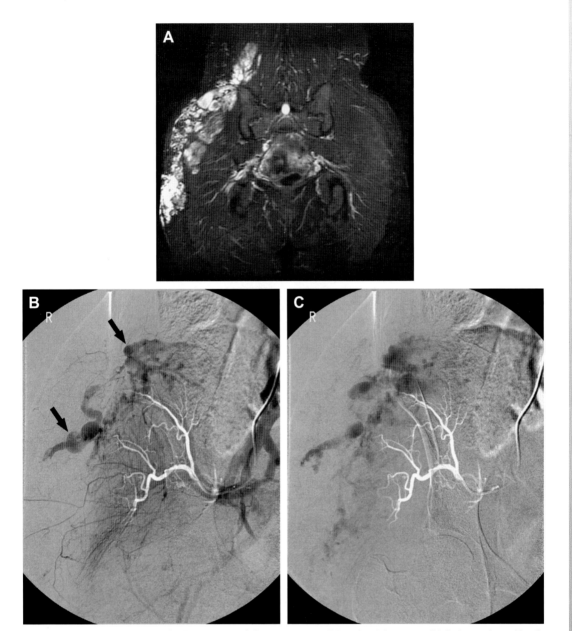

Fig. 27. Additional angiographic findings in VMs. (*A*) Large VM involving the right upper thigh, buttock, and lumbar region. (*B*) Selective superior gluteal digital subtraction arteriogram in late arterial phase with an early arterial phase mask demonstrating early opacification of dilated venous spaces (*arrows*) in the same patient. (*C*) Later venous phase images in the same patient reveal continued transit of contrast, further delineating the extent of the VM.

have been reported.[163] Overall, polidocanol seems to have relatively high efficacy in the treatment of VMs and, combined with its relatively low complication rate, may make this agent the sclerosant of choice.[161] There is a clear need, however, for prospective trials in this regard.[141]

Ethanolamine oleate is a salt of unsaturated fatty acids and, like other sclerosants, has been used previously in the treatment of gastroesophageal varices and works by two simultaneous mechanisms. The oleic portion of this agent induces a dose-related inflammatory response within the intima and penetrates the vascular wall, leading to a dose-related extravascular inflammatory reaction and activating coagulation. The ethanolamine portion suppresses fibrin clot organization. In combination, the agent allows fibrosis and sclerosis to replace the lesion that may progress over time and appear in delayed manner.[164–166] Ethanolamine oleate may have

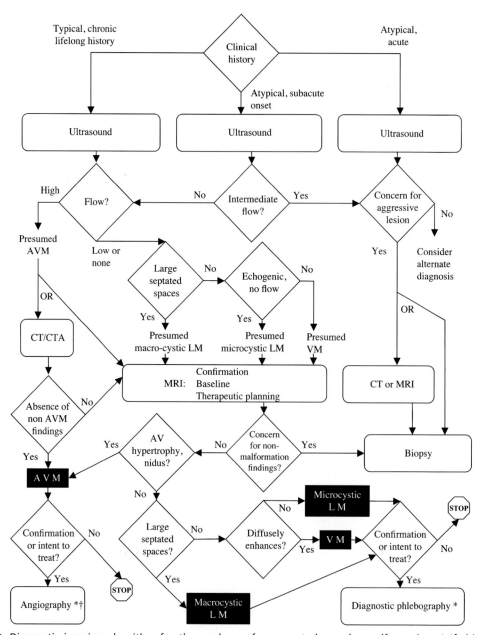

Fig. 28. Diagnostic imaging algorithm for the work-up of a suspected vascular malformation. * If this study does not confirm the suspected diagnosis, biopsy may be indicated. † One may consider performing CT angiography as confirmation or in advance of arteriography for treatment planning if not already performed in the work-up.

less of a penetrative effect beyond the vascular wall, particularly where a nerve runs along the lesion in question, and may have a wider safety margin than ethanol.[167] Ethanolamine oleate has been used in both high-flow[167,168] and low-flow vascular malformations[104,136,165,169] and is thought to have a low incidence of distal embolization.[168] This sclerosant has been known to cause intravascular hemolysis, renal insufficiency, and hepatotoxicity in higher doses, however, and prophylactic haptoglobin administration may be necessary.[101,136,167] To avoid this complication, some have recommended using no more than 1 mL of 5% ethanolamine solution[170] and diluting the solution to 2.5% or 1.25% with the added benefit of less local irritation.[165]

Alcoholic solution of zein is composed of zein solution, sodium amidotrizoate, oleum papaveris,

Table 6
Indications for intervention in venous malformations

Author	Absolute Indications	Relative Indications
Lee[a,123]	Hemorrhage	Disabling pain or discomfort of a progressive nature
	Secondary complications of venous hypertension	Functional disability or impairment affecting daily activity and the quality of life
	Lesion located at life- or limb-threatening region (eg, proximity to the airway)	Cosmetically severe deformity accompanying physical or psychologic disability and negative impact on the quality of life
	Lesions threatening vital functions (eg, seeing, hearing, eating, or breathing)	Vascular-bone syndrome with rapid progress of long bone growth discrepancy accompanied by significant pelvic tilt or compensatory scoliosis
		Lesions located at a region with a high risk of complication (eg, hemarthrosis, deep vein thrombosis)
		Lesions with recurrent infection or sepsis
Tan[141]	Hemorrhage	Nonsevere cosmetic deformity
	Disabling pain necessitating the use of oral analgesia	
	Functional impairment secondary to swelling or pain	
	Tissue loss or ulceration	
	Severe cosmetic deformity	
Dubois[37]	Pain	
	Functional problems	
	Aesthetic problems	

[a] *Data from* Lee BB. New approaches to the treatment of congenital vascular malformations (CMVs): a single center experience. Eur J Vasc Endovasc Surg 2005;30:184–97.

and propylene glycol. The zein solution is made of a water-insoluble prolamine from corn gluten used to form the hard clear shells for coating foods and pharmaceutical products, creating a very viscous solution. Once administered, alcoholic solution of zein requires approximately 10 to 15 minutes to solidify. The agent then remains relatively static in the lesion without passing into venous outflow and is allowed to exert a sustained sclerosant effect leading to necrosis, thrombosis, and fibrosis over the extended dwell time.[171,172] Alcoholic solution of zein is then degraded into amino and glutamic acids over approximately 11 days. Alcoholic solution of zein has been used to good effect within VMs.[171,173–175] The material also has been used in LMs and AVMs.[174,176,177] The disadvantages of alcoholic solution of zein include its relative unavailability, usual need for general anesthesia, and possible delayed extrusion of the embolic material to the skin surface.[171,176] As such it is no longer considered a first-line agent.

Sodium morrhuate is sodium salt of fatty acids in cod liver oil that was originally used to treat arthritic joints and varicose veins as a sclerosant, and has been used within VMs.[137] It has been found, however, to be 1.5 to 4 times less effective than STS.[150]

Historically, many other sclerosing or fixative agents have been used either within VMs or for other pathologic cystic phenomena including hypertonic 50% dextrose, hypertonic saline, acetic acid, methylmethacrylate, triamcinolone, bleomycin, and tetracycline.[178,179]

Patient Preparation

Once the clinical and imaging work-up has been completed, the diagnosis of VM has been made, and the patient has met the institutionally accepted set of criteria or indications for sclerotherapy, treatment should begin with a final in-person office consultation with the radiologist performing the procedure. This office visit should occur in a quiet, relaxed, and undisturbed setting well away from the inherently distracting interruption-prone environment of a typical angiointerventional unit. This visit should include a directed medical history and physical examination supplemented by comparative lesion to normal-side tape-measurements and medical photography of the lesion for baseline assessment. The discussion with the patient should include patient-specific indications, technique, and complications of sclerotherapy; expected level of pain and swelling postprocedure; and the probable need for additional sessions of therapy. Particularly if the visit is the patient's first time being presented with the diagnosis and options of therapy, it is recommended that the patient not make a commitment to proceed with therapy immediately, but rather to "go home and think about it" and notify the interventional radiologist as to their remaining questions or wishes to proceed with or defer therapy. This ensures both parties that the patient, now informed of the benign nature of the disease process, has had sufficient time to be objective about the level and impact on quality of life of their symptoms, and has had time to think about the cost/benefit ratio of therapy. If the informed patient wishes to proceed with therapy, a further visit can be scheduled to obtain informed witnessed consent and pertinent laboratory studies and to make arrangements for preprocedure anesthesia and postprocedure physiotherapy consultations, if deemed necessary.

Direct Percutaneous Phlebography Technique

Direct percutaneous phlebography and sclerotherapy should be performed in an angiography suite equipped with digital angiographic capabilities, real-time ultrasound, and an "in-room" ability to review and correlate with prior MR imaging or angiographic imaging. Except for the rare instance where diagnostic imaging is equivocal for VMs and direct diagnostic phlebography is performed as a purely diagnostic test, the patient usually requires at least conscious sedation and possibly local or regional block or general anesthesia. With increasing use of less toxic sclerosants, some authors use general anesthesia in only a minority of cases,[141,157] whereas some use no sedation in most cases.[161] The patient is then positioned to allow best access to the lesion, and draped and prepared in a sterile fashion leaving all relevant access points to the lesion exposed.

A standard instrument tray is assembled with the addition of clearly labeled syringes or containers of saline, iodinated contrast, and sclerosants. A 20- to 27-gauge needle with short low-volume connector tubing or a butterfly needle is connected to a saline-filled syringe by a three-way stopcock. Whether for purely diagnostic purposes or as a prelude to sclerotherapy, the direct percutaneous phlebogram classically begins with the percutaneous introduction of the needle into the substance of the VM under real-time ultrasound guidance[37,162] with or without fluoroscopic correlation.[180] Occasionally, if very superficial, the lesion can be entered by palpation alone.[141] If sclerotherapy is contemplated in a superficial malformation, it is recommended that the needle be advanced through normal adjacent tissue en route to the lesion to avoid blood loss or extravasation along the tract during and after sclerotherapy.[137] If the lesion is in close proximity to a nerve, a needle approach as far away as possible from the nerve is recommended and, if sclerotherapy is contemplated, intraprocedural nerve monitoring is recommended.[106] As the needle is slowly advanced toward and into the malformation, the syringe is gently and continuously aspirated on, until a flashback of blood is observed signifying intraluminal position of the needle.[9,37,141] Once the flashback is observed, the needle tip is stabilized, and very minimal contrast is gently injected to confirm intraluminal and intralesional positioning. Then, low frame-rate digital subtraction phlebography or venography is performed during gentle contrast injection to confirm the presence or absence of VM and to establish that stable intraluminal access has been achieved (**Fig. 29**).[37,141]

Lesion Morphology: Implications on Technique and Prognosis

Before the injection of sclerosant, certain morphologic characteristics of the VM must be considered. The phlebogram should be evaluated for internal architecture characteristics, flow rate, type of venous drainage, involvement of adjacent structures, and overall volume of contrast distribution relative to the known imaging appearance.[9]

Similar to the MR imaging–based morphology classification schemes developed by Goyal and coworkers[110] and Fayad and coworkers[106] that correlated imaging characteristics to treatment options and outcomes, several phlebography-based morphologic classifications have also been developed to provide a framework on which to base intrasclerotherapeutic technical decisions, postprocedure management, and prediction of outcomes. Dubois and coworkers[37] describe three

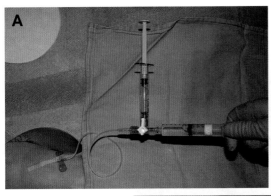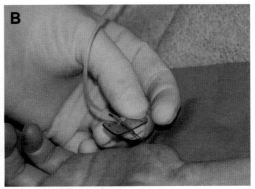

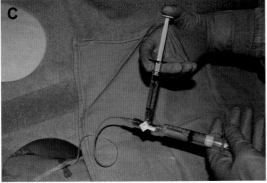

Fig. 29. Diagnostic direct percutaneous phlebography technique. (*A*) Typical three-way stopcock assembly allowing for saline aspiration (*horizontal syringe*) as lesion is entered. (*B*) Flashback of blood created on needle entry into the vascular spaces of the VM. (*C*) Administration of contrast (*vertical syringe*) into the lesion for diagnostic phlebography.

basic phlebographic patterns within VMs. Cavitary pattern lesions are thought to be the most common and demonstrate late venous drainage without evidence of abnormal veins. Spongy pattern VMs consist of multiple "honeycomb" cavities with late venous drainage. Dysmorphic pattern lesions when injected on phlebography rapidly fill dysmorphic veins (**Fig. 30**). The author of this scheme states that better results of sclerotherapy have been observed with cavitary lesions and dysmorphic lesions; however, the latter category is prone to recurrence. Spongy pattern malformations are more difficult to treat, especially if intramuscular.[37]

Dubois and coworkers[171] and Puig and coworkers[3,131] separately further categorize VMs based on their venous drainage pattern into one of three or four categories, respectively. Discussed in a combination, type I VMs demonstrate a well-circumscribed or isolated lesion without visible draining veins. Type II VMs have the body of the lesion drain into normal veins and venous system. Type III lesions drain the malformation by ectatic or dysplastic veins. Type IV VMs[3,131] are comprised entirely of venous ectasia or dysplasia (**Figs. 31 and 32**). The authors of this

classification state that the risk of complications and central or downstream embolization of sclerosant and secondary phlebitis is much greater in type III and IV lesions[131,171] and, as a result, approximately 33% to 60% of patients with this pattern may be excluded from sclerotherapy.[131] All of this information should be incorporated into the decision to continue onto sclerotherapy and whether ancillary maneuvers are necessary (see **Table 5**).

Traditional Sclerotherapy Technique: Administration of Sclerosant

For the period of sclerosant administration, removal of the saline syringe and addition of a second three-way stopcock with dual sclerosant syringes facilitates easy syringe exchanges that do not disturb the often precarious needle position within the canalicular channels of the VM (**Fig. 33**).[137] Once the VM has been adequately opacified with iodinated contrast and note is made of both volume of distribution and rate of flow, the chosen sclerosant is gently injected into the lesion at a corresponding rate and volume that gradually displaces the contrast from the region of the VM being treated

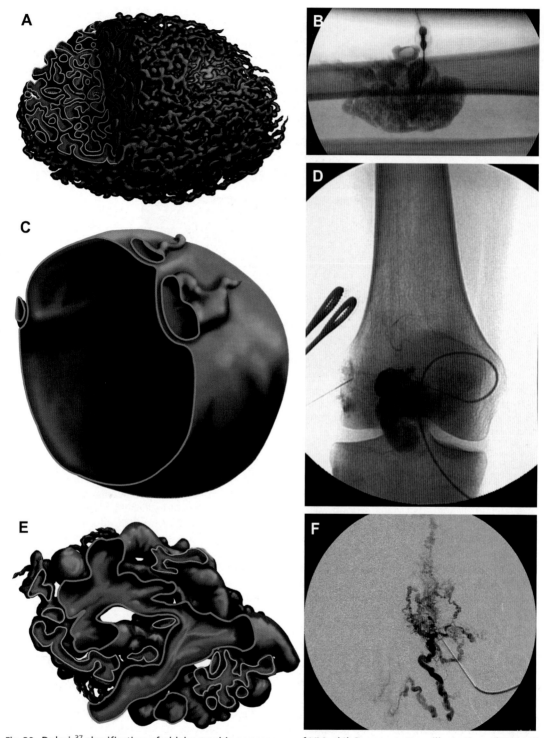

Fig. 30. Dubois[37] classification of phlebographic appearance of VMs. (*A*) Spongy pattern illustration of VM with "honeycomb" cavities and late venous drainage. (*Modified from* Legiehn GM, Heran MK. Classification, diagnosis, and interventional radiologic management of vascular malformations. Orthop Clin North Am 2006;37:435–74; with permission.) (*B*) Spongy pattern on phlebography. (*C*) Cavitary pattern illustration. This pattern is thought to be the most commonly seen in VMs. (*D*) Cavitary pattern VM on phlebography. (*E*) Dysmorphic pattern illustration revealing varying sized dysmorphic veins. (*F*) Phlebography of dysmorphic lesion revealing rapid filling of numerous dysmorphic veins.

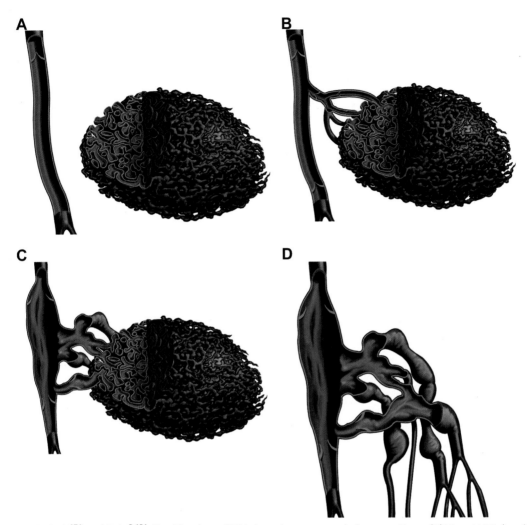

Fig. 31. Dubois[171] and Puig[3,131] Classification of VMs based on venous drainage pattern. (*A*) Type I VM showing negligible venous drainage into normal venous circulation. (*B*) Type II VM anatomy revealing normal venous outflow into general venous circulation. (*C*) Type III anatomy demonstrates drainage from the VM by way of abnormally ectatic or dysplastic veins. (*D*) Type IV lesions are composed entirely of ectatic or dysplastic veins. (*From* Legiehn GM, Heran MK. Classification, diagnosis, and interventional radiologic management of vascular malformations. Orthop Clin North Am 2006;37:435–74; with permission.)

(**Figs. 34 and 35**).[9,137,141] Intermittent aspiration should be performed to ensure a flashback of red blood is present, indicating maintenance of intravascular position and incomplete occlusion of the channel in question.[137] As venospasm and vascular occlusion occur within the regions of the lesion that come into contact with the sclerosant, new pathways or territories may appear. Sclerosant delivery may be continued, or may require additional contrast to define better a new territory before continuing. Careful observation and monitoring is required during sclerosant delivery to assess for extravasation; overly rapid efflux of sclerosant into the venous outflow; resistance to injection; cessation of flashback of red blood; signs of major patient distress; or signs of skin blanching, which

may indicate chemical toxicity or ischemia to the skin. Any one of these findings should prompt immediate cessation of further injection of sclerosant.[110,141,181] If palpable, the operator should observe the degree of induration of the lesion over the course of sclerotherapy[148,182] and limit administration as the lesion becomes firm. The vascular territory defined by phlebography on any given needle pass may only represent a portion of the lesion; repeated comparison should be made with the MR image or ultrasound in deciding if multiple needle placements for sclerotherapy are warranted (**Fig. 36**).[120,141,183] The procedure is terminated once an adequate volume of the VM is treated, if maximum allowable sclerosant dose is reached,[141] or if the presence of intravascular or extravascular

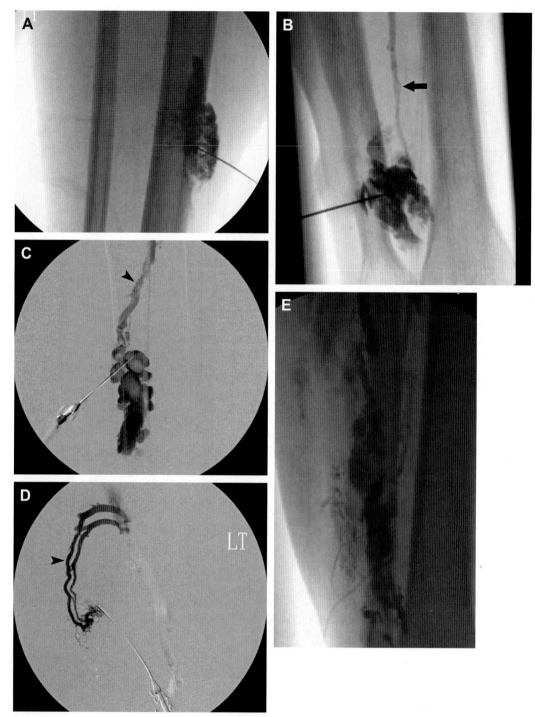

Fig. 32. Phlebographic examples of VMs based on venous drainage pattern. (*A*) Type I VM with no discernible venous drainage. (*B*) Type II lesion within the forearm with drainage by a normal vein (*arrow*). (*C, D*) Type III VMs on digital subtraction phlebography revealing abnormally rapid drainage by abnormally dilated veins (*arrowheads*). (*E*) Type IV VM composed entirely of ectatic and dysplastic veins.

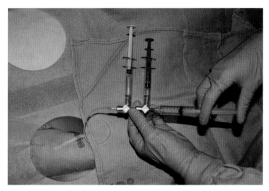

Fig. 33. Initial sclerotherapy technique. After diagnostic phlebography, the saline syringe is removed and replaced with an additional stopcock and dual sclerosant syringes to be administered for sclerotherapy.

contrast obscures visibility of the lesion such that safe intraluminal sclerosant delivery cannot be ensured. The maximum allowable doses for ethanol is 1 mL/kg[134]; however, this dosage is rarely if ever reached. The maximum manufacturer's recommended dose of STS (for varicose veins) is 3 mL of 3% solution; however, some authors recommend a greater maximal allowable dose.[141] Quoted maximal doses for polidocanol (for varicose veins) are 2 mg/kg/d,[163,184,185] or 6 mL of 3% polidocanol solution.[161] Some advocate a maximum of up to 300 mg or 10 mL of 3% polidocanol solution, however, in the treatment of VMs.[157]

Technical Challenges and Modifications to Sclerotherapy Technique

Because all sclerosants are radiolucent, opacifying agents can be added to the sclerosant to facilitate visualization before injection into the lesion. Dilution to any degree, however, can decrease sclerosant effectiveness.[186] Commonly, 3% STS can be diluted with contrast in a 2:1 ratio, allowing visualization while maintaining sufficient sclerosant effect[141]; however ratios of as low as 1:2 have been described.[148] Care must be taken when mixing ethanol with certain contrast agents because some can cause crystallization or precipitation and should not be injected.[187] Ethanol has been mixed with ethiodized oil in a 9:1 ethanol to oil ratio for better visualization and does not precipitate (**Fig. 37**).[183] The resultant admixture does not dilute as with other contrast agents once in the vascular pool but rather remains coalesced into small droplets that can be followed as they migrate through the lesion, with cessation of movement thought to indicate vascular occlusion. The greater viscosity of this mixture also increases dwell time within the lesion and resultant sclerosant effect. In the small volumes of ethiodized oil used, pulmonary oil embolization has not been demonstrated.[183]

An alternate form of fluoroscopic visualization of a sclerosing agent without the addition of iodinated contrast is first to opacify the lesion as per routine. Before adding the sclerosant, a digital roadmap image is then acquired, followed by administration of sclerosant under this "blank" roadmap. The region in which contrast is displaced by sclerosant appears white with the outwardly moving "front" of contrast in the lesion appearing dark. This technique allows accurate assessment of relative volume and degree of filling of the lesion (**Fig. 38**).

MR imaging may offer a new and developing alternative method of real-time image guidance

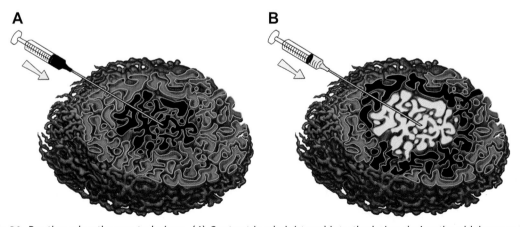

Fig. 34. Routine sclerotherapy technique. (*A*) Contrast is administered into the lesion during the phlebogram to demonstrate volume and distribution within the lesion. (*B*) While under close fluoroscopic observation, radiolucent sclerosant is slowly administered through the same site displacing the contrast peripherally within the lesion. (*Modified from* Legiehn GM, Heran MK. Classification, diagnosis, and interventional radiologic management of vascular malformations. Orthop Clin North Am 2006;37:435–74; with permission.)

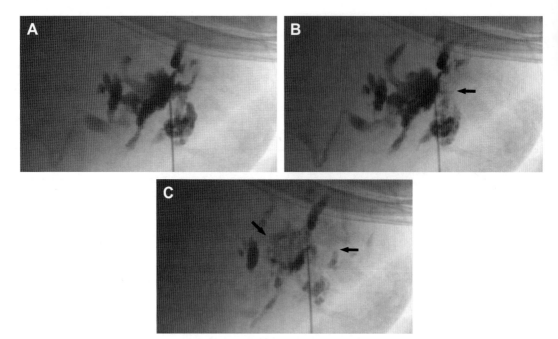

Fig. 35. Phlebographic observations during sclerotherapy. (*A*) Contrast opacified VM on phlebography. (*B*) Initial entry of radiolucent sclerosant displaces contrast from the intraluminal spaces closest to the needle entry site (*arrow*). (*C*) Continued sclerosant administration further displaces contrast from the lesion confirming continued intraluminal delivery of the agent (*arrows*).

for sclerotherapy of VMs. Fast imaging steady-state procession (FISP) MR imaging fluoroscopy has provided safe guidance and monitoring of injection for patients undergoing ethanolamine or STS sclerotherapy with acceptable procedures times, therapeutic outcome, and low complication rates.[104,105] Another method of MR imaging guidance for sclerotherapy begins with the opacification of a VM with dilute gadolinium under FISP MR imaging fluoroscopic control rendering it hyperintense. A gadolinium-sclerosant mixture is then administered under reverse FISP MR imaging

fluoroscopy that can be monitored as the lesion is gradually rendered hypointense.[103]

To enhance visualization and control, tourniquets or pneumatic cuffs (inflated to approximately 60 mm Hg in adults) are commonly placed proximal to the lesion.[9,101,120,141,154,156,183] This has diagnostic benefits of greater distention of the intravascular component of the lesion, greater lesion conspicuity on ultrasound, and greater ease and stability of needle access for phlebography and sclerotherapy. In the case of head and neck lesions, positive end-expiratory

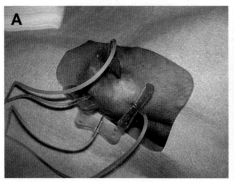
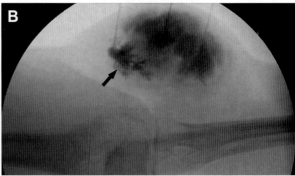

Fig. 36. Multisite access for sclerotherapy. (*A*) Multiple butterfly needles positioned within a VM for sclerotherapy. (*B*) Contrast administration through a third needle site before sclerotherapy reveals an additional region (*arrow*) of the spongy type VM not adequately filled by the previous needle placements.

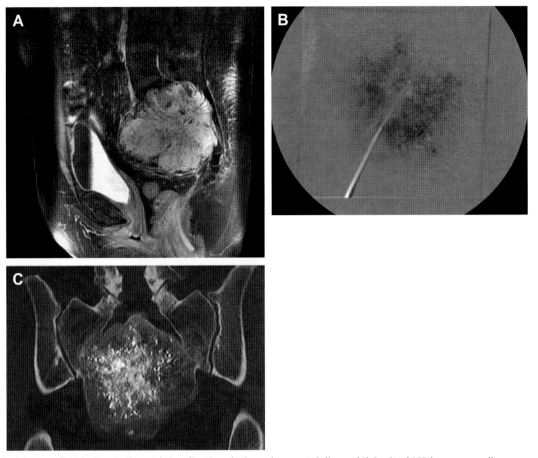

Fig. 37. Use of ethiodized oil to aid visualization during sclerosant delivery. (*A*) Sagittal MR image revealing symptomatic large exophytic intraosseous VM within the sacrum. (*B*) Direct puncture of the VM and administration of Lipiodol ethanol sclerosant admixture. Small radiodense droplets are identified within the sclerosant mixture allowing better detection of distribution and rate of flow during sclerotherapy and also increase viscosity of the solution. (*C*) Coronal CT reconstruction on follow-up reveals presence of Lipiodol within the lesion demarcating treatment zone.

pressure can be used to increase venous pressure and improve filling within the lesion.[148] Overly rapid efflux of contrast (or sclerosant) by draining veins, as is commonly seen in type 3 and 4 VMs, may be prevented or reduced with additional tourniquets, cuffs, or even direct application of manual pressure.[37] This can be accomplished with an instrument applied to the skin over the point of the draining vein as seen on fluoroscopy (**Figs. 39 and 40**).[120] Tourniquets also have the therapeutic benefit of slowing lesion flow and sclerosant transit, thereby increasing dwell time and sclerosant effect; however, they should be used cautiously and sparingly. Overzealous use of tourniquets can result in tissue ischemia, sclerosant extravasation, and sclerosant reflux into the normal capillary or arterial system, sometimes with devastating consequences.

The two most important variables predicting successful sclerotherapy (ie, sclerosant concentration

and dwell time) are inherently optimized in the newly reported techniques of foam sclerotherapy for VMs. Originally conceived in 1944 by Orbach[188], it was not until the 1990s that Cabrera and coworkers[189,190] put forth the use of a therapeutic foam of STS or polidocanol within varicose veins. The rationale of greater efficacy of a given sclerosant in foam versus liquid form is that a foam largely displaces blood from the target vessel, remains undiluted, and persists in the vessel to maximize its sclerosant effect.[154] This greater therapeutic effect has been supported in the recent literature.[191–193] A number of techniques to produce foam were developed; however, the technique first described by Tessari[191] in 2000 has become the dominant method because of its quality of foam, simplicity, and low cost.[154] In this technique, a syringe containing 1 mL of 1% to 3% sclerosant is connected to a syringe containing 4 to 5 mL room air by way of a three-way stopcock. Ten rapid passages

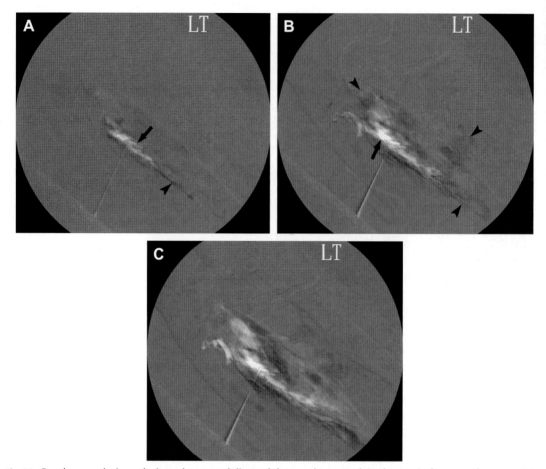

Fig. 38. Roadmap technique during sclerosant delivery. (*A*) A roadmap mask is obtained after opacification of the VM with contrast on phlebography. Initial sclerosant injection displaces contrast, creating a "white" region (*arrow*) corresponding to intraluminal sclerosant. A "front" of contrast is displaced into previously unopacified regions, creating a "dark" appearance on roadmap technique (*arrowhead*). (*B*) Further sclerosant administration results in a larger treatment zone seen as white (*arrow*) with further displacement of contrast outward (*arrowheads*). (*C*) Continued sclerosant delivery results in near complete treatment of the lesion.

through the stopcock are made, the stopcock is maximally narrowed, and a further 10 passages are made (**Fig. 41**). The resulting foam has duration of approximately 3 to 4 minutes[154] and should be administered through as short a catheter system as possible because the silicone in most catheters interferes with the polar molecules maintaining the foam state. Such foams have been identified 30 days after treatment.[154] The first treatment of a VM using a sclerosant in microfoam form was described by Cabrera and coworkers[161] in 2003 and used a range of 0.25% to 4% polidocanol carbon dioxide mixture. Since then, a variety of 3 to 6:1 room air to sclerosant Tessari admixtures using STS or polidocanol have been administered under solely ultrasound guidance for the treatment of VMs.[141,154,158] Administration of the foam results in a highly echogenic appearance distributed within the treated portions of the malformation (**Fig. 42**).[156]

To maximize contact further between sclerosant and endothelial wall and minimize dilutional effects with the blood pool, some authors have advocated aspirating the phlebographic contrast before administering the sclerosant.[186] This is not, however, always possible. Manual compression of a malformation after needle placement to allow expression of blood to lower the intravascular volume and sclerosant dilutional effects has also been described.[137]

A novel double-needle technique has been described by Puig and coworkers[194] whereby a second needle is positioned some distance from the initial sclerotherapy needle. Sclerosant is injected through the first needle and, as intralesional pressure increases, the combination of contrast,

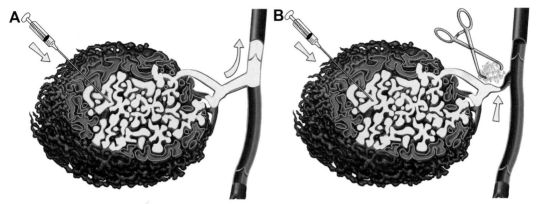

Fig. 39. Maneuvers to decrease venous outflow during sclerotherapy. (*A*) Illustration of rapid passage of sclerosant from the VM into the venous outflow that may result in local or systemic complications. (*B*) Manual compression of the venous outflow (or use of tourniquets) results in maintenance of sclerosant in the lesion with greater dwell time and lower risk of complications. (*Modified from* Legiehn GM, Heran MK. Classification, diagnosis, and interventional radiologic management of vascular malformations. Orthop Clin North Am 2006;37:435–74; with permission.)

blood, and sclerosant transits along the path of least resistance exiting out the second needle. Using this technique, the path and distribution of sclerosant can be closely monitored before exiting the second needle and, as a result, the passage of sclerosant into systemic circulation can be avoided. Equally important, the release or venting of intralesional pressure by the second needle prevents administered sclerosant from reaching an intraluminal pressure that it might otherwise extravasate or flow into adjacent normal vessels causing local tissue damage (**Fig. 43**).[194]

To address concerns regarding local discomfort during the sclerotherapy, 1% lidocaine can be administered into the vascular spaces either prophylactically before sclerosant delivery or at any time during the procedure.[120]

Completing the Sclerotherapy Procedure

Once administration of sclerosant has been completed and the lesion has been treated to the previously described end points, tourniquets or pneumatic cuffs, if used, can be left in place for 2 to 10 minutes to maximize dwell time and sclerosant effect.[141,156,157] The sclerosant needles should be left in situ while the tourniquet or cuff is in position to avoid a significant increase in pressure within the lesion that could lead to extravasation and necrosis.[141] If there is fear of an overly large volume of sclerosant exiting into the general circulation by draining veins on deflation of the tourniquet or cuff, the lesion can be aspirated through the sclerosant needle used to deliver the agent before deflation.[157] If it is suspected that a quantity of sclerosant has entered into the

normal deep venous system, limb elevation and flushing of the system with an intravenous infusion more distally may lessen local injury. After final evaluation of the site by palpation and inspection for signs that may portend skin necrosis, such as blanching, ecchymoses, or retarded capillary refill, the needles can be removed (**Fig. 44**). To allow vascular wall apposition and reduce intralesional volume and dilution effects, compression can be applied to the lesion immediately afterward. Direct compression can be applied merely for several minutes within the procedure room.[150,195] Many advocate some form of sustained compression with a dressing for 24 hours[120,156] to 3 to 7 days,[141,162] however, supplemented with elevation of the involved limb for 24 hours.[120] To commence anti-inflammatory therapy, ketorolac, 10 mg, can be administered parentally in the case room. If a significant quantity of ethanol was used as the sclerosant, some have advocated drawing a serum ethanol level.[195] Immediately before the patient leaves the procedure room, a final examination of cutaneous and vascular integrity of the treated region should be performed and documented, including a perfunctory sensory motor function assessment if possible based on the patient's level of consciousness.

Immediate Postprocedure Management

The course and intensity of observation and medical management of the treated VM patient varies greatly based on the type and quantity of sclerosant used, and the size and location of the lesion. Because there is inevitably pain and swelling within the adequately treated region

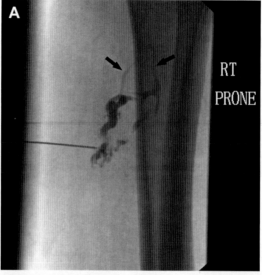

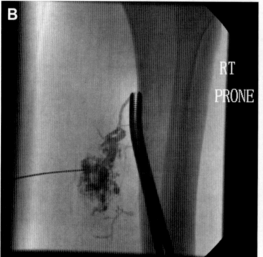
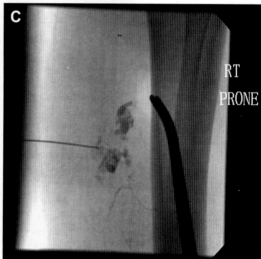

Fig. 40. Use of manual compression during sclerotherapy. (*A*) Phlebogram before sclerotherapy reveals gross underopacification of the VM caused by rapid efflux of contrast though at least two small veins (*arrows*) that enter larger deep veins. (*B*) Compression of venous outflow results in better opacification of lesion and no venous outflow. (*C*) Sclerotherapy can safely proceed, with deopacification of the lesion seen as sclerosant is delivered.

postsclerotherapy,[181] analgesics or anti-inflammatory agents are nearly always necessary. Analgesic agents, whether in hospital or after discharge, can range from acetaminophen, 325 mg, to oxycodone, 5 mg.[105,141] Anti-inflammatory agents, such as ketorolac, 10 mg, or ibuprofen, 400 mg, can be continued while in hospital and the patient can be discharged on ibuprofen, 400 mg.[141] Although steroids are not routinely incorporated into a postprocedure prophylactic anti-inflammatory regimen,[120,141] stronger sclerosants, larger treatment areas, or proximity to vital structures may necessitate their use. A number of authors have suggested steroid use,[37,120,195] with dosages up to 0.1 mg/kg intravenous

dexamethasone for 3 days, then tapered over 5 days for ethanol-treated head and neck lesions.[195] Barring complications, total duration of hospital stay can vary from 6 hours to several days.[156,195] A low-molecular-weight heparin regimen should be considered preprocedure and postprocedure if sclerotherapy is performed in conjunction with surgery.[33,70] Doppler ultrasound of the affected region should be performed if there are concerns regarding deep venous thrombosis during or after hospitalization. Given the propensity for the treated VM to form scar and retract,[125] lesions in critically mobile areas require initiation of some form of physiotherapy regimen that should be arranged before discharge from hospital.[9] Patients

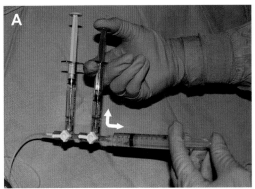
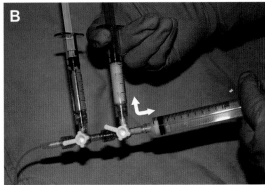

Fig. 41. Tessari technique of foam creation for sclerotherapy. (*A*) Air and sclerosant, most commonly STS or polidocanol, are agitated by repeated rapid passage between two syringes through a stopcock. (*B*) A relatively stable foam is created that has greater surface contact within the malformation when used for sclerotherapy.

must be counseled or reminded of the routine expected levels of swelling and discomfort associated with the recovery period and to have a low threshold to contact the on-call interventional radiology service with any concerns.

Patient Follow-up

The optimal spacing between sclerotherapy sessions, should the lesion require, ranges from 3 weeks to 3 months[37,141,195] and may be preceded by an additional ultrasound examination[156,161] to evaluate the level of flow and regional involution to direct further therapy. Routine ultrasound evaluation of all patients at 1 month can be performed[156] and provides the opportunity to reassess the patient and assess level of satisfaction and need for further therapy. Although some have advocated MR imaging follow-up as early as 1 to 3 months,[157] significant inflammatory changes within the lesion as a result of sclerotherapy need to resolve and involute before management decisions can be based on its findings. Except in very specific circumstances, MR imaging follow-up should occur 6 full months after the last sclerotherapy session.[37] MR imaging evaluation should demonstrate decreased lesion size, decreased T1 and T2 signal intensity, and decreased enhancement in successfully treated regions, and allows for specific targeting of unchanged regions on future sclerotherapy sessions if necessary (**Fig. 45**).[9,37] After the MR imaging, a further in-person patient visit can then be scheduled, preferably in a multidisciplinary setting,

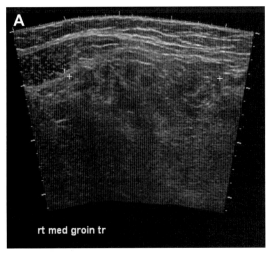
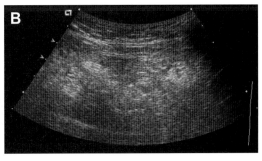

Fig. 42. Sonographic monitoring during foam sclerotherapy. (*A*) Ultrasound before sclerotherapy reveals a predominantly hypoechoic heterogenous mass. (*B*) After the administration of foam sclerosant, the treated regions within the lesion immediately become diffusely hyperechoic.

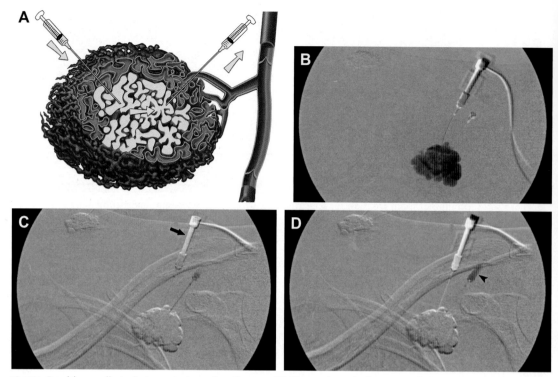

Fig. 43. Double-needle technique during sclerotherapy. (*A*) Illustration of sclerosant administration by one needle and decompression of the lesion by the second venting needle. This lowers the risks of local sclerosant extravasation or systemic embolization. (*Modified from* Legiehn GM, Heran MK. Classification, diagnosis, and interventional radiologic management of vascular malformations. Orthop Clin North Am 2006;37:435–74; with permission.) (*B*) Digital subtraction contrast opacification of a Type I VM through a first needle after placement of a second venting needle. (*C*) After a roadmap mask, sclerosant is administered through the first needle in which contrast is displaced from the hub resulting in a "white" appearance (*arrow*). (*D*) Further sclerosant delivery through the first needle enters the lesion and then displaces contrast within the lesion into the previously unopacified second needle, resulting in a "black" appearance at the second needle hub (*arrowhead*).

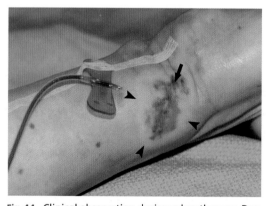

Fig. 44. Clinical observation during sclerotherapy. During and after sclerotherapy, the skin must be closely observed for sign of impending skin ischemia or necrosis, such as bruising or ecchymoses (*arrow*), poor capillary refill, or areas of skin blanching (*arrowheads*). This patient went on to have an uneventful procedure recovery.

where lesion tape-measurements, medical photography, review of imaging, and a discussion of the patient's status and expectations can guide further management if necessary (**Fig. 46**).

Therapeutic Issues Specific to Venous Malformation Syndromes

The management of Klippel-Trénaunay patients is largely noninterventional. Using the CEAP classification and grading system of chronic venous disease of the lower limbs,[196] surgical intervention has been performed on C_3 to C_6 lesions[197] and has consisted of marginal or lateral vein stripping or resection or varicosity avulsions or excision and venous reconstruction or bypass.[130,197] Klippel-Trénaunay patients present a unique therapeutic challenge, having high-volume venous trunks over an extensive area associated with venous incompetence that would normally require prohibitively large volumes of sclerosant with a high probability of major systemic sclerosant

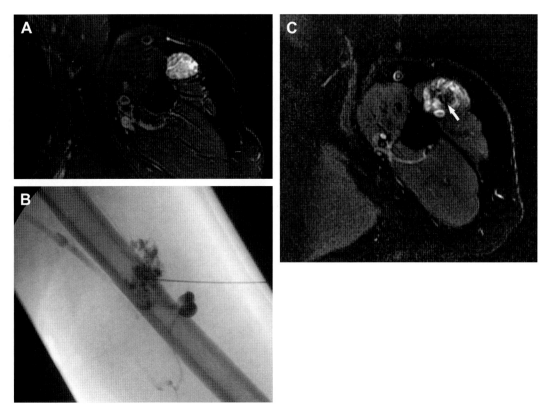

Fig. 45. Imaging follow-up postsclerotherapy with MR imaging. (*A*) Small VM within the deltoid region before sclerotherapy. (*B*) Technically limited sclerotherapy of a portion of the lesion. (*C*) Interval appearance of decreased signal within the central portions of the undertreated VM (*arrow*) that corresponds exactly with the treated portions in (*B*).

embolic complications. Polidocanol foam sclerotherapy for Klippel-Trénaunay syndrome, first described in 2003,[161] was found to be particularly effective in these patients because it greatly increased the effective surface area of sclerosant contact, and while displacing blood, remains undiluted and persists in the vessel.[154,158,161,198] There

are differences in patient selection and basic technique within this population of truncular malformations as opposed to conventional extratruncular lesions previously described. Patients should be evaluated on the basis of their baseline CEAP classification, with C_4 or greater lesions described as candidates for sclerotherapy.[158] Patients should

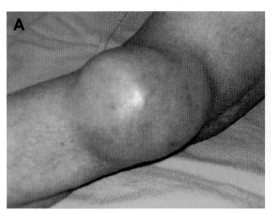
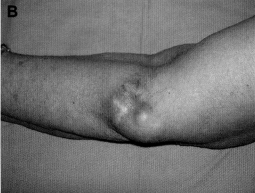

Fig. 46. Clinical follow-up postsclerotherapy. (*A*) Large VM before sclerotherapy. (*B*) Significant reduction in size after two sessions of ethanol sclerotherapy.

be excluded if there is aplasia or obstruction of the deep venous system or if there is a history of deep venous thrombosis.[158] Hematologic evaluation, including plasma fibrinogen level, platelet count, and prothrombin time, can be obtained before and 24 to 48 hours after therapy.[161] Because of the large volume venous channels, 0.25% to 0.5% polidocanol should be used[161]; however, concentrations of up to 4% have been used.[158] A total of 10 to 25 mL of 3:1 air to sclerosant foam and 20 to 80 mL carbon dioxide microfoam has been injected into the anomalous venous channels under continuous sonographic guidance.[158,161] As described generally for all malformation patients by Cabrera and coworkers,[161] after administration of 20 to 25 mL of foam, aspiration is performed to assess level of dilution. Overdilution caused by high capacity or inflow was evident with a red aspirate and remedied with limb elevation or afferent arterial trunk compression. Subsequent injection might on occasion be performed more briskly to displace blood more effectively. Aspiration productive of pink or white solution indicates little or no dilution of sclerosant and a more effective technique. Except for a study where only one to four sessions of therapy were required,[198] a large number of treatment session are often necessary, with nearly all patients receiving from 5 to more than 21 treatments[158,161] at 15- to 30-day intervals.[158,161]

Optimal treatment of glomuvenous malformations is still relatively unknown. Sclerotherapy may be less effective in shrinking glomuvenous malformations than in conventional VMs,[49] and also comparatively less effective at reducing discoloration; it may optimally better serve as an adjunct to surgical treatment rather than as a stand-alone therapy.[199]

Complications of Sclerotherapy

Complications resulting from sclerotherapy of VMs can be classified as minor and major, or local and systemic. Minor local complications include erythema, swelling, pain, and tenderness. Skin blistering can resolve completely or evolve into hyperpigmentation, skin ulceration, and necrosis; however, these complications are still considered to be minor in the literature (**Fig. 47**).[124,141] Major local complications can include transient or permanent nerve impairment or paralysis, thrombophlebitis, deep venous thrombosis, muscular contracture,[106] and compartment syndrome. Major systemic complications of sclerotherapy for VMs, both observed and theoretic, include hemolysis, renal toxicity, pulmonary embolism, ocular disturbances, anaphylactic reactions, hypotension, bradyarrhythmia, and cardiopulmonary collapse.[37] Because most patients undergo multisession therapy, per patient complication rates are always significantly higher than per session rates.

VM morphology can influence type and rate of complications.[9] Types I and II VMs demonstrate a 92.3% and 93.8% positive predictive value of complication-free sclerotherapy.[131] Approximately 50% of type III and IV lesions are not treated because of fear of sequelae of systemic embolization of sclerosant. Superficial lesions have greater risk of skin necrosis by reflux through skin capillaries,[124,137] especially if visibly blue-tinged. Deep intramuscular lesions have a higher rate of contracture posttherapy.[106] MR imaging grade of the lesion does not seem to have value in predicting rate of complications.[110]

Choice of sclerosant is the most important variable in the quoted rates of complications. Ethanol is probably the most commonly used sclerosant in

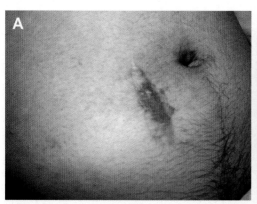
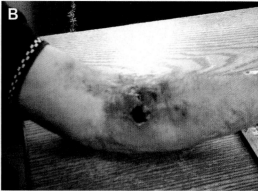

Fig. 47. Complications of sclerotherapy. (*A*) Sclerotherapy of a large diffuse anterior abdominal and flank VM resulting in a focal area of skin blistering and subsequent region of hyperpigmentation (shown here) in a site of previous surgical scar. (*B*) Ulceration and skin necrosis within a treatment region after ethanol sclerotherapy. The lesion completely healed with topical and systemic antibiotics without the need for skin grafting.

the treatment of VMs and, although probably the most efficacious, is clearly associated with the highest rates of complication.[9,141,157] In by far the largest reported series using ethanol in 87 patients over 379 sessions,[124] minor and major complications occurred in 12.4% of sessions and 27.9% of patients. A total of 8.8% of sessions resulted in erythema, blistering, or localized skin or subcutaneous ulceration or necrosis that resolved with conservative management. A total of 1.5% resulted in deeper injury requiring surgical intervention. Transient and permanent nerve injury occurred as a consequence of 0.8% and 0.5% of sessions, respectively. Deep venous thrombosis and pulmonary embolism occurred in 1.25% and 0.25% of sessions, respectively. Minor limited chronic musculoskeletal symptoms occurred in 8% of patients, requiring conservative therapy, whereas 1.1% of patients experienced contracture requiring surgical correction. No evidence of transient pulmonary hypertension was identified in the 379 sessions. Other series using exclusively ethanol as the sclerosant for VMs quote complication rates that are consistent with those mentioned previously.[110,121,128,183,195]

Significantly lower complication rates are observed with STS sclerotherapy compared with ethanol. In the largest series to date using exclusively tetradecyl sulfate foam in 72 patients over 226 sessions,[141] no major complications were observed. Minor complications occurred in 3.1% of sessions and 9.7% of patients. Complications included ulceration or skin necrosis in 2.2% of sessions or 6.9% of patients and either transient sensory deficit or urticaria, each occurring in 0.44% of sessions and 1.4% of patients. Other than venous thrombosis leading to monocular blindness from treatment of a juxtaocular lesion in a single patient,[148] other studies using tetradecyl sulfate have observed comparably low purely minor complication rates ranging from 0% to 14%.[120,148,150]

Even lower complication rates have been observed with polidocanol sclerotherapy of VMs. Pain and marked swelling are the most commonly encountered complications, occurring in 82% and 75% of patients, respectively. A total of 22% of treated patients can exhibit local erythema and induration.[156] Transient hyperpigmentation has been observed in 8% with epidermal necrosis or skin blistering occurring in 0% to 0.7%.[156,157,161,162] Skin necrosis (6%–7% of patients) or inadvertent intra-arterial injection has been observed, resulting in necrosis or nerve impairment (4% of patients).[154,161] Transient limb numbness, hypotension, and bradyarrhythmias,[157] and reversible cardiac arrest,[163] have

been described during the treatment of VMs with polidocanol. Sclerofoam has been observed traversing a patent foramen ovale (that is present in 20%–25% of adults) and may be responsible for rare transient ocular disturbances described in the varicosity literature. No definite right-to-left shunting complications have yet been described, however, during polidocanol foam treatment of VMs.[154]

Ethanolamine oleate therapy results in mild erythema and inflammation in most patients for up to 72 hours with no significant reports of necrosis or nerve impairment.[104,136,165] Similarly, in the largest series using alcoholic solution of zein for sclerotherapy of VMs,[171] pain, swelling at the injection site, and low-grade fever were the most common complications. A total of 5% of patients experienced skin necrosis and focal extrusion of the alcoholic solution of zein contents, however, and 2.6% developed superficial thrombophlebitis. No significant complications have been reported in smaller series.[173,175]

Therapeutic Efficacy of Sclerotherapy

Many clinical and imaging variables enter into the equation of determining degree of therapeutic benefit after sclerotherapy of a VM, making comparison between conservative, surgical, and various interventional radiologic treatment arms difficult. Most studies evaluating efficacy are retrospective and without objective pain scoring systems, which then introduce patient and investigator bias. Clinical outcomes are commonly divided into relatively arbitrary categories, such as excellent, good, fair, poor, or worse, based on reported patient symptoms that may also incorporate imaging based on change in lesion size. Relatively objective prelesion and postlesion size measurements obtained clinically and by imaging, however, are not necessarily well correlated with reduction in malformation-associated symptoms.[141] It is also known that malformation size can be dynamic, and can change with dependent positioning and exercise at times of maximum symptoms and is difficult to assess by static resting state MR imaging. The total number of studies evaluating sclerotherapy of VMs is still relatively small and there are no prospective randomized trials between sclerosants or techniques. There are very few studies that correlate lesion morphology or location with outcome. Because of these issues, it is not surprising that no sclerosant or technique has yet proved itself to be clearly superior.[9]

Despite these shortcomings, certain general trends predicting benefit can be derived based on lesion morphologic characteristics. As previously described by Dubois and coworkers,[37] better results of sclerotherapy have been observed with cavitary lesions and dysmorphic VMs; however, dysmorphic lesions are more prone to recurrence. Spongy pattern malformations are more difficult to treat, especially if intramuscular. With respect to the MR imaging grading system described by Goyal and coworkers,[110] a lower grade was clearly correlated with better response during ethanol sclerotherapy. Within grade 1 lesions, 71% had excellent response and none had a poor response. Grade 2A lesions demonstrated 22% excellent and 33% poor response. Grade 2B lesions had 27% excellent and 60% poor response. Grade 3 lesions revealed a not surprising 0% excellent response and 57% poor response.

Quality of life assessments have been performed in patients undergoing ethanol sclerotherapy compared with matched controls, and have determined that most patients had decreased symptoms and did well posttherapy.[128] Poorest outcomes were in those patients in whom the VM occupied an entire muscle or compartment.

Predictions of recovery period and therapeutic effect after sclerotherapy for VMs have been reported based on the level of swelling postethanol treatment.[181] In patients in whom there was marked swelling posttreatment, 80% had a prolonged recovery period and 100% had marked therapeutic effect. In those without marked swelling, 6% had prolonged recovery and 76% had therapeutic effect.

In the largest of series using purely ethanol sclerotherapy for VMs,[124] 87 patients receiving on average three sessions of therapy over 8.2 months, with an average follow-up of 18.2 months, and greater than 24 months in 72, technical success was observed in 95% of sessions with no evidence of recurrence. Fair to good outcomes as defined earlier[121] were observed in 95.4%, and poor in 4.6%. Other studies using ethanol report good to excellent results in 53% to 100%.[110,128,181,183,195] In the largest series using purely STS sclerotherapy,[141] 72 patients received an average of 3.1 sessions, with an average follow-up of 41 months. A total of 15% of patients became asymptomatic, 28% had a good response, 24% were improved, 28% were unchanged, and 5.6% worsened. Pretherapy and posttherapy MR imaging performed in approximately half the patients revealed the VM had decreased in size in 54%, was unchanged in 31%, and had increased in size in 14%. Size reduction did not seem to correlate with symptomatic improvement. Other studies using STS alone or in conjunction with other therapies demonstrate patient benefit with moderate or excellent results in 68% to 86%.[120,148,150] Clinically significant therapeutic benefit of polidocanol sclerotherapy, as defined in a number of studies, ranges from 78% to 100%.[154,156,157,161,162] Ethanolamine oleate therapy within VMs has produced significant response in 87.5% to 100%.[104,136,165] In the largest series using alcoholic solution of zein,[171] excellent results were present in 74% of patients, with complete cure in 50% of cases. Other smaller alcoholic solution of zein series state complete therapy with sclerotherapy alone in 38% to 100% of patients.[173,175]

Outcomes of Sclerotherapy in Klippel-Trénaunay Syndrome

Reports of efficacy and complications of sclerotherapy in Klippel-Trénaunay patients are largely imbedded in larger series of treatment for venous or vascular malformations as a whole,[137,141,150,154,161,162,198] making overall outcomes more difficult to glean from the literature. In the only dedicated series describing sclerotherapy for Klippel-Trénaunay syndrome,[158] 100% of seven C_4 to C_6 patients experienced improvement in signs and symptoms after 2% to 4% polidocanol foam sclerotherapy with no major complications. Five of seven patients were very satisfied with the cosmetic result. In the largest number of patients treated in any one study,[161] 15 Klippel-Trénaunay patients underwent polidocanol foam sclerotherapy, with most requiring 6 to 20 sessions of therapy. A total of 87% demonstrated good to excellent results, with the remainder demonstrating moderate improvement. No patients became worse. Better outcomes were noted with treatment spaced at 15- versus 30-day intervals. Complications included temporary hyperpigmentation in 13% and skin necrosis in 7%. Other studies using various sclerosants suggest varying degrees of benefit.[137,141,150,154,162,198] A 1% polidocanol treatment in a 5-year-old Klippel-Trénaunay patient resulted in reversible cardiac arrest.[163]

REFERENCES

1. Vikkula M, Boon LM, Mulliken JB. Molecular genetics of vascular malformations. Matrix Biol 2001; 20(5–6):327–35.
2. Eifert S, Villavicencio JL, Kao TC, et al. Prevalence of deep venous anomalies in congenital vascular malformations of venous predominance. J Vasc Surg 2000;31(3):462–71.
3. Puig S, Casati B, Staudenherz A, et al. Vascular low-flow malformations in children: current concepts for classification, diagnosis and therapy. Eur J Radiol 2005;53(1):35–45.

4. Boon LM, Mulliken JB, Vikkula M, et al. Assignment of a locus for dominantly inherited venous malformations to chromosome 9p. Hum Mol Genet 1994;3(9):1583–7.

5. Vikkula M, Boon LM, Mulliken JB. Molecular basis of vascular anomalies. Trends Cardiovasc Med 1998;8:218–92.

6. Brouillard P, Vikkula M. Vascular malformations: localized defects in vascular morphogenesis. Clin Genet 2003;63:340–51.

7. Dowd CF, Cullen SP, Hoffman WY, et al. Radiographic misdiagnosis confounds evaluation of vascular anomalies. Paper presented at: 15th Congress of the International Society for the Study of Vascular Anomalies. Wellington, New Zealand, February 22–25, 2004.

8. Wu JK, Lane TS, Roberts CT, et al. Accuracy in terminology, diagnosis and management for referrals to a vascular anomalies center. Paper presented at: 15th Congress of the International Society for the Study of Vascular Anomalies. Wellington, New Zealand, February 22–25, 2004.

9. Legiehn GM, Heran MK. Classification, diagnosis, and interventional radiologic management of vascular malformations. Orthop Clin North Am 2006; 37(3):435–74, vii–viii.

10. Marler JJ, Mulliken JB. Vascular anomalies: classification, diagnosis, and natural history. Facial Plast Surg Clin North Am 2001;9(4):495–504.

11. Tasnadi G. Epidemiology and etiology of congenital vascular malformations. Semin Vasc Surg 1993;6(4):200–3.

12. Nagy M, Brodsky L. Multidisciplinary approach to management of hemangiomas and vascular malformations. Facial Plast Surg Clin North Am 2001; 9(4):551–9.

13. Hein KD, Mulliken JB, Kozakewich HP, et al. Venous malformations of skeletal muscle. Plast Reconstr Surg 2002;110(7):1625–35.

14. Lee BB, Bergan JJ. Advanced management of congenital vascular malformations: a multidisciplinary approach. Cardiovasc Surg 2002;10(6):523–33.

15. Mulliken JB, Glowacki J. Hemangiomas and vascular malformations in infants and children: a classification based on endothelial characteristics. Plast Reconstr Surg 1982;69:412–20.

16. Fishman SJ, Mulliken JB. Hemangiomas and vascular malformations of infancy and childhood. Pediatr Clin North Am 1993;40(6):1177–200.

17. Virchow R. Angiome. In: Virchow R, editor, Die krankhaften geschwulste, vol. 3. Berlin: August Hirschwald; 1863. p. 306–25.

18. Wegener G. Ueber lymphangiome. Arch Klin Chir 1877;20:641–707.

19. DeTakats G. Vascular anomalies of the extremities. Report of five cases. Surg Gynecol Obstet 1932;55: 227–37.

20. Watson WL. Blood and lymph vessel tumors: a report of 1,056 cases. Surg Gynecol Obstet 1940; 71:569–88.

21. Belov S. Anatomopathological classification of congenital vascular defects. Semin Vasc Surg 1993;6: 219–24.

22. Malan E. Malformations (angiodysplasias). Milan (Italy): Carlo Erba Foundation; 1974.

23. Degni M, Gerson L, Ishikawa K, et al. Classification of the vascular diseases of the limbs. J Cardiovasc Surg (Torino) 1973;14:109–16.

24. Degni M, Gerson L, Ishikava K, et al. [Classification of vascular diseases of the limbs]. Minerva Cardioangiol 1973;21(2):162–7 [in Italian].

25. Burrows PE, Muliken JB, Fellows KE, et al. Childhood hemangiomas and vascular malformations: angiographic differentiation. AJR Am J Roentgenol 1983;141:483–8.

26. Belov S. Classification, terminology and nosology of congenital vascular defects. In: Belov S, Loose DA, Weber J, editors. Vascular malformations. Proceedings of the 7th Meeting of the International Workshop on Vascular Malformations. Reinbek (Germany): Einhorn-Presse Verlag; 1989. p. 25–8.

27. Belov S. Classification of congenital vascular defects. Int Angiol 1990;9:141–6.

28. Jackson IT, Carreno R, Potparic Z, et al. Hemangiomas, vascular malformations, and lymphovenous malformations: classification and methods of treatment. Plast Reconstr Surg 1993;91: 1216–30.

29. Enjolras O. Classification and management of the various superficial vascular anomalies: hemangioma and vascular malformation. J Dermatol 1997; 24:701–10.

30. Garzon MC, Huang JT, Enjolras O, et al. Vascular malformations: part I. J Am Acad Dermatol 2007; 56(3):353–70 [quiz: 371–4].

31. North PE, Mihm MC Jr. Histopathological diagnosis of infantile hemangiomas and vascular malformations. Facial Plast Surg Clin North Am 2001;9(4): 505–24.

32. Kilpatrick SE. Diagnostic musculoskeletal surgical pathology: clinicoradiologic and cytologic correlations. Philadelphia: Saunders; 2004.

33. Mazoyer E, Enjolras O, Laurian C, et al. Coagulation abnormalities associated with extensive venous malformations of the limbs: differentiation from Kasabach-Merritt syndrome. Clin Lab Haematol 2002;24(4):243–51.

34. Clearkin KP, Enzinger FM. Intravascular papillary endothelial hyperplasia. Arch Pathol Lab Med 1976;100(8):441–4.

35. Mulliken JB, Fishman SJ, Burrows PE. Vascular anomalies. Curr Probl Surg 2000;37:519–84.

36. Vikkula M, Boon LM, Carraway KL III, et al. Vascular dysmorphogenesis caused by an activating

mutation in the receptor tyrosine kinase TIE2. Cell 1996;87(7):1181–90.

37. Dubois J, Soulez G, Oliva VL, et al. Soft-tissue venous malformations in adult patients: imaging and therapeutic issues. Radiographics 2001;21(6):1519–31.

38. North PE, Waner M, Mizeracki A, et al. GLUT1: a newly discovered immunohistochemical marker for juvenile hemangiomas. Hum Pathol 2000;31(1):11–22.

39. Adegboyega PA, Qiu S. Hemangioma versus vascular malformation: presence of nerve bundle is a diagnostic clue for vascular malformation. Arch Pathol Lab Med 2005;129(6):772–5.

40. Kahn HJ, Bailey D, Marks A. Monoclonal antibody D2-40, a new marker of lymphatic endothelium, reacts with Kaposi's sarcoma and a subset of angiosarcomas. Mod Pathol 2002;15(4):434–40.

41. Fukunaga M. Expression of D2-40 in lymphatic endothelium of normal tissues and in vascular tumours. Histopathology 2005;46(4):396–402.

42. Galambos C, Nodit L. Identification of lymphatic endothelium in pediatric vascular tumors and malformations. Pediatr Dev Pathol 2005;8(2):181–9.

43. Debelenko LV, Perez-Atayde AR, Mulliken JB, et al. D2-40 immunohistochemical analysis of pediatric vascular tumors reveals positivity in kaposiform hemangioendothelioma. Mod Pathol 2005;18(11):1454–60.

44. Tille JC, Pepper MS. Hereditary vascular anomalies: new insights into their pathogenesis. Arterioscler Thromb Vasc Biol 2004;24(9):1578–90.

45. Moore KL. The developing human. Philadelphia: Saunders; 1982.

46. Luttun A, Carmeliet G, Carmeliet P. Vascular progenitors: from biology to treatment. Trends Cardiovasc Med 2002;12(2):88–96.

47. Risau W. Mechanisms of angiogenesis. Nature 1997;386(6626):671–4.

48. Risau W, Sariola H, Zerwes HG, et al. Vasculogenesis and angiogenesis in embryonic-stem-cell-derived embryoid bodies. Development 1988;102(3):471–8.

49. Boon LM, Mulliken JB, Enjolras O, et al. Glomuvenous malformation (glomangioma) and venous malformation: distinct clinicopathologic and genetic entities. Arch Dermatol 2004;140(8):971–6.

50. Gallione CJ, Pasyk KA, Boon LM, et al. A gene for familial venous malformations maps to chromosome 9p in a second large kindred. J Med Genet 1995;32(3):197–9.

51. Zietz S, Happle R, Hohenleutner U, et al. The venous nevus: a distinct vascular malformation suggesting mosaicism. Dermatology 2008;216(1):31–6.

52. Ramsauer M, D'Amore PA. Getting Tie(2)d up in angiogenesis. J Clin Invest 2002;110(11):1615–7.

53. Brouillard P, Vikkula M. Genetic causes of vascular malformations. Hum Mol Genet 2007;16(Spec No. 2):R140–9.

54. Li LY, Barlow KD, Metheny-Barlow LJ. Angiopoietins and Tie2 in health and disease. Pediatr Endocrinol Rev 2005;2(3):399–408.

55. Wang QK. Update on the molecular genetics of vascular anomalies. Lymphat Res Biol 2005;3(4):226–33.

56. Loughna S, Sato TN. Angiopoietin and Tie signaling pathways in vascular development. Matrix Biol 2001;30:319–25.

57. Calvert JT, Riney TJ, Kontos CD, et al. Allelic and locus heterogeneity in inherited venous malformations. Hum Mol Genet 1999;8(7):1279–89.

58. Davis J, Aldrich TH, Jones PF, et al. Isolation of angiopoietin-1, a ligand for the TIE2 receptor, by secretion-trap expression closing. Cell 1996;87:1161–9.

59. Suri C, Jones PF, Patan S, et al. Requisite role of angiopoietin-1, a ligand for the TIE2 receptor, during embryonic angiogenesis. Cell 1996;87:1171–80.

60. Sato TN, Qin Y, Kozak CA, et al. Tie-1 and tie-2 define another class of putative receptor tyrosine kinase genes expressed in early embryonic vascular system. Proc Natl Acad Sci U S A 1993;90(20):9355–8.

61. Sato TN, Tozawa Y, Deutsch U, et al. Distinct roles of the receptor tyrosine kinases Tie-1 and Tie-2 in blood vessel formation. Nature 1995;376:70–4.

62. Maisonpierre PC, Suri C, Jones PF, et al. Angiopoietin-2, a natural antagonist for Tie2 that disrupts in vivo angiogenesis. Science 1997;277:55–60.

63. Hellstrom M, Kalen M, Lindahl P, et al. Role of PDGF-B and PDGFR-beta in recruitment of vascular smooth muscle cells and pericytes during embryonic blood vessel formation in the mouse. Development 1999;126(14):3047–55.

64. Brouillard P, Boon LM, Mulliken JB, et al. Mutations in a novel factor, glomulin, are responsible for glomuvenous malformations (glomangiomas). Am J Hum Genet 2002;70(4):866–74.

65. Miettinen M, Paal E, Lasota J, et al. Gastrointestinal glomus tumors: a clinicopathologic, immunohistochemical, and molecular genetic study of 32 cases. Am J Surg Pathol 2002;26(3):301–11.

66. Miettinen M, Lehto VP, Virtanen I. Glomus tumor cells: evaluation of smooth muscle and endothelial cell properties. Virchows Arch B Cell Pathol Incl Mol Pathol 1983;43(2):139–49.

67. Dervan PA, Tobbia IN, Casey M, et al. Glomus tumours: an immunohistochemical profile of 11 cases. Histopathology 1989;14(5):483–91.

68. Chen YG, Liu F, Massague J. Mechanism of TGFbeta receptor inhibition by FKBP12. EMBO J 1997;16(13):3866–76.

69. Tian XL, Kadaba R, You SA, et al. Identification of an angiogenic factor that when mutated causes susceptibility to Klippel-Trenaunay syndrome. Nature 2004;427(6975):640–5.

70. Enjolras O, Ciabrini D, Mazoyer E, et al. Extensive pure venous malformations in the upper or lower limb: a review of 27 cases. J Am Acad Dermatol 1997;36(2 Pt 1):219–25.

71. Dubois J, Garel L. Imaging and therapeutic approach of hemangiomas and vascular malformations in the pediatric age group. Pediatr Radiol 1999;29:879–93.

72. Abernethy LJ. Classification and imaging of vascular malformations in children. Eur Radiol 2003; 13(11):2483–97.

73. Redondo P. [Vascular malformations (I). Concept, classification, pathogenesis and clinical features]. Actas Dermosifiliogr 2007;98(3):141–58 [in Spanish].

74. Nicolaides AN, Breddin HK, Carpenter P, et al. Thrombophilia and venous thromboembolism. International consensus statement. Guidelines according to scientific evidence. Int Angiol 2005; 24(1):1–26.

75. Klippel LM, Trenaunay P. Du naevus variqueux ostéohypertrophique. Archives générales de médecine (Paris) 1900;185:641–72.

76. Maari C, Frieden IJ. Klippel-Trenaunay syndrome: the importance of geographic stains in identifying lymphatic disease and risk of complications. J Am Acad Dermatol 2004;51(3):391–8.

77. Muliken JB, Young AE. Vascular birthmarks: hemangiomas and malformations. Philadelphia: WB Saunders; 1988.

78. Servelle M. Klippel and Trenaunay's syndrome: 768 operated cases. Ann Surg 1985;201(3):365–73.

79. Gloviczki P, Hollier LH, Telander RL, et al. Surgical implications of Klippel-Trenaunay syndrome. Ann Surg 1983;197(3):353–62.

80. Gloviczki P, Stanson AW, Stickler GB, et al. Klippel-Trenaunay syndrome: the risks and benefits of vascular interventions. Surgery 1991;110(3): 469–79.

81. Dogan R, Dogan OF, Oc M, et al. A rare vascular malformation, Klippel-Trenaunay syndrome: report of a case with deep vein agenesis and review of the literature. J Cardiovasc Surg (Torino) 2003; 44(1):95–100.

82. Bean WB. Blue rubber bleb nevi of the skin and gastrointestinal tract: vascular spiders and related lesions of the skin. Springfield (IL): Charles Thomas; 1958. p. 178–85.

83. Garzon MC, Huang JT, Enjolras O, et al. Vascular malformations. Part II: associated syndromes. J Am Acad Dermatol 2007;56(4):541–64.

84. Redondo P. [Vascular malformations (II). Diagnosis, pathology and treatment]. Actas Dermosifiliogr 2007;98(4):219–35 [in Spanish].

85. Boyd JB, Mulliken JB, Kaban LB, et al. Skeletal changes associated with vascular malformations. Plast Reconstr Surg 1984;74:789–97.

86. Pearse HE, Morton JJ. The stimulation of bone growth by venous stasis. J Bone Joint Surg Am 1930;12:97–111.

87. Bergula AP, Huang W, Frangos JA. Femoral vein ligation increases bone mass in the hindlimb suspended rat. Bone 1999;24(3):171–7.

88. de Greef C, Flandroy P, Mathurin P, et al. [Low flow venous malformations in children]. Phlebologie 1992;45(4):477–81 [in French].

89. Kanterman RY, Witt PD, Hsieh PS, et al. Klippel-Trenaunay syndrome: imaging findings and percutaneous intervention. AJR Am J Roentgenol 1996; 167(4):989–95.

90. Enjolras O, Wassef M, Merland JJ. [Maffucci syndrome: a false venous malformation? A case with hemangioendothelioma with fusiform cells]. Ann Dermatol Venereol 1998;125(8):512–5 [in French].

91. Jackson JBS. A boneless arm. Boston Med Surg Journal 1838;18:368–9.

92. Gorham LW, Stout AP. Massive osteolysis (acute spontaneous absorption of bone, phantom bone, disappearing bone): its relation to hemangiomatosis. J Bone Joint Surg Am 1955;37-A(5):985–1004.

93. Johnson PM, Mc CJ. Observations on massive osteolysis: a review of the literature and report of a case. Radiology 1958;71(1):28–42.

94. Moller G, Priemel M, Amling M, et al. The Gorham-Stout syndrome (Gorham's massive osteolysis): a report of six cases with histopathological findings. J Bone Joint Surg Br 1999;81(3):501–6.

95. Moller G, Gruber H, Priemel M, et al. [Gorham-Stout idiopathic osteolysis: a local osteoclastic hyperactivity?]. Pathologe 1999;20(3):177–82 [in German].

96. Paltiel HJ, Burrows PE, Kozakewich HP, et al. Soft-tissue vascular anomalies: utility of US for diagnosis. Radiology 2000;214:747–54.

97. Latifi HR, Siegel MJ. Color Doppler flow imaging of pediatric soft tissue masses. J Ultrasound Med 1994;13(3):165–9.

98. Trop I, Dubois J, Guibaud L, et al. Soft-tissue venous malformations in pediatric and young adult patients: diagnosis with Doppler US. Radiology 1999;212:841–5.

99. Sintzoff SA Jr, Gillard I, Van Gansbeke D, et al. Ultrasound evaluation of soft tissue tumors. J Belge Radiol 1992;75(4):276–80.

100. Bastarrika G, Redondo P, Sierra A, et al. New techniques for the evaluation and therapeutic planning of patients with Klippel-Trenaunay syndrome. J Am Acad Dermatol 2007;56(2):242–9.

101. Hyodoh H, Hori M, Akiba H, et al. Peripheral vascular malformations: imaging, treatment approaches, and therapeutic issues. Radiographics 2005; 25(25):S159–71.

102. Konez O, Burrows PE. Magnetic resonance of vascular anomalies. Magn Reson Imaging Clin N Am 2002;10(2):363–88, vii.

103. Hayashi N, Masumoto T, Okubo T, et al. Hemangiomas in the face and extremities: MR-guided sclerotherapy: optimization with monitoring of signal intensity changes in vivo. Radiology 2003;226(2):567–72.

104. Lewin JS, Merkle EM, Duerk JL, et al. MR imaging-guided percutaneous sclerotherapy: preliminary experience with 14 procedures in three patients. Radiology 1999;211(2):566–70.

105. Boll DT, Merkle EM, Lewin JS. Low-flow vascular malformations: MR-guided percutaneous sclerotherapy in qualitative and quantitative assessment of therapy and outcome. Radiology 2004;233:376–84.

106. Fayad LM, Hazirolan T, Bluemke D, et al. Vascular malformations in the extremities: emphasis on MR imaging features that guide treatment options. Skeletal Radiol 2006;35(3):127–37.

107. Vilanova JC, Barceló J, Smirniotopoulos JG, et al. Hemangioma from head to toe: MR imaging with pathologic correlation. Radiographics 2004;24:367–85.

108. Meyer JS, Hoffer FA, Barnes PD, et al. Biological classification of soft tissue vascular anomalies: MR correlation. AJR Am J Roentgenol 1991;157:559–64.

109. Konez O. Vascular anomalies. emedicine.com. Modified March 23, 2007. Available at: www.emedicine.com/radio/topic896.htm. Accessed May 13, 2008.

110. Goyal M, Causer PA, Armstrong D. Venous vascular malformations in pediatric patients: comparison of results of alcohol sclerotherapy with proposed MR imaging classification. Radiology 2002;223(3):639–44.

111. Burrows PE, Laor T, Paltiel H, et al. Diagnostic imaging in the evaluation of vascular birthmarks. Dermatol Clin 1998;16(3):455–88.

112. Robertson RL, Robson CD, Barnes PD, et al. Head and neck vascular anomalies of childhood. Neuroimaging Clin N Am 1999;9(1):115–32.

113. Kern S, Niemeyer C, Darge K, et al. Differentiation of vascular birthmarks by MR imaging. Acta Radiol 2000;41:453–7.

114. van Rijswijk CS, van der Linden E, van der Woude HJ, et al. Value of dynamic contrast-enhanced MR imaging in diagnosing and classifying peripheral vascular malformations. AJR Am J Roentgenol 2002;178(5):1181–7.

115. Stepansky F, Hecht EM, Rivera R, et al. Dynamic MR angiography of upper extremity vascular disease: pictorial review. Radiographics 2008;28(1):e28.

116. Polak JF, Fox LA. MR assessment of the extremity veins. Semin Ultrasound CT MR 1999;20(1):36–46.

117. Herborn CU, Goyen M, Lauenstein TC, et al. Comprehensive time-resolved MRI of peripheral vascular malformations. AJR Am J Roentgenol 2003;181(3):729–35.

118. Ohgiya Y, Hashimoto T, Gokan T, et al. Dynamic MRI for distinguishing high-flow from low-flow peripheral vascular malformations. AJR Am J Roentgenol 2005;185(5):1131–7.

119. Korosec FR, Frayne R, Grist TM, et al. Time-resolved contrast-enhanced 3D MR angiography. Magn Reson Med 1996;36(3):345–51.

120. O'Donovan JC, Donaldson JS, Morello FP, et al. Symptomatic hemangiomas and venous malformations in infants, children and young adults: treatment with percutaneous injection of sodium tetradecyl sulfate. AJR Am J Roentgenol 1997;169(3):723–9.

121. Lee BB, Kim DI, Huh S, et al. New experiences with absolute ethanol sclerotherapy in the management of a complex form of congenital venous malformation. J Vasc Surg 2001;33(4):764–72.

122. Lee BB, Kim YW, Seo JM, et al. Current concepts in lymphatic malformation. Vasc Endovascular Surg 2005;39(1):67–81.

123. Lee BB. New approaches to the treatment of congenital vascular malformations (CMVs): a single centre experience. Eur J Vasc Endovasc Surg 2005;30(2):184–97.

124. Lee BB, Do YS, Byun HS, et al. Advanced management of venous malformation with ethanol scherotherapy: mid-term results. J Vasc Surg 2003;37(3):533–8.

125. Donnelly LF, Adams DM, Bisset GS III. Vascular malformations and hemangiomas: a practical approach in a multidisciplinary clinic. AJR Am J Roentgenol 2000;174(3):597–608.

126. Buckmiller LM. Update on hemangiomas and vascular malformations. Curr Opin Otolaryngol Head Neck Surg 2004;12(6):476–87.

127. Rinker B, Karp NS, Margiotta M, et al. The role of magnetic resonance imaging in the management of vascular malformations of the trunk and extremities. Plast Reconstr Surg 2003;112(2):504–10.

128. Rautio R, Saarinen J, Laranne J, et al. Endovascular treatment of venous malformations in extremities: results of sclerotherapy and the quality of life after treatment. Acta Radiol 2004;45(4):397–403.

129. Villavicencio JL. Primum non nocere: is it always true? The use of absolute ethanol in the management of congenital vascular malformations. J Vasc Surg 2001;33(4):904–6.

130. Lee BB. New approach to the combined form of congenital vascular malformation: venolymphatic malformation. Presented at the Eastern Vascular Society 18th Annual Meeting. Pittsburgh (PA), May 5–7, 2005.

131. Puig S, Aref H, Chigot V, et al. Classification of venous malformations in children and implications for sclerotherapy. Pediatr Radiol 2003;33(2):99–103.

132. Upton J, Coombs CJ, Mulliken JB, et al. Vascular malformations of the upper limb: a review of 270 patients. J Hand Surg [Am] 1999;24:1019–35.

133. Lee BB, Do YS, Yakes W, et al. Management of arteriovenous malformations: a multidisciplinary approach. J Vasc Surg 2004;39(3):590–600.

134. Yakes WF, Rossi P, Odink H. How I do it. Arteriovenous malformation management. Cardiovasc Intervent Radiol 1996;19(2):65–71.

135. Do YS, Yakes WF, Shin SW, et al. Ethanol embolization of arteriovenous malformations: interim results. Radiology 2005;235(2):674–82.

136. Choi YH, Han MH, O-Ki K, et al. Craniofacial cavernous venous malformations: percutaneous sclerotherapy with use of ethanolamine oleate. J Vasc Interv Radiol 2002;13(5):475–82.

137. de Lorimier AA. Sclerotherapy for venous malformations. J Pediatr Surg 1995;30(2):188–93.

138. Shin BS, Do YS, Lee BB, et al. Multistage ethanol sclerotherapy of soft-tissue arteriovenous malformations: effect on pulmonary arterial pressure. Radiology 2005;235(3):1072–7.

139. Yakes WF, Haas DK, Parker SH, et al. Symptomatic vascular malformations: ethanol embolotherapy. Radiology 1989;170(3 Pt 2):1059–66.

140. Yakes WF, Krauth L, Ecklung J, et al. Ethanol endovascular management of brain arteriovenous malformations: initial results. Neurosurgery 1997;40(6):1145–52.

141. Tan KT, Kirby J, Rajan DK, et al. Percutaneous sodium tetradecyl sulfate sclerotherapy for peripheral venous vascular malformations: a single-center experience. J Vasc Interv Radiol 2007;18(3):343–51.

142. Mason KP, Michna E, Zurakowski D, et al. Serum ethanol levels in children and adults after ethanol embolization or sclerotherapy for vascular anomalies. Radiology 2000;217(1):127–32.

143. Yakes WF, Luethke JM, Parker SH, et al. Ethanol embolization of vascular malformations. Radiographics 1990;10(5):787–96.

144. Stefanutto TB, Halbach V. Bronchospasm precipitated by ethanol injection in arteriovenous malformation. AJNR Am J Neuroradiol 2003;24(10):2050–1.

145. Behnia R. Systemic effects of absolute alcohol embolization in a patient with a congenital arteriovenous malformation of the lower extremity. Anesth Analg 1995;80(2):415–7.

146. Yakes WF, Baker R. Cardiopulmonary collapse: sequelae of ethanol embolotherapy [abstract]. Radiology 1993;189(P):145.

147. Garel L, Mareschal JL, Gagnadoux MF, et al. Fatal outcome after ethanol renal ablation in child with end-stage kidneys. AJR Am J Roentgenol 1986;146:593–4.

148. Siniluoto TM, Svendsen PA, Wikholm GM, et al. Percutaneous sclerotherapy of venous malformations of the head and neck using sodium tetradecyl sulphate (sotradecol). Scand J Plast Reconstr Surg Hand Surg 1997;31(2):145–50.

149. Anavi Y, Har-El G, Mintz S. The treatment of facial haemangioma by percutaneous injections of sodium tetradecyl sulfate. J Laryngol Otol 1988;102(1):87–90.

150. Woods JE. Extended use of sodium tetradecyl sulfate in treatment of hemangiomas and other related conditions. Plast Reconstr Surg 1987;79(4):542–9.

151. Govrin-Yehudain J, Moscona AR, Calderon N, et al. Treatment of hemangiomas by sclerosing agents: an experimental and clinical study. Ann Plast Surg 1987;18(6):465–9.

152. Baurmash H, DeChiara S. A conservative approach to the management of orofacial vascular lesions in infants and children: report of cases. J Oral Maxillofac Surg 1991;49(11):1222–5.

153. Cho KJ, Williams DM, Brady TM, et al. Transcatheter embolization with sodium tetradecyl sulfate: experimental and clinical results. Radiology 1984;153(1):95–9.

154. Pascarella L, Bergan JJ, Yamada C, et al. Venous angiomata: treatment with sclerosant foam. Ann Vasc Surg 2005;19:457–64.

155. Guex JJ. Indications for the sclerosing agent polidocanol (aetoxisclerol dexo, aethoxisklerol kreussler). J Dermatol Surg Oncol 1994;19(10):959–61.

156. Jain R, Bandhu S, Sawhney S, et al. Sonographically guided percutaneous sclerosis using 1% polidocanol in the treatment of vascular malformations. J Clin Ultrasound 2002;30(7):416–23.

157. Mimura H, Kanazawa S, Yasui K, et al. Percutaneous sclerotherapy for venous malformations using polidocanol under fluoroscopy. Acta Med Okayama 2003;57(5):227–34.

158. Nitecki S, Bass A. Ultrasound-guided foam sclerotherapy in patients with Klippel-Trenaunay syndrome. Isr Med Assoc J 2007;9(2):72–5.

159. Cacciola E, Giustolisi R, Musso R, et al. Activation of contact phase of blood coagulation can be induced by the sclerosing agent polidocanol: possible additional mechanism of adverse reaction during sclerotherapy. J Lab Clin Med 1987;109(2):225–6.

160. Suzuki N, Nakao A, Nonami T, et al. Experimental study on the effects of sclerosants foresophageal varices on blood coagulation, fibrinolysis and systemic hemodynamics. Gastroenterol Jpn 1992;27(3):309–16.

161. Cabrera J, Cabrera JJ, Garcia-Olmedo MA, et al. Treatment of venous malformations with sclerosant in microfoam form. Arch Dermatol 2003;139(11):1409–16.

162. Yamaki T, Nozaki M, Sasaki K. Color duplex-guided sclerotherapy for the treatment of venous malformations. Dermatol Surg 2000;26(4):323–8.

163. Marrocco-Trischitta MM, Guerrini P, Abeni D, et al. Reversible cardiac arrest after polidocanol sclerotherapy of peripheral venous malformation. Dermatol Surg 2002;28(2):153–5.

164. Ethamolin, clinical pharmacology. Available at: http://www.rxlist.com/cgi/generic/ethamolin_cp.htm. Accessed February 2, 2008.

165. Johann AC, Aguiar MC, do Carmo MA, et al. Sclerotherapy of benign oral vascular lesion with ethanolamine oleate: an open clinical trial with 30 lesions. Oral Surg Oral Med Oral Pathol Oral Radiol Endod 2005;100(5):579–84.

166. Connor WE, Hoak JC, Warner ED. Massive thrombosis produced by fatty acid infusion. J Clin Invest 1963;42:860–6.

167. Hyodoh H, Fujita A, Hyodoh K, et al. High-flow arteriovenous malformation of the lower extremity: ethanolamine oleate sclerotherapy. Cardiovasc Intervent Radiol 2001;24(5):348–51.

168. Mitsuzaki K, Yamashita Y, Utsunomiya D, et al. Balloon-occluded retrograde transvenous embolization of a pelvic arteriovenous malformation. Cardiovasc Intervent Radiol 1999;22(6):518–20.

169. Gabal AM. Percutaneous technique for sclerotherapy of vertebral hemangioma compressing spinal cord. Cardiovasc Intervent Radiol 2002;25(6): 494–500.

170. Matsumoto K, Nakanishi H, Koizumi Y, et al. Sclerotherapy of hemangioma with late involution. Dermatol Surg 2003;29(6):668–71 [discussion: 671].

171. Dubois JM, Sebag GH, De Prost Y, et al. Soft-tissue venous malformations in children: percutaneous sclerotherapy with Ethibloc. Radiology 1991;180: 195–8.

172. Kauffmann GW, Rassweiler J, Richter G, et al. Capillary embolization with Ethibloc: new embolization concept tested in dog kidneys. AJR Am J Roentgenol 1981;137(6):1163–8.

173. Gorriz E, Carreira JM, Reyes R, et al. Intramuscular low flow vascular malformations: treatment by means of direct percutaneous embolization. Eur J Radiol 1998;27(2):161–5.

174. Kuhne D, Helmke K. Embolization with Ethibloc of vascular tumors and arteriovenous malformations in the head and neck. Neuroradiology 1982;23(5): 253–8.

175. Riche MC, Hadjean E, Tran-Ba-Huy P, et al. The treatment of capillary-venous malformations using a new fibrosing agent. Plast Reconstr Surg 1983; 71(5):607–14.

176. Dubois J, Garel L, Abela A, et al. Lymphangiomas in children: percutaneous sclerotherapy with an alcoholic solution of zein. Radiology 1997;204(3): 651–4.

177. Herbreteau D, Riche MC, Enjolras O, et al. Percutaneous embolization with Ethibloc of lymphatic cystic malformations with a review of the experience in 70 patients. Int Angiol 1993;12(1):34–9.

178. Coetzee PF, Ionescu GO, Fourie P, et al. Results of intralesional bleomycin injection treatment for congenital vascular anomalies. Paper presented at: 15th Congress of the International Society for the Study of Vascular Anomalies. Wellington, New Zealand, February 22–25, 2004.

179. Garcia-Marin V, Ravina J, Trujillo E, et al. Symptomatic cavernous hemangioma of the occipital condyle treated with methacrylate embolization. Surg Neurol 2001;56(5):301–3.

180. Donnelly LF, Bissett III GS, Adams DM. Combined sonographic and fluoroscopic guidance: a modified technique for percutaneous sclerosis of low-flow vascular malformations. AJR Am J Roentgenol 1999;173(3):655–7.

181. Donnelly LF, Bisset GS 3rd, Adams DM. Marked acute tissue swelling following percutaneous sclerosis of low-flow vascular malformations: a predictor of both prolonged recovery and therapeutic effect. Pediatr Radiol 2000;30(6):415–9.

182. Holt PD, Burrows PE. Interventional radiology in the treatment of vascular lesions. Facial Plast Surg Clin North Am 2001;9(4):585–99.

183. Suh JS, Shin KH, Na JB, et al. Venous malformations: sclerotherapy with a mixture of ethanol and lipiodol. Cardiovasc Intervent Radiol 1997;20(4):268–73.

184. Rosenberg LZ. Sclerotherapy. emedicine.com. Available at: http://www.emedicine.com/plastic/topic437.htm. Accessed February 3, 2008. 2006.

185. Feied CF, Jackson JJ, Bren TS, et al. Allergic reactions to polidocanol for vein sclerosis: two case reports. J Dermatol Surg Oncol 1994;20(7):466–8.

186. Deveikis JP. Percutaneous ethanol sclerotherapy for vascular malformations in the head and neck. Arch Facial Plast Surg 2005;7(5):322–5.

187. Wysoki MG, White RI Jr. Crystallization when mixing contrast materials with ethanol for embolization of venous malformations. J Vasc Interv Radiol 2001;12(2):264.

188. Orbach EJ. Sclerotherapy of varicose veins: utilization of intravenous air block. Am J Surg 1944;66(3): 362–6.

189. Cabrera J, Cabrera J Jr. Nuevo método de esclerosis en las varices tronculares. Patol Vasc 1995;4: 55–73.

190. Cabrera J, Cabrera J Jr, Garcia-Olmedo MA, et al. Elargissement des limites de la sclerotherapie: nouveaux produits sclerosants. Phlebologie 1997; 2:181–8.

191. Tessari L. Nouvelle technique d'obtention de la sclero-mousse. Phlebologie 2000;53:129–33.

192. Frullini A, Cavezzi A. Sclerosing foam in the treatment of varicose veins and telangiectases: history

and analysis of safety and complications. Dermatol Surg 2002;28(1):11–5.

193. Hamel-Desnos C, Desnos P, Wollmann JC, et al. Evaluation of the efficacy of polidocanol in the form of foam compared with liquid form in sclerotherapy of the greater saphenous vein: initial results. Dermatol Surg 2003;29(12):1170–5 [discussion: 1175].

194. Puig S, Aref H, Brunelle F. Double-needle sclerotherapy of lymphangiomas and venous angiomas in children: a simple technique to prevent complications. AJR Am J Roentgenol 2003;180(5): 1399–401.

195. Lee CH, Chen SG. Direct percutaneous ethanol instillation for treatment of venous malformation in the face and neck. Br J Plast Surg 2005;58(8):1073–8.

196. Beebe HG, Bergan JJ, Bergqvist D, et al. Classification and grading of chronic venous disease in the lower limbs: a consensus statement. Eur J Vasc Endovasc Surg 1996;12(4):487–91 [discussion: 491–82].

197. Noel AA, Gloviczki P, Cherry KJ Jr, et al. Surgical treatment of venous malformations in Klippel-Trenaunay syndrome. J Vasc Surg 2000;32(5): 840–7.

198. Bergan J, Pascarella L, Mekenas L. Venous disorders: treatment with sclerosant foam. J Cardiovasc Surg (Torino) 2006;47(1):9–18.

199. Mounayer C, Wassef M, Enjolras O, et al. Facial glomangiomas: large facial venous malformations with glomus cells. J Am Acad Dermatol 2001; 45(2):239–45.

Musculoskeletal Interventional Radiology: Radiofrequency Ablation

Emily Ward, MBBChBAO, MRCPI[a], Peter L. Munk, MD, CM, FRCPC[b],
Faisal Rashid, MBBS, FRANZCR[b],
William C. Torreggiani, MBBCh, MRCPI, FRCR, FFRRCSI[a,*]

KEYWORDS

- Radiofrequency ablation
- Catheter ablation • Ultrasound • Computerized tomography
- Osteoid osteoma • Metastases

Radiofrequency ablation (RFA) involves the use of electrodes to heat abnormal tissue to a high enough temperature that it results in cell death. Thermal ablation of tumors is, however, nothing new. The first described use of heat as a method of treating tumors came from the early Greeks and Egyptians who used cautery as a method of killing abnormal cells.[1] Thermal ablation has been studied in many forms, including microwave, laser, high-intensity focused ultrasound, and cryotherapy (freezing below $-20°C$). RFA has emerged as the most commonly used method for thermal ablation in bone, soft tissues, kidney, liver, and heart. Radiofrequency energy is a low-voltage, high-frequency form of electrical energy that results in a homogeneous destruction of tissue. The relative safety of this type of energy source has contributed to the widespread adoption of RFA as a therapeutic modality in a variety of conditions within the human body. RFA continues to increase in popularity and has many different uses, ranging from its ability to destroy aberrant conduction pathways in the treatment of arrhythmias[2] to the treatment of small tumors of the kidney,[3,4] colorectal metastases,[5] primary lung cancers,[6,7] and primary liver tumors.[8] Traditionally the role of RFA primarily was to treat lesions that

were deemed to be inoperable or to use when surgery was associated with high perioperative mortality. However, it is now gaining acceptance as an attractive primary therapeutic option, especially when the lesion is small (less than 4 cm) in size.[9] In the musculoskeletal system, RFA is now increasingly used to treat a variety of lesions ranging from osteoid osteomas to metastasis. In some cases it is now being combined with other interventional techniques such as intraosseous cement injection to enhance its effect and range of uses.

PRINCIPAL OF RADIOFREQUENCY ABLATION

Injury to cells from exposure to heat will begin at $42°C$ with the time of heat exposure required to achieve cell death varying depending on tissue type and condition.[10] As the temperature is increased above $42°C$, the exposure time necessary to produce cell death decreases exponentially. At $42°C$, 3 to 50 hours may be required to produce a cytodestructive response, whereas at $46°C$, this could be achieved in only 8 minutes and in only 2 minutes at $51°C$.[10–12] Malignant cells are more resilient to destruction from freezing than normal cells, but interestingly they are more

[a] Department of Radiology, Adelaide and Meath Hospitals (incorporating the National Children's Hospital) (AMNCH), Tallaght, Dublin 24, Ireland
[b] Department of Radiology, Musculoskeletal Division, Vancouver General Hospital, 899 West 12th Avenue, Vancouver, BC V5Z 1M9, Canada
* Corresponding author.
E-mail address: William.torreggiani@amnch.ie (W.C. Torreggiani).

Radiol Clin N Am 46 (2008) 599–610
doi:10.1016/j.rcl.2008.02.006
0033-8389/08/$ – see front matter © 2008 Elsevier Inc. All rights reserved.

susceptible to damage from heating,[13] and it is on this principle that RFA is based.

When radiofrequency is applied to tissue, a high-frequency alternating current moves from the tip of an electrode into the tissue surrounding that electrode. The current causes the ions in the tissue to change direction and align in the direction of the current. This change in movement causes friction, and heat is generated. When the temperature exceeds 60°C, the cells die, resulting in tissue necrosis. However, a typical RFA treatment results in local tissue temperatures that exceed 100°C. This high temperature also destroys tissue microvasculature, thereby leading to local vessel thrombosis. Because of the high temperature achieved, the radiofrequency current reliably heats and kills the cells and tissues through which it passes. The tissues immediately surrounding the electrode are heated by the radiofrequency current to a relatively uniform temperature. The heat emitted from this tissue then spreads out to create an enlarging area of ablated tissue. The temperature of the tissue surrounding the electrode falls rapidly as the distance from the electrode increases.[14] Spread of heat into the adjacent tissues is also dependent on composition of the adjacent tissue. For example, a large vessel within the ablation zone may dissipate the heat away from the target zone and is therefore an important consideration in planning RFA.

PHYSICS OF RADIOFREQUENCY ABLATION

RFA causes coagulative necrosis by the application of a high-frequency alternating current through an electrode into the targeted lesion. The current moves from the tip of the electrode into the tissue surrounding the electrode causing rapid vibrations of ions and subsequent production of heat. In other words, it is not the probe that emits heat but the cells themselves. In areas in which heating is sufficient, cytodestruction occurs, which results in necrosis of tissue in the area surrounding the electrode.[15] The conductive heat emitted from the tissue radiates out from the electrode. The final size of the region of heat-ablated tissue is proportional to the square of the radiofrequency current, also known as the radiofrequency power density.[16] The radiofrequency power/current delivered via a monopolar electrode decreases in proportion to the square of the distance from the electrode.[17] Therefore, the tissue temperature decreases rapidly with increasing distance away from the electrode.[14,15] If the tip of the electrode is placed within the center of the targeted lesion, this principal helps to focus heat on this lesion while decreasing damage to adjacent normal tissue.

There is a relatively uniform zone of radiant/conductive heat within the first few millimeters of electrode-tissue interface around the electrode. However, the tissues at the boundary of the ablated zone undergo less uniform heat with the most peripheral region of the ablation zone undergoing partial necrosis, resulting in a small transitional peripheral zone extending from the inner region of cell death through an area of cell damage to outer normal tissue. For this reason, it is important that during treatment of a lesion, that the ablation zone is bigger than the actual size of the lesion to be ablated to account for this transitional zone.

TECHNIQUE

RFA generally is performed under the guidance of either ultrasound or, more commonly, computerized tomography (CT). For lesions involving the osseous skeleton such as osteoid osteomas and metastases, CT allows precise localization of the tumor and enables visualization of the radiofrequency electrode within the lesion (Fig. 1). Ultrasound-guided ablation of osseous lesions is difficult because many osseous lesions are either invisible or difficult to see unless there is a sizeable soft tissue mass. Ultrasound-guided RFA is, however, feasible when the lesion to be ablated lies within muscle or soft tissue and in such cases, RFA may be performed under real time allowing accurate and precise localization of the radiofrequency needle (Fig. 2). In all cases, it is necessary to ensure that the procedure has been discussed fully with the patient to explain its merits and possible complications. Careful preprocedural planning is required to map out the lesion and determine a safe access route that avoids important structures such as the neurovascular bundle. If it is anticipated that any potentially important structure may be damaged, it is important that the patient be informed of this beforehand. Depending on the clinical position of the tumor, muscle necrosis may occur, and if adjacent to a joint, articular cartilage may also be damaged. Adjacent organs such as bladder, liver, or other structures may also be affected, and this must be factored into planning of the lesion treatment. In selected instances, damage to important structures such as a nerve may be acceptable if no other successful palliative maneuver can reasonably be performed.

Before embarking on RFA, it is also important to ascertain if the treatment is appropriate for the particular patient. For example, a vertebral metastasis may be better treated by surgery, radiation, vertebroplasty, or even chemotherapy depending on the histologic subtype of the lesion as well as

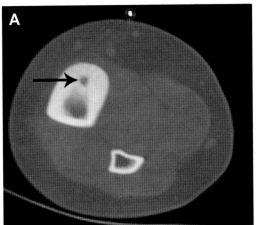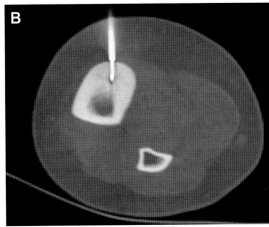

Fig. 1. (*A*) Classical osteoid osteoma of the anterior tibia shows typical nidus (*arrow*) with a markedly thickened anterior cortex of the tibia. (*B*) Single tip radiofrequency electrode has been advanced into the nidus of the osteoid osteoma allowing successful radiofrequency ablation of the lesion.

its location and patient suitability. In most cases, RFA may be performed under local anesthetic and conscious sedation. The exceptions to this include patient preference, patients who are likely to find it difficult to remain still without general anesthetic, and ablation of lesions that are likely to cause pain when stimulated such as osteoid osteomas. Such case probably are best performed under general anesthetic, although there is not uniform agreement on this in the literature, with some investigators preferring local anesthetic and conscious sedation in all cases.

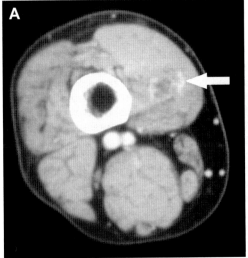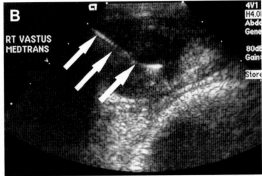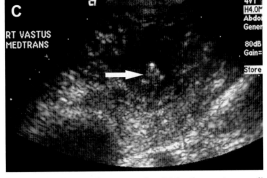

Fig. 2. Ultrasound-guided radiofrequency ablation of a symptomatic renal metastasis within the vastus medialis muscle. (*A*) Contrast-enhanced CT shows an enhancing mass within the vastus medialis muscle consist a metastasis (*arrow*). (*B*) Under real-time ultrasound guidance the radiofrequency electrode (*arrows*) can be seen clearly to enter the metastasis within the vastus medialis muscle. (*C*) The deployed wires from the radiofrequency probe may be seen within the metastasis (*arrow*).

After appropriate sedation or anesthetic as deemed appropriate, the skin is prepped and draped in the usual fashion, using a sterile technique. A small incision is made in the skin with a scalpel, and the radiofrequency probe is selected. The size of the radiofrequency probe is dependent largely on the size of the lesion to be ablated. Most vendors now supply a range of sizes of probes allowing for lesions up to 5 cm to be ablated. In general, the ablation zone should be larger than the tumor, and one should allow about 1 cm extra diameter to ensure adequate ablation. Ablation zones are based on the theoretic model of a sphere. It is therefore important that the needle tip is placed in the center of the theoretic sphere to ensure as accurate an ablation zone as possible. It should also be remembered that most tumors and lesions are irregular in shape, and it is their longest diameter that should be used. In addition to this, it is important that imaging is performed before RFA to assess if there is any adjacent large vessel that may contribute to flow-related cooling of the ablation zone. Finally, it is important to assess with imaging that the ablation zone does not involve any critical structures such as adjacent bowel, which could result in delayed bowel perforation caused by heat damage of the bowel wall. Once these criteria have been satisfied, the radiofrequency electrode is advanced under imaging so that the tip of the needle is within the center of the lesion. Sometimes it is not possible to get the electrode exactly within the center of a lesion, and one must make allowances for this and ensure that the zone of ablation is sufficient to kill the entire lesion to be treated. Any viable tumor tissue left untreated may lead to recurrence and its associated symptomatology. As with RFA in other parts of the body, RFA in the musculoskeletal system may employ more than one ablation in various locations around a lesion so that the combined overlap of the ablated zone may cover a lesion larger than 5 cm. This may be relevant particularly to lesions that are "long" rather than "round." The main disadvantage of multiple ablations is that this significantly increases the time required to treat a particular lesion leading to both potential patient discomfort as well as operator fatigue.

Unlike RFA of many intra-abdominal lesions, RFA in the osseous skeleton requires that access be created through a channel into the lesion. When the lesion has a large soft tissue component, this is easy and simply requires direct pressure to the electrode. However, when there is no soft tissue component and the lesion lies under the cortex of the bone, the bone may be difficult to penetrate, and a drill may be required to access the lesion with the electrode. This is particularly so with osteoid osteomas where the lesion often is associated with a thick sclerotic hard periosteal reaction.

When a channel has to be drilled through the bone, there are a variety of needles or intraosseous needles available for this purpose. At the authors' institution, the intraosseous needle is routinely used. For the purposes of RFA after tract formation, a gauge of at least 16 is required to allow the electrode to fit through the channel that has been created. After drilling into the bone, there is an option to obtain a tissue biopsy at this stage. After this, it is important that the guide cannula remains in place without moving its position over the hole that has just been created in the bone (**Fig. 3**). This allows the electrode to pass easily through the guide cannula and directly into the target lesion within the bone. When trying to penetrate or drill into the bone, there are a number of methods to achieve this purpose. If the bone has a thin cortex and is soft, it may be possible to use manual pressure to advance the needle into the bone. However, when the bone cortex is thick, an electrical drill is required. We have adopted a hand-held commercial drill to drill into the bone (**Fig. 4**). This allows a versatile, reliable, and cheap method to access the bone. However, the type of drill used is dependent largely on the individual operator.

Once a channel has been drilled through the bone into the lesion, the electrode may then be placed through this channel into the lesion. Once the electrode tip is in the correct location, the inner individual wires (or struts) are then deployed. This is usually done by simply pressing downward on the outside component of the probe, although some probes require a rotating motion to deploy the active wires. When there is no soft tissue component within a lesion, it may not be possible to deploy the wires within the adjacent dense bone. This occurs typically when treating osteoid osteomas, and in such cases, it is important that the tip of the electrode is an active component. Although this results in a smaller field of ablation, in the case of an osteoid osteoma, it is the nidus of the osteoid osteoma that requires ablation, and this usually is small enough in size to be fully ablated without the need for the wires to be deployed.

Once the electrode is in place and the wires deployed as appropriate, the radiofrequency generator is attached to the needle electrode, and two grounding pads are placed on the patient (usually on each of the patient's thighs). An algorithm then is applied based on the manufacturer's guidelines, lesion type, and the radiologist's experience,

A 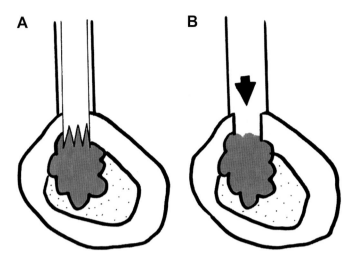 B

Fig. 3. Schematic bone biopsy needle and cannula before radiofrequency ablation. (*A*) A guiding cannula is placed onto the surface of the bone overlying the lesion to be treated. A biopsy needle is then drilled into the lesion and a sample obtained and removed. (*B*) The guiding cannula is then left in place allowing a channel (*arrow*) through which the radiofrequency electrode may pass. (*Courtesy of* Lorie Marchinkow, Vancouver, BC, Canada.)

which ensures that the correct RF energy is applied to the target lesion.

Once ablation of a tumor or lesion is achieved, it is a useful maneuver to ablate the tract through which ablation has taken place. This is performed

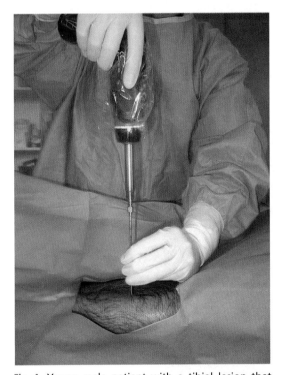

Fig. 4. Young male patient with a tibial lesion that required a channel to be drilled through the thick cortex of the tibia. A 16-gauge intraosseous needle was drilled through a guiding cannula using a hand-held commercial drill. After this a radiofrequency electrode was passed through the channel created into the osseous lesion allowing successful RFA to take place.

by gradually pulling out the electrode needle through the tract with the tip of the electrode remaining active. The rationale for tract ablation is to prevent potential seeding of tumor.

RFA may be combined with the intralesional injection of cement in a similar fashion to vertebroplasty. This is done immediately after RFA. A hollow needle is advanced into the lesion, and polymethylmethacrylate (acrylic bone cement) mixed with tantalum powder for radiopacity is then injected to fill the cavity. This is performed under CT or fluoroscopic guidance. This procedure has benefits both in terms of pain relief as well as strengthening and stabilizing a lytic lesion that may be prone to pathologic fracture.

Size of ablation zones can be extended by preprocedural transarterial embolization, which effectively decreases the heat sump effect around the ablation area.[18,19] There is a risk, however, that the ablation zone may not only become larger but become unevenly distributed. Increased tumor kill must therefore be weighed against potential thermal injury to adjacent normal structures.[18] Other techniques aimed at facilitating more extensive coagulation necrosis include cooling of the exposed tip of the radiofrequency electrodes through internal water irrigation, which has the advantage of avoiding tissue charring around the cooled needle tip. This mechanism produces even thermal tumor destruction with larger volumes of necrosis.[20] The main disadvantage of this method is that larger-diameter probes are generally required to carry out the procedure.

INDICATIONS

Although the main application for RFA in the musculoskeletal system worldwide has been treatment of osteoid osteomas,[18] increasingly over recent years other lesions have also been found suitable for treatment.[21] In particular there has been much interest in the treatment of metastatic bone disease for the purposes of palliation.[22–24] Experience with this technique is somewhat limited but growing, with an increasing number of reports now appearing in the literature. Ablation can be performed with either straight probes, probe clusters, or umbrella configuration probes either alone or in combination with saline infusion,[25] depending on the size and configuration of the lesion to be treated. Lesions that are very sclerotic are not usually amenable to treatment, whereas lytic lesions with a significant soft tissue component are more suitable. The best therapeutic effect is achieved by including in the ablation field the interface between the tumor and the normal adjacent bone or tissue. Principles of ablation, described initially in the nonmusculoskeletal literature of which there is considerable more experience in treating tumors of the kidney and liver metastases,[26,27] apply in a similar way in the musculoskeletal system.

A lack of ablation of the lesion–bone interface in the musculoskeletal system is likewise, therefore, usually associated with recurrence and a poor clinical outcome. In some cases, more than one RFA application may be needed, and this is especially true for metastases, in which lesions may be large or in which there is more than one lesion present. In addition, some lesions may contain areas of necrosis or hemorrhage, particularly centrally, and there is little benefit in treating this portion of the tumor. The same applies for tumors containing myxoid material, which generally is not poorly responsive to RFA.

Increasingly, reports have appeared in the literature describing the combination of RFA with percutaneous injection of cement (**Fig. 5**).[28–33] This is particularly valuable in weight-bearing areas such as the acetabulum in which ablation alone may not be sufficient to relieve pain if inadequate structural support in the area is present. The acetabulum is an important example of an anatomic site in which the introduction of cement provides the structural support promoting weight

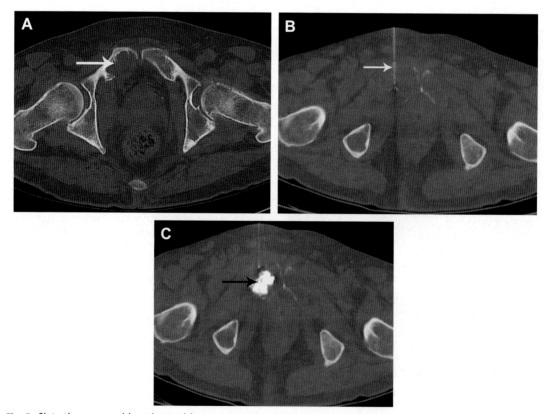

Fig. 5. Sixty-three-year-old patient with symptomatic metastases involving the right pubic bone. (*A*) There is a large lytic metastasis involving the right pubic bone (*arrow*). There are scattered metastases within the rest of the pelvis. (*B*) A radiofrequency electrode has been advanced into the lesion and the wires fully deployed. (*C*) After ablation of the lesion, intralesional cement was injected into the ablated cavity. The patient had good palliative pain relief after the procedure.

bearing through the treated area. Currently it is unclear whether the combination of RFA with cement injection is of significant additional benefit than using one treatment alone. For instance, in the acetabulum, good clinical results usually can be anticipated from cement injection alone. Furthermore, variable analgesic reduction has been reported with the combined technique.[23,29] Theoretically, RFA may permit more extensive destruction of tumor, rendering it necrotic, whereas systemic embolization of live tumor cells on injection of cement may be prevented via both the thrombosis of the paravertebral and intervertebral veins[33] and tissue necrosis itself. Although these advantages remain conjectural and undoubtedly will be better understood as further experience accrues, the effect of combined therapy already has been reported to be greater than or equal to either cement injection or RFA alone in pain alleviation in bone metastases in at least two large series.[29,30,32] Regardless, the minimally invasive nature and potential for day care treatment are definite advantages.[33]

RADIOFREQUENCY ABLATION IN PRIMARY BONE TUMORS

It is worth individually discussing osteoid osteomas in some detail, because it is this lesion in which RFA has performed spectacularly well and helped propel the use of RFA in the musculoskeletal system. Osteoid osteoma is a benign bone lesion of unknown etiology. It can occur in any bone, but it tends to affect the appendicular skeleton with the proximal femur being the most common site. Osteoid osteoma most commonly affects young patients, typically in the second decade, and the male to female ratio is 2:1. These benign lesions account for approximately 10% of benign bone tumors.[34] Osteoid osteomas have no malignant potential.[35] The tumor seldom increases in size but may occasionally regress spontaneously. The typical osteoid osteoma has a nidus measuring less than 2 cm in diameter, and it may be associated with overlying bone sclerosis (see **Fig. 1**; **Figs. 6 and 7**). The classical clinical presentation is with dull pain at the tumor site. This is classically worse at night. The pain is dramatically relieved with treatment with nonsteroidal anti-inflammatory medication, typically aspirin. Plain film is the initial examination of choice, and the diagnosis often can be made on this alone. The typical radiologic appearance of an osteoid osteoma is that of an ovoid or spherical radiolucent nidus surrounded by an area of bone sclerosis. The amount of surrounding sclerosis is variable around the nidus and may even be absent. CT can be used for more exact localization. Radionuclide scanning shows significantly increased uptake within the lesion. It shows high sensitivity but low specificity. The treatment options available for osteoid osteomas that do not show spontaneous regression or are causing significant symptoms include percutaneous RFA of the central nidus or surgical resection. In the past, surgical removal was the treatment of choice. However, this required a hospital stay of several days and limitation of weight bearing in the postoperative period. RFA is the other main

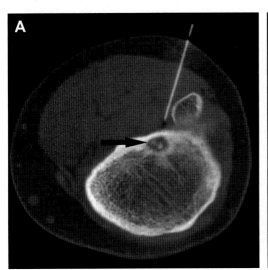 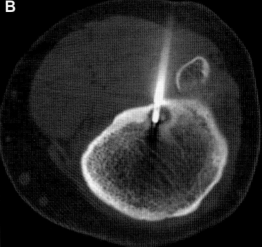

Fig. 6. (*A*) Typical CT appearances of an osteoid osteoma show a typical nidus with a lucent cavity and central dense area (*arrow*). A guide needle has been advance onto the posterior cortex of the tibia to localize the lesion before drilling into it. (*B*) A radiofrequency electrode has been placed into the nidus of the lesion after drilling of a tract through the tibial cortex.

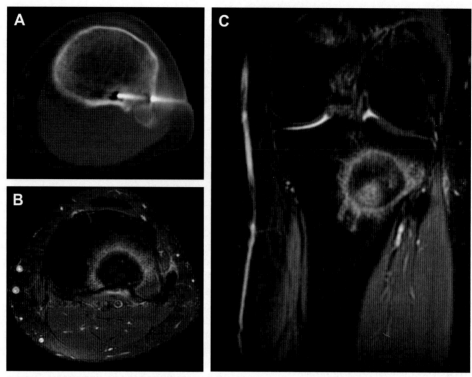

Fig. 7. Thirty-two-year-old male patient with osteoid osteoma of the posterior tibia. (*A*) CT-guided radiofrequency ablation shows electrode with its tip within the nidus of the osteoid osteoma. (*B*) Transverse and (*C*) coronal contrast-enhanced T1-weighted sequences with fat suppression show circular area of nonenhanced bone in keeping with ablation zone. Note peripheral enhancement at the transition zone between ablated bone and normal bone.

treatment option. It is suitable for the treatment of most osteoid osteomas and has a shorter recovery time. Success rates have been reported as high as 97% (primary success rate) and 100% (secondary success rate).[36] In most studies, there have been few complications with patients resuming normal activities within 24 hours. Most investigators now recommended RFA to be the procedure of choice in treating osteoid osteomas.

Although RFA has been described predominantly in treating osteoid osteomas, there are increasing reports of other primary bone tumors treated successfully by RFA. Recently, RFA has been shown to be effective in the treatment of chondroblastomas.[35] These are rare benign bone tumors occurring in the cartilage. Although surgery has previously been the treatment of choice, it can be difficult and lead to significant morbidity because of the epiphyseal location of chondroblastomas. In their report, Petsas and colleagues [37] describe two subarticular femoral head chondroblastomas that were treated successfully with RFA. Although this form of treatment seems easier than surgery, it is in itself not without its problems. Because chondroblastomas tend to occur in the

epiphysis of weight-bearing joints and therefore lie close to the articular cartilage, the cartilage may get damaged, resulting in an increased risk of treatment failure and postprocedural complications. Some of these complications were encountered by Tins and colleagues[38] who reported that four chondroblastomas were ablated successfully, but complications were encountered in two of these cases.

BONE METASTASES

In the United States, of the estimated 1.2 million new cases of neoplasm diagnosed yearly, more than 50% of these patients will in time have metastases to the skeleton.[39] Pain from skeletal metastases is the most frequently reported symptom and can be caused by mechanical or chemical factors.[40] Although external beam radiation remains the gold standard treatment for painful bony metastases, up to 20% or 30% of patients do not experience symptom relief.[41] RFA has been performed on patients to treat and palliate painful osseous bony metastatic disease successfully for years.[42] Multiple studies have found this to be an effective method of managing refractory cases.[21,41] However, because metastases usually are multiple, prudent patient selection is required to select patients that will truly benefit from RFA. At all times, it should be kept in mind that RFA is a relatively expensive and sometimes time-consuming technique and its use should always be based as best as possible on principles of cost effectiveness and best practice.

COMBINED RFA AND CEMENTOPLASTY IN METASTATIC DISEASE

More recently there have been case reports and subsequently studies that have explored the use of RFA in combination with cementoplasty for the treatment of painful bony metastases (see **Fig. 5**). The main indication for cementoplasty is to attempt to control the pain as well as stabilization of lytic metastasis. Treatment of vertebral body fractures secondary to osteoporosis or metastatic disease has to date shown excellent results both regarding improvement in mobility and relief of pain.[24,43–45] In one study of the combined use of RFA with cementoplasty, technical success was achieved in 100% of cases. These investigators found initial pain relief was seen in 100% with a mean duration of pain relief being 7.3 months. Analgesic reduction was achieved in 41%. The main complications encountered were hematomata. In this study, the combination of RFA with cementoplasty was found to be safe and effective.[29] A further case report in the *Journal of Vascular and Interventional Radiology* [31] described a pathologic fracture secondary to osteolytic metastases from a melanoma primary tumor that was treated with a combination of RFA followed immediately by percutaneous injection of polymethylmethacrylate. The patient tolerated both procedures well. Pain was relieved and mobility re-established. The investigators felt this approach should be considered as an alternative treatment method in palliative care situations to improve quality of life. A further report in *Surgical Neurology* describes a case of vertebral metastases treated with RFA and vertebroplasty without complications. The patient was discharged home the same day without complaints. These investigators also described how RFA could also minimize procedure-related complications during the cementoplasty. In properly selected patients, they felt the RFA might increase the duration of local spinal stabilization afforded by vertebroplasty alone.

FOLLOW-UP IMAGING

If imaging is performed within a short time after RFA, it is quite common to see gas bubbles in the lesion. This must not be confused with infection because it may lead to unnecessary treatment with antibiotics or even surgery. Gas after RFA is believed to result from a combination of instrumentation and tissue necrosis. It is seen easily on CT as small focal areas of air attenuation within the ablation zone. The air is much harder to recognize on ultrasound scan where it appears as an area of dirty shadowing. Unless a patient has other symptoms to suggest infection, the air can be safely ignored and will usually resolve in after a few days.

MR imaging, unlike CT and ultrasonography is generally not useful in guiding treatment for RFA; however, it may be an invaluable modality in staging lesions before RFA as well as in the follow-up of ablated lesions. During follow-up with MR imaging, imaging is best performed after the administration of intravenous contrast where it is extremely helpful in delineating the extent of the ablation zone to determine completeness of the ablation (**Fig. 8**).[46,47] Ablated tissue shows no enhancement, because it is dead. Some enhancement can, however, be seen in the periphery of the ablated area, and this should not be mistaken for tumor. It is important to ensure that the pretreatment images are also viewed in conjunction with the postablation imaging to ensure accurate analysis of postoperative imaging.

CLINICAL FOLLOW-UP

It is important that radiologist involve themselves not just with the imaging follow-up but also the clinical follow-up of patients undergoing RFA. Before the procedure, patients should be given a realistic expectation of symptom improvement that they will achieve after RFA. Although the majority of patients will show improvement in pain with adequate ablation,[21,23,24,48] a significant minority will not show appreciable improvements in their symptomatology. Pain relief is generally considered by the patient as the marker of success. In the case of osteoid osteomas, pain relief often is instant and carries a cure rate of approximately 97% of cases with a secondary cure rate of 100%.[36] In this group of patients, the pain typically has been present for many months or even years causing significant problems for the patient, and the relief of the pain can be very rewarding for both the patient and the radiologist. In cases in which pain relief has not been achieved after RFA of any musculoskeletal lesion , the cause of this may relate to a number of reasons. Poor technique, inadequate ablation, and technical faults may all result in failure. Sometimes the cause of

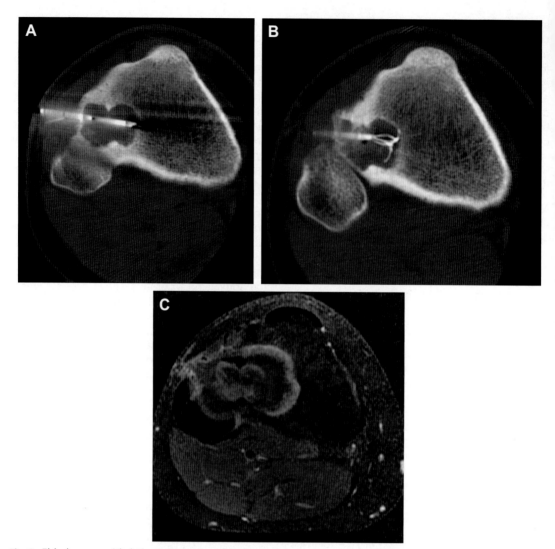

Fig. 8. Elderly man with lytic metastasis within the proximal tibia. (*A*) Radiofrequency electrode can be seen within the lytic lesion before deployment of its wires. (*B*) The wires of the electrode can be seen deployed within the lesion. Because of the irregular cavity of the metastasis, there is not uniform deployment of the wires. (*C*) Contrast-enhanced T1-weighted MR image with fat suppression in the transverse plain shows that the zone of ablation has exceeded the size of the treated lesion indicating a technically successful ablation.

failure may be because the actual cause of the patient's pain is from something other than the ablated lesion. This can usually be avoided if the radiologist has discussed with the patient their symptomatology and correlated this with their imaging before performing RFA. For example, a patient with a lytic lesion at the first lumbar level may have an associated disc protrusion at a lower level causing their pain, and this could probably be predicted with an accurate clinical history and examination correlated to high-quality imaging. After RFA, patients often will have a flare of pain in the 6- to 24-hour period after the ablation as the local anesthetic and sedation wears away.

Thankfully however, this pain usually recedes quickly after that time.

FUTURE DIRECTIONS

The utility of RFA in the musculoskeletal system has not been explored fully. Many centers are still completely unaware of the potential role that RFA may play in the treatment of musculoskeletal metastases, particularly as part of pain palliation. It is likely that with time and as clinicians become aware of these techniques, there will be a significant growth of these procedures. It is partly the responsibility for the radiologist to make the medical community aware of the role RFA may contribute in the treatment of patients. Newer techniques such as the combination of cementoplasty with RFA may further help enhance the success and clinical outcomes of RFA. For certain lesions such as osteoid osteomas, there are clear advantages over surgery with good scientific evidence of the superiority of RFA over surgery.

It is important that as we look to the future, as musculoskeletal radiologists, we maximize our efforts that the procedures we do are audited, analyzed, and, when possible, included in part of a scientific study. The era of evidence-based medicine is upon us, and although many individuals have single cases of which they are proud, a more scientific and nonbiased approach will be needed to firmly establish the role of RFA within the bigger medical community.

Currently, RFA of skeletal metastases is predominantly performed as a palliative procedure. It is our vision that as techniques and knowledge improve, RFA will one day be able to cure patients of their disease. This may be achieved using a combination of RFA with molecular-directed therapies and novel chemotherapies. The future for RFA in the musculoskeletal system is bright. We should embrace its potential and drive it forward to maximize its potential benefits in the future.

SUMMARY

RFA of musculoskeletal lesions has undergone major progress over the last 10 years. Techniques and outcomes have continually improved as experience and new technologies have come on board. The range of indications continues to expand with novel indications being continually described in the literature. Although RFA of osteoid osteomas is now accepted generally as the treatment of choice for these lesions, much work needs to be done to scientifically support the expanding role of RFA in the palliative treatment of bone metastases. Pain palliation as well as prophylactic treatment of bone metastases may increase the quality of life for patients, and it is important that the medical community are made aware of the availability of these techniques.

REFERENCES

1. LeVeen R. Laser hyperthermia and radiofrequency ablation of hepatic lesions. Seminars in Interventional Radiology 1997;14:313–4.
2. Andrew P, Montenero AS. Atrial flutter: a focus on treatment options for a common supraventricular tachyarrhythmia. J Cardiovasc Med (Hagerstown) 2007;8:558–67.
3. Park S, Cadeddu JA. Outcomes of radiofrequency ablation for kidney cancer. Cancer Control 2007; 14:205–10.
4. Lovisolo JA, Legramandi CP, Fonte A. Thermal ablation of small renal tumors–present status. Scientific World Journal 2007;7:756–67.
5. Leen E, Horgan PG. Radiofrequency ablation of colorectal liver metastases. Surg Oncol 2007;16: 47–51.
6. Matsuoka T, Okuma T. CT-guided radiofrequency ablation for lung cancer. Int J Clin Oncol 2007;12: 71–8.
7. Ambrogi MC, Dini P, Melfi F, et al. Radiofrequency ablation of inoperable non-small cell lung cancer. J Thorac Oncol 2007;2:S2–3.
8. Pereira PL. Actual role of radiofrequency ablation of liver metastases. Eur Radiol 2007;17:2062–70.
9. McDougal WS. Radiofrequency ablation of renal cell carcinoma. BJU Int 2007;99:1271–2.
10. Dickson JA, Calderwood SK. Temperature range and selective sensitivity of tumors to hyperthermia: a critical review. Ann N Y Acad Sci 1980;335: 180–205.
11. Hill R. Hyperthermia. In: Hunt J, editor. The basic science of oncology. New York: Pergamon Press; 1987. p. 337–57.
12. Haines DE, Watson DD, Halperin C. Characteristics of heat transfer and determination gradient and viability threshold during radiofrequency fulgaration of isolated perfused canine right ventricle. Circulation 1987;76:278–83.
13. Bischof J, Christov K, Rubinsky B. A morphological study of cooling rate response in normal and neoplastic human liver tissue: cryosurgical implications. Cryobiology 1993;30:482–92.
14. Curley SA. Radiofrequency ablation of malignant liver tumors. Oncologist 2001;6:14–23.
15. Davis KW, Choi JJ, Blankenbaker DG. Radiofrequency ablation in the musculoskeletal system. Semin Roentgenol 2004;39:129–44.
16. Curley SA, Izzo F, Delrio P, et al. Radiofrequency ablation of unresectable primary and metastatic hepatic malignancies: results in 123 patients. Ann Surg 1999;230:1–8.
17. Frezza EE. Therapeutic management algorithm in cirrhotic and noncirrhotic patients in primary or secondary liver masses. Dig Dis Sci 2004;49:866–71.
18. Munk PL, Legiehn GM. Musculoskeletal interventional radiology: applications to oncology. Semin Roentgenol 2007;42:164–74.
19. Nakai M, Sato M, Sahara S, et al. Radiofrequency ablation in a porcine liver model: effects of transcatheter arterial embolization with iodized oil on ablation time, maximum output, and coagulation

diameter as well as angiographic characteristics. World J Gastroenterol 2007;13:2841–5.

20. Khatri VP, McGahan J. Non-resection approaches for colorectal liver metastases. Surg Clin North Am 2004;84:587–606.

21. Kojima H, Tanigawa N, Kariya S, et al. Clinical assessment of percutaneous radiofrequency ablation for painful metastatic bone tumors. Cardiovasc Intervent Radiol 2006;29:1022–6.

22. Georgy BA, Wong W. Plasma-mediated radiofrequency ablation assisted percutaneous cement injection for treating advanced malignant vertebral compression fractures. AJNR Am J Neuroradiol 2007;28:700–5.

23. Callstrom MR, Charboneau JW, Goetz MP, et al. Painful metastases involving bone: feasibility of percutaneous CT- and US-guided radio-frequency ablation. Radiology 2002;224:87–97.

24. Gronemeyer DH, Schirp S, Gevargez A. Image-guided radiofrequency ablation of spinal tumors: preliminary experience with an expandable array electrode. Cancer J 2002;8:33–9.

25. Buy X, Basile A, Bierry G, et al. Saline-infused bipolar radiofrequency ablation of high-risk spinal and paraspinal neoplasms. AJR Am J Roentgenol 2006;186:S322–6.

26. Ogan K, Jacomides L, Dolmatch BL, et al. Percutaneous radiofrequency ablation of renal tumors: technique, limitations, and morbidity. Urology 2002;60: 954–8.

27. Goldberg SN, Gazelle GS, Compton CC, et al. Treatment of intrahepatic malignancy with radiofrequency ablation: radiologic-pathologic correlation. Cancer 2000;88:2452–63.

28. Nakatsuka A, Yamakado K, Maeda M, et al. Radiofrequency ablation combined with bone cement injection for the treatment of bone malignancies. J Vasc Interv Radiol 2004;15:707–12.

29. Toyota N, Naito A, Kakizawa H, et al. Radiofrequency ablation therapy combined with cementoplasty for painful bone metastases: initial experience. Cardiovasc Intervent Radiol 2005;28: 578–83.

30. van der Linden E, Kroft LJ, Dijkstra PD. Treatment of vertebral tumor with posterior wall defect using image-guided radiofrequency ablation combined with vertebroplasty: preliminary results in 12 patients. J Vasc Interv Radiol 2007;18:741–7.

31. Schaefer O, Lohrmann C, Herling M, et al. Combined radiofrequency thermal ablation and percutaneous cementoplasty treatment of a pathologic fracture. J Vasc Interv Radiol 2002;13:1047–50.

32. Halpin RJ, Bendok BR, Sato KT, et al. Combination treatment of vertebral metastases using image-guided percutaneous radiofrequency ablation and

vertebroplasty: a case report. Surg Neurol 2005; 63:469–74 [discussion: 474–5].

33. Schaefer O, Lohrmann C, Markmiller M, et al. Technical innovation. Combined treatment of a spinal metastasis with radiofrequency heat ablation and vertebroplasty. AJR Am J Roentgenol 2003;180:1075–7.

34. Bloem JL, Kroon HM. Osseous lesions. Radiol Clin North Am 1993;31:261–78.

35. Rosenthal DI, Hornicek FJ, Wolfe MW, et al. Percutaneous radiofrequency coagulation of osteoid osteoma compared with operative treatment. J Bone Joint Surg Am 1998;80:815–21.

36. Martel J, Bueno A, Ortiz E. Percutaneous radiofrequency treatment of osteoid osteoma using cool-tip electrodes. Eur J Radiol 2005;56:403–8.

37. Petsas T, Megas P, Papathanassiou Z. Radiofrequency ablation of two femoral head chondroblastomas. Eur J Radiol 2007;63:63–7.

38. Tins B, Cassar-Pullicino V, McCall I, et al. Radiofrequency ablation of chondroblastoma using a multi-tined expandable electrode system: initial results. Eur Radiol 2006;16:804–10.

39. Swanson KC, Pritchard DJ, Sim FH. Surgical treatment of metastatic disease of the femur. J Am Acad Orthop Surg 2000;8:56–65.

40. Dupuy DE, Goldberg SN. Image-guided radiofrequency tumor ablation: challenges and opportunities–part II. J Vasc Interv Radiol 2001;12:1135–48.

41. Callstrom MR, Charboneau JW. Image-guided palliation of painful metastases using percutaneous ablation. Tech Vasc Interv Radiol 2007;10:120–31.

42. Posteraro AF, Dupuy DE, Mayo-Smith WW. Radiofrequency ablation of bony metastatic disease. Clin Radiol 2004;59:803–11.

43. Weill A, Chiras J, Simon JM, et al. Spinal metastases: indications for and results of percutaneous injection of acrylic surgical cement. Radiology 1996;199:241–7.

44. Kaufmann TJ, Jensen ME, Schweickert PA, et al. Age of fracture and clinical outcomes of percutaneous vertebroplasty. AJNR Am J Neuroradiol 2001; 22:1860–3.

45. Levine SA, Perin LA, Hayes D, et al. An evidence-based evaluation of percutaneous vertebroplasty. Manag Care 2000;9(3):56–60, 63.

46. Solbiati L, Goldberg SN, Ierace T, et al. Hepatic metastases: percutaneous radio-frequency ablation with cooled-tip electrodes. Radiology 1997;205:367–73.

47. Goldberg SN, Gazelle GS, Solbiati L, et al. Ablation of liver tumors using percutaneous RF therapy. AJR Am J Roentgenol 1998;170:1023–8.

48. Goetz MP, Callstrom MR, Charboneau JW, et al. Percutaneous image-guided radiofrequency ablation of painful metastases involving bone: a multicenter study. J Clin Oncol 2004;22:300–6.

Percutaneous Vertebral Augmentation: Vertebroplasty, Kyphoplasty and Skyphoplasty

Wilfred C.G. Peh, MBBS, MHSM, MD, FRCPE, FRCPG, FRCR[a],*,
Peter L. Munk, MD, CM, FRCPC[b], Faisal Rashid, MBBS, FRANZCR[b],
Louis A. Gilula, MD, FACR[c]

KEYWORDS
- Hemangioma • Metastases • Kyphoplasty • Osteoporosis
- Percutaneous vertebral augmentation • Skyphoplasty
- Spine compression fracture
- Spine interventional procedure
- Vertebral augmentation • Vertebroplasty

Percutaneous vertebroplasty, first described in 1987, is an imaging-guided procedure that entails the percutaneous injection of radiopaque polymethylmethacrylate (PMM) cement into a painful compressed vertebra. This procedure was originally described to treat painful aggressive vertebral hemangiomas.[1,2] It is most frequently used today for treatment of painful vertebral fractures caused by osteoporosis.[3–24] The second most common use is for treatment of painful vertebral fractures caused by metastatic disease. In the United States, osteoporosis affects more than 10 million people and, according to estimates, results in more than 700,000 vertebral compression fractures annually.[25] Vertebroplasty and other percutaneous vertebral augmentation procedures have now become accepted as treatment options in patients with intractable back pain due to osteoporotic vertebral compression fractures. When performed by experienced practitioners in carefully selected patients, percutaneous vertebroplasty has been found to be a safe, inexpensive, and highly effective procedure. A nationwide Medicare database survey from 2001 to 2003 found that radiologists performed the majority of Medicare-reimbursed vertebroplasty procedures in the United States (70%), with a large minority (25%) being performed by orthopedic surgeons, neurosurgeons, and anesthesiologists. During this period, radiologists had the greatest increase in volume of vertebroplasties compared with other specialties.[26]

Kyphoplasty, a modification of vertebroplasty, aims to restore vertebral height and improve kyphosis, as well as provide the pain relief achieved with percutaneous vertebroplasty. Introduced in 2001, kyphoplasty employs a height-restoration device, known as a balloon tamp, which resembles an angioplasty balloon.[27] The balloon tamp, when inflated, aims to restore the

[a] Department of Diagnostic Radiology, Alexandra Hospital, 378 Alexandra Road, Singapore 159964, Republic of Singapore
[b] Department of Radiology, University of British Columbia, Vancouver General Hospital, 899 West 12th Avenue, Vancouver, BC V5Z 1M9, Canada
[c] Mallinckrodt Institute of Radiology, Washington University Medical Center, 510 South Kingshighway Blvd., St. Louis, MO 63110, USA
* Corresponding author. Department of Diagnostic Radiology, Alexandra Hospital, 378 Alexandra Road, Singapore 159964, Republic of Singapore.
E-mail address: wilfred@pehfamily.per.sg (W.C.G. Peh).

Radiol Clin N Am 46 (2008) 611–635
doi:10.1016/j.rcl.2008.05.005
0033-8389/08/$ – see front matter © 2008 Elsevier Inc. All rights reserved.

original shape of the vertebral body and create a cavity into which cement is injected. Kyphoplasty is as useful as percutaneous vertebroplasty for producing rapid relief of pain resulting from vertebral compression fracture. Both procedures depend on mechanical stabilization of the fracture produced by PMM cement injection into the fractured vertebra.[27–37]

Skyphoplasty is similar to kyphoplasty but uses a new device that uses, in place of an inflatable balloon, a stiff plastic tube deployed through the cannula inside the vertebral body and compressed in an accordion fashion into a popcornlike crenulated configuration (**Fig. 1**), thereby creating a cavity. The device is then removed and the cavity is filled with PMM cement using a cement application device similar to that employed in kyphoplasty (**Fig. 2**). This device shows promise for treatment of vertebral compression fractures, according to early reports.

PATIENT SELECTION
Indications

The goal of percutaneous vertebroplasty is to provide pain relief and to strengthen bone in patients with vertebral body compression fractures. Selected patients should have severe focal midline pain at or adjacent to the level of the fracture, without definite radicular signs and symptoms. These patients should also have undergone a period of conservative management, typically lasting 6 to 12 weeks.[18–20,23,38] Exceptions are patients with thoracic spine fractures with pain radiating to the ribs, and fractures at the level of the conus medullaris, where pain may sometimes radiate to the hips without evidence of cord compression.[18]

Well-recognized causes of compression fractures that warrant vertebroplasty are osteoporosis, myeloma, metastasis, and painful aggressive vertebral hemangioma.[1,2,5–20,39–45] Vertebroplasty has been found to be useful in treating multiple myeloma of the cervical spine in a small series of patients.[46] Fuwa and colleagues[47] recently described successful treatment of a symptomatic

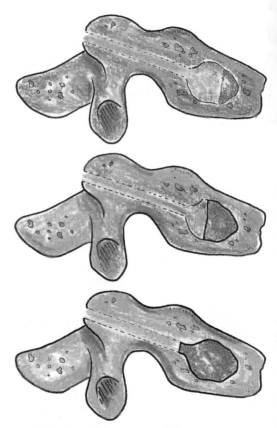

Fig. 2. Injection of bone cement (*red*) into the cavity formed by the SKy bone expander.

vertebral neural arch hemangioma using a technique termed pediculoplasty. Less common indications for vertebroplasty in such conditions as spinal pseudarthrosis, intravertebral vacuum phenomena (**Fig. 3**), Langerhans cell histiocytosis, osteogenesis imperfecta, and Paget's disease have also been reported.[48–53] Painful Schmorl nodes refractory to medical or physical therapy have been suggested as a new indication.[54]

Contraindications

Generally accepted contraindications to vertebroplasty are uncontrollable bleeding, unstable fracture due to posterior element involvement, lack of a definable level of vertebral collapse, infection, and a nonpainful fracture. Relative contraindications include patient inability to lie prone for the expected duration of the procedure, lack of surgical backup or patient monitoring facilities, and the presence of neurologic signs and symptoms caused by vertebral body collapse or tumor extension.[20,23] Multilevel vertebroplasty should be avoided in patients with low cardiopulmonary reserve (eg, chronic obstructive airways disease or

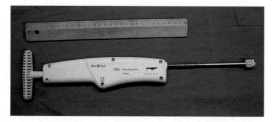

Fig. 1. SKy bone expander for cavity creation in skyphoplasty. The polymer has been compressed in an accordion fashion into a crenulated configuration.

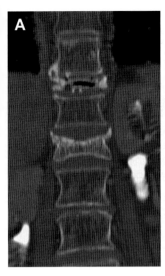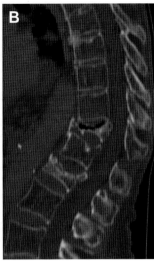

Fig. 3. Coronal (*A*) and sagittal (*B*) reconstructed CT images demonstrating two vertebral compression fractures. The superior fracture demonstrates greater height reduction and an intravertebral vacuum cleft. (*From* Heran MK, Legiehn GM, Munk PL. Current concepts and techniques in percutaneous vertebroplasty. Orthop Clin North Am 2006;37:411; with permission.)

congestive cardiac failure) as these patients may be at high risk for symptomatic pulmonary fat embolism.[55]

Vertebroplasty has been reported to be safely performed in patients with malignant compression fractures with epidural involvement and also in patients with spinal canal compromise.[56,57] Very severe vertebral compression fractures may be technically difficult to perform but are not a contraindication to the procedure.[58] Vertebroplasty for treatment of burst fractures has been reported.[59,60] Recently, vertebroplasty has been performed in patients with severe noncompression osteoporotic vertebral pain. These patients had MR imaging features of vertebral bone marrow edema, seen as T1-hypointense and T2-hyperintense signal changes. Vertebroplasty was found to be useful in treating these patients.[61] Vertebroplasty combined with pedicular instrumentation has been advocated for a selected group of osteoporotic and cancer patients with disabling back pain due to vertebral body osteolysis, microfractures, and compression fractures.[62]

PRELIMINARY ASSESSMENT

It is important to interview the patient and carefully review all the patient's clinical charts and radiological images. Radiographs show the degree of vertebral compression (**Fig. 4**), any osteolysis, extent

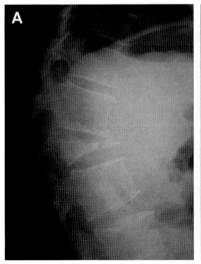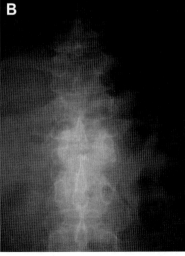

Fig. 4. Lateral (*A*) and frontal (*B*) radiographs demonstrate a focal kyphotic deformity about a severe vertebral compression fracture (vertebra plana). (*From* Heran MK, Legiehn GM, Munk PL. Current concepts and techniques in percutaneous vertebroplasty. Orthop Clin North Am 2006;37:413; with permission.)

of pedicle involvement, and fracture or cortical destruction. CT can be used to detect destruction of the vertebral body posterior cortical wall; to determine extension of bone tumor or retropulsion of bone fragment into the epidural space or intervertebral foramen; to assess the vertebral body shape;[18,19] to provide information about the pedicular size and presence of posterior element involvement; and to aid in estimating the needle path and size.[18–20]

Bone scintigraphy and MR imaging helps identify acute or healing fractures, particularly in patients with multiple levels of compression (ie, suitable sites for vertebroplasty).[63–65] Uemura and colleagues[66] found that vertebral body contrast enhancement during preprocedural MR imaging was indicative of a painful lesion and that extensive contrast enhancement predicted better pain relief after vertebroplasty. In patients with multiple compression fractures, MR imaging can be useful in selection of the one or two acute fractures. MR imaging also is excellent at showing the extent of marrow involvement by tumor (**Fig. 5**). Where MR imaging is not possible, such as in cases involving a pacemaker or a recently placed stent, bone scintiscan may show intense uptake at the site of acute or subacute fracture.[24] Most practitioners agree that a trial period of 6 to 12 weeks of conservative medical treatment should be instituted before vertebroplasty is considered.[20,67] Chronic fractures can also be treated using vertebroplasty, although complete relief of pain is more likely in treating less mature fractures.[68,69]

TECHNICAL CONSIDERATIONS

The American College of Radiology document *Standard for the Performance of Vertebroplasty* provides important information about this procedure and is highly recommended.[70] Although actual techniques vary among practitioners, depending on such factors as training, personal preference, and equipment availability, the basic principles for vertebroplasty are common to all. For thoracic and lumbar vertebroplasty, the patient is positioned prone or slightly prone oblique (**Fig. 6**). The patient's vital signs, such as blood pressure, EKG, heart rate, and pulse oximetry, are monitored continuously. A prophylactic broad-spectrum antibiotic is usually administered intravenously at the start of the procedure. Most patients receive intravenous sedatives and analgesics during the procedure.[20] Assisted sedation using continuous propofol infusion titrated to the patient's need has been found to be a safe and easy method for pain-free percutaneous vertebroplasty, with age being an important factor to titrate propofol dose.[71]

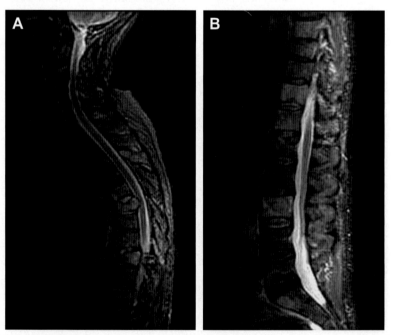

Fig. 5. (*A and B*) Sagittal short tau inversion recovery MR images demonstrating multiple vertebral metastases and pathologic compression fractures. (*From* Heran MK, Legiehn GM, Munk PL. Current concepts and techniques in percutaneous vertebroplasty. Orthop Clin North Am 2006;37:413; with permission.)

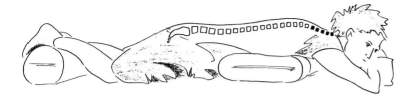

Fig. 6. Patient positioning for vertebroplasty. Padding flattens the spinal curvature while maximizing patient comfort. (*From* Heran MK, Legiehn GM, Munk PL. Current concepts and techniques in percutaneous vertebroplasty. Orthop Clin North Am 2006;37:415; with permission.)

The entire procedure should be performed under strict aseptic conditions. Biplane fluoroscopy or high-quality C-arm fluoroscopy is used for guiding the needle insertion. Biplane fluoroscopy is preferred because it requires less imaging time and makes possible simultaneous visualization in two orthogonal planes. An alternative is to use two C-arm fluoroscopes, which also allows simultaneous anteroposterior and lateral views while reducing procedure time.[72] CT fluoroscopy in combination with C-arm fluoroscopy has been described as an alternative technique.[5,9,73] Conventional fluoroscopy has the advantage of enabling visualization of the entire vertebral body area and adjacent tissues during injection for detecting early cement leakage, while CT fluoroscopy usually does not allow a large enough field of view to see this entire area. However, others have found CT-guided percutaneous vertebroplasty to be efficacious in treating patients with osteoporosis and malignancy. CT guidance reduces the risks of complications and facilitates the detection of small cement leakages.[73,74]

Local anesthetic is administered to the skin, subcutaneous tissues, and periosteum for both short- and longer-term pain relief. Many different types of needles and needle kits are commercially available. The needle set consists of a large bore needle, usually 10 to 13 gauge, together with one or more accompanying stylets (**Fig. 7**). A diamond-shaped multibeveled stylet can be used to penetrate the cortex and then used to enter the pedicle. Once the pedicle is traversed, this multibeveled needle can be replaced by a single-beveled stylet that allows some steering of the needle direction. Other practitioners prefer to use just a single diamond-shaped needle, as it is less expensive.[20] A unipedicular approach performed through an individualized needle insertion angle that had been evaluated using axial MR imaging before vertebroplasty has been described recently.[75]

Under imaging guidance, the needle is guided through the center of the pedicle and then into the vertebral body (**Fig. 8**). Some practitioners use a small orthopedic hammer to tap in the needle in an attempt to better control the needle insertion. Otherwise, the needle is inserted by hand using a clockwise turning motion. One major reason for using a hammer is to drive a needle through very hard bone, such as a treated metastatic vertebra.[20] To ensure that the needle is correctly positioned, it is important to frequently switch between the frontal and lateral projections during fluoroscopy. Using fluoroscopic control, the pedicle of interest is profiled over the superior, middle, or inferior portion of the vertebral body to be entered (**Fig. 9**). Once the needle has just entered the posterior cortex of the lamina and pedicle, the needle is stabilized and the C-arm then turned to the lateral position to profile the vertebral body of interest in a true lateral projection. The needle is then directed more carefully toward the vertebral body.[20] Once the needle reaches the posterior portion of the vertebral body, frontal fluoroscopy is used to verify that the medial pedicle cortex has not been traversed. Lateral fluoroscopy is then used to monitor advancement of this needle to the anterior vertebral body. Ideally, the needle tip should be placed in the anterior one-fourth to one-third of the vertebral body, as close as possible to the midline (**Fig. 10**). The needle tip is then checked for midline location in the frontal

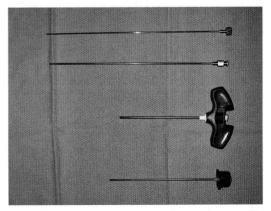

Fig. 7. Disassembled components of a standard needle/trocar unit used in vertebroplasty. 14-gauge biopsy needle set (top 2 objects). Vertebroplasty set (bottom 2 objects).

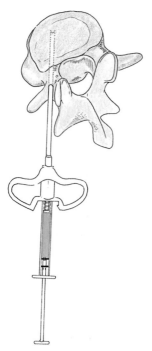

Fig. 8. A standard transpedicular puncture during vertebroplasty with a medial needle trajectory through the pedicle.

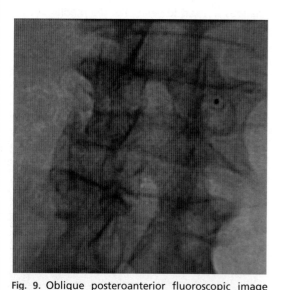

Fig. 9. Oblique posteroanterior fluoroscopic image demonstrating ideal pedicle visualization. The pedicle is seen en face projected over the vertebral body. Note the 22-gauge spinal needle, which has been passed to contact the periosteum of the superior portion of the pedicle. (*From* Heran MK, Legiehn GM, Munk PL. Current concepts and techniques in percutaneous vertebroplasty. Orthop Clin North Am 2006;37:416; with permission.)

position.[20] If biopsy is indicated, it can be performed with the stylet removed as the needle passes through the pedicle into the midthird of the vertebral body (ie, before the final needle position). Modification of the "bull's-eye" technique allows multiple biopsy cores to be taken from the same entry site, with the advantage of eliminating the need for additional needles. This technique also enables the largest cores to be obtained as the vertebroplasty needle is used, and not a smaller needle placed through the vertebroplasty needle.[76]

After the needle tip is positioned in the desired location, the stylet is removed. Intraosseous "blush" venography, using 0.5 to 1 mL of a nonionic contrast agent, may then be performed. Intraosseous venography helps determine whether the needle tip is positioned within a direct venous anastomosis to the central or epidural veins (**Fig. 11**). Intraosseous venography also shows vertebral segment vascularity and the site of the draining veins, hence providing additional information for planning and monitoring the injection of cement.[77] The practice of performing intraosseous venography during vertebroplasty is controversial with many authorities feeling it may have little value.[78–81]

There are various types of cement (methylmethacrylate powder) currently in use. These products differ in their polymerization times, and the practitioner performing the procedure should be very familiar with the polymerization times of the particular type of powder to be used. Opacification of the cement is required. For that, practitioners use tungsten, tantalum powder,[6,7,11] or commercially prepared sterile barium. The cost of obtaining sterile barium for vertebroplasty can be substantially reduced by in-hospital dry-heat sterilization.[82] Commercial preparations of cement with increased barium sulfate content specifically designed for use in vertebroplasty are on the market. Cortoss (Orthovita, Malvern, Pennsylvania) is a recently developed bisphenol-A–glycidyldimethacrylate resin. In a study of 34 patients with 42 vertebral lesions, Cortoss vertebroplasty has been found to provide comparable efficacy and safety to conventional PMM cement.[83] A liquid methylmethacrylate polymer is added to the powder and mixed to a toothpastelike consistency. To ensure a controlled cement injection, one method found to be cost-effective is the use of a reusable flange converter with a hub lock for injection in conjunction with a metallic screw-plunger device with a rubber tip taken from the plastic plunger of the 10-mL syringe.[84] The polymerization time of PMM cement can be extended by cooling the mixture in an iced bath of sodium chloride solution.[85]

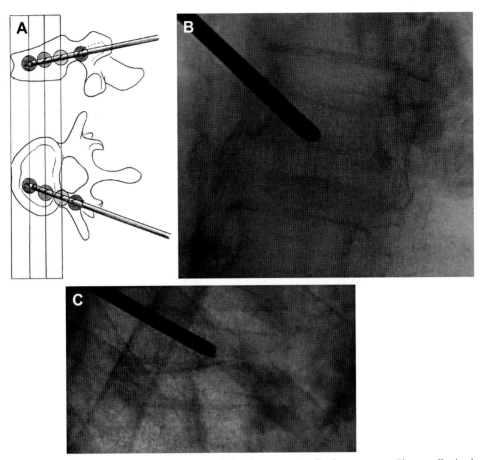

Fig. 10. (*A*) An ideal needle trajectory and endpoint following a transpedicular puncture. The needle tip should lie at the junction of the anterior and middle thirds of the vertebral body. (*B*) Posteroanterior and (*C*) lateral fluoroscopic images during vertebroplasty. The tip of the needle should be in the midline on the frontal projection and adjacent to the equatorial plane (above or below) on the lateral to minimize extravasation into the basivertebral venous plexus. (*From* Heran MK, Legiehn GM, Munk PL. Current concepts and techniques in percutaneous vertebroplasty. Orthop Clin North Am 2006;37:417; with permission.)

Lateral fluoroscopic imaging must be used to monitor the injection of PMM cement. Having a "last image hold" option on a second television screen allows early identification of any leakage and progression of cement toward the posterior vertebral wall.[20] Clinicians should look out for leakage into the surrounding soft tissue structures, particularly the veins and epidural space. If leakage occurs, pressure on the injecting syringe is released and the injection is stopped for 1 to 2 minutes to allow the cement to harden and plug the leak. Stoppage of injection for needle repositioning may also be necessary.[20] Otherwise, injection of cement is terminated when it reaches the posterior one-quarter of the vertebral body. Ideally, the cement column should extend between the superior and inferior endplates, and between both pedicles (**Fig. 12**). Such cement filling should help prevent later collapse of the treated vertebral body. If a fracture cleft is present, one should aim to fill the cleft with cement.[20]

Most practitioners aim to obtain satisfactory cement placement into the vertebral body using a single unipedicular approach, with advantages of reduced procedure time and decreased patient discomfort. If cement does not fill both sides of the vertebral body, the contralateral pedicle may need to be injected. It has been shown that there is no difference in clinical outcomes between the unipedicular and bipedicular approaches.[86] Bilateral pedicular needle placement may be necessary for optimal opacification of the H-shaped pattern of severe vertebral collapse.[58] Rarely, the paravertebral, parapedicular, or costovertebral approaches may be used for needle placement, especially if the pedicle is too small or too damaged for safe needle placement (**Fig. 13**). The safe performance of vertebroplasty through the

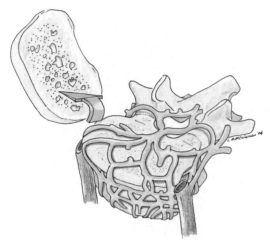

Fig. 11. The vertebral venous plexus. (*From* Heran MK, Legiehn GM, Munk PL. Current concepts and techniques in percutaneous vertebroplasty. Orthop Clin North Am 2006;37:421; with permission.)

osteolysed pedicle in metastatic disease has been described.[87] Transpedicle body augmenter vertebroplasty, using a porous titanium spacer, has been found to be safe and effective in patients with spinal tumors and avoids the possible dangers of cement leakage and tumor displacement into the spinal canal.[88] This method has also been shown to be useful in treating patients with painful osteoporotic compression fractures.[89] The intercostal approach has been used for the thoracic vertebra while the transoral route has

been described for C2 vertebra injection.[90–92] The percutaneous approach has been described for treatment of a C2 fracture due to multiple myeloma.[93] Vertebroplasty using a transdiscal route in a patient who had previously undergone transpedicular instrumentation has also been described.[94]

POTENTIAL HAZARDS

Adverse events and complications related to vertebroplasty and other vertebral augmentation procedures have been reported. However, fortunately, with meticulous technique and use of high-quality fluoroscopy, such events and complications are rare.

The complications of percutaneous vertebroplasty can be classified into those directly related to cement leakage from the vertebral body (**Fig. 14**) and those not due to cement leakage.[95] Cement leakage occurs frequently, with incidences of 30% to 72.5% on radiographs[6,7,9,13,14,58,96] and higher incidences of 87.9% to 93% on CT.[97,98] Cement leakage may track into various structures, such as the spinal canal, neural foramina, intervertebral disc, paravertebral soft tissues, and such vascular structures as the prevertebral veins, epidural veins, inferior vena cava, and aorta.[6,7,58,95,99] As cement leakage produces the main clinical complications of this procedure, special efforts should be made to avoid and prevent leaks. The vast majority of leaks seen are small, asymptomatic, and of no clinical consequence.

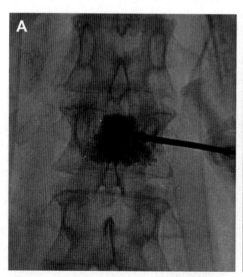
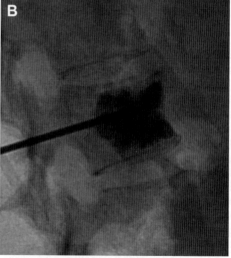

Fig. 12. (*A*) Posteroanterior and (*B*) lateral images during verteboplasty via a right transpedicular puncture demonstrating ideal cement distribution with opacification between the superior and inferior endplates and no cement within the posterior quarter of the vertebral body. (*From* Heran MK, Legiehn GM, Munk PL. Current concepts and techniques in percutaneous vertebroplasty. Orthop Clin North Am 2006;37:420; with permission.)

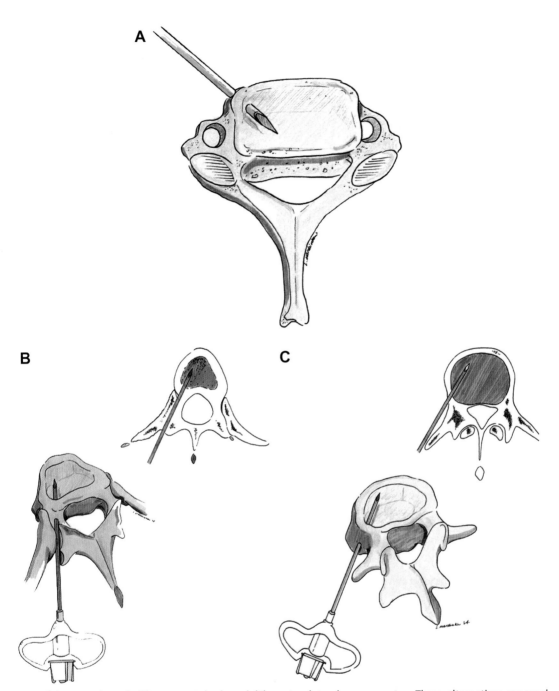

Fig. 13. (*A*) Anterolateral, (*B*) costovertebral, and (*C*) posterolateral access routes. These alternatives are used when transpedicular access is not feasible. (*From* Heran MK, Legiehn GM, Munk PL. Current concepts and techniques in percutaneous vertebroplasty. Orthop Clin North Am 2006;37:419; with permission.)

The most dreaded complication of percutaneous vertebroplasty is probably inadvertent cement extravasation into the spinal canal and neural foramina. This complication is often due to destruction of the posterior cortex of the vertebral body and of the medial or inferior cortex of the pedicle.[95,100,101] This complication may rarely necessitate emergency surgical decompression if clinical symptoms develop.[102,103] Cement leakage is less well tolerated in the narrow neural foramen than in the spinal canal.[6,7,15,95] For patients who develop radicular pain due to foraminal leakage, the immediate periradicular placement of a cooling system consisting of lidocaine followed by

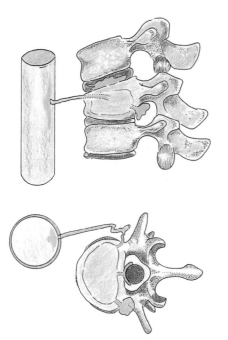

Fig. 14. Cement extravasation to the intervertebral disk, the neural exit foramina, and the epidural venous plexus. (*From* Heran MK, Legiehn GM, Munk PL. Current concepts and techniques in percutaneous vertebroplasty. Orthop Clin North Am 2006;37:424; with permission.)

pressurized saline perfusion may be needed. This is based on the reasoning that the resultant nerve root injury mechanism may be more related to heat or chemical irritation than compression.[104] Alternatively, steroid and local anesthetic may be injected adjacent to the cement and affected nerve.

Cement leakage into the adjacent paravertebral soft tissues is almost always asymptomatic, although transient femoral neuropathy related to cement leakage into the psoas muscle has been reported.[7,99] Most practitioners agree that leakage into the intervertebral disc, a frequent occurrence, is of no major clinical consequence (**Fig. 15**).[7,8,13,58] Using CT, Pitton and colleagues[105] found the incidence of intradiscal cement leak to be 55.6%. Jung and colleagues[106] found that the incidence of cement leakage in osteoporotic compression fractures with or without intravertebral clefts were similar, while Krauss and colleagues[107] found that patients with intravertebral clefts had a significantly lower risk of cement leakage during vertebroplasty. Deramond and colleagues[11] postulated that intradiscal leakage of PMM may have mechanical consequences on adjacent vertebrae, particularly those with osteoporosis. Lin and colleagues[108] have shown that leakage of PMM into the disc during vertebroplasty increases the risk of fracture of adjacent vertebral bodies. However, Pitton and colleagues[105] subsequently showed that the rates of secondary adjacent and nonadjacent fractures are quite similar, and that intradiscal leakages had no specific impact on the occurrence of adjacent secondary fractures.

Small perivertebral venous leakages are usually not clinically significant (**Fig. 16**).[10,11,13] Asymptomatic extension into the inferior vena cava may occur.[6,99] If the venous system is opacified by cement, vertebroplasty should be stopped because of the risk of massive pulmonary embolism.[10,11,16–18,65] Asymptomatic pulmonary embolization may occur in up to 4.0% to 6.8% of

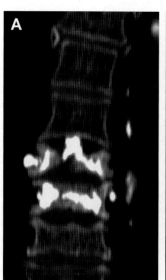
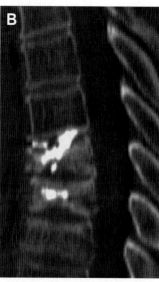

Fig. 15. (*A*) Coronal and (*B*) sagittal reconstructed CT images demonstrate cement extravasation into the intervertebral disk.

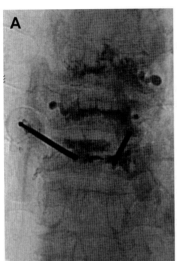 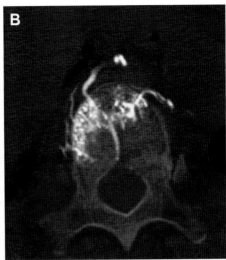

Fig. 16. (A) Posteroanterior fluoroscopic image and (B) axial CT image demonstrating numerous curvilinear regions of perivertebral venous contrast extravasation. (From Heran MK, Legiehn GM, Munk PL. Current concepts and techniques in percutaneous vertebroplasty. Orthop Clin North Am 2006;37:425; with permission.)

patients after vertebroplasty[109–112] Pulmonary embolectomy is one of the recommended treatment options for symptomatic cement embolization.[113–115] Paradoxical cerebral PMM embolism due to right-to-left shunt through a patent foramen ovale has been reported.[116] It has been shown in a cadaveric study that percutaneous vertebroplasty produces higher intravertebral pressures in vertebrae with simulated osteolytic metastasis, with the conclusion that the generated pressure is high enough to cause embolic phenomena.[117] Komemushi and colleagues[118] showed that carbon dioxide was frequently retained in the renal vein after the gas was injected into the vertebra during intraossoeus venography using carbon dioxide as a contrast agent. A rare complication of multiple cardiac perforations and pulmonary embolism caused by cement leakage after percutaneous vertebroplasty has recently been reported.[119] Local metastasis occurring in the needle track after vertebroplasty has also been reported.[120]

An increase in local pain and fever may occur following the procedure, but usually lasts less than 72 hours.[6,10] Postvertebroplasty secondary infection has been reported but should be preventable with a strictly aseptic technique and prophylactic antibiotics.[121] Epidural abscess developing as a complication of vertebroplasty, and requiring surgical drainage, has occurred.[122] The use of polymerase chain reaction has been used to diagnose the infecting organism in a patient who developed vertebral infection following vertebroplasty.[123] A case of life-threatening aortic aneurysm that occurred as a result of pyogenic spondylitis developing secondary to

vertebroplasty has been published. The patient underwent successful resection of all infected tissue with replacement of the descending thoracic aorta with a vascular graft.[124] For infected vertebroplasty, it is recommended that initial conservative management consists of needle biopsy and antibiotics. If this fails, then surgical debridement should be done to remove the infected tissue and cement, and to stabilize the spine.[125]

Vertebroplasty may be associated with a risk of adjacent vertebral body fracture although this remains an issue of debate and controversy.[126–129] The altered load transfer that results from increased stiffness due to the rigid cement fixation is thought to increase pressure on the adjacent intervertebral disc and vertebrae, thereby producing fractures.[130–133] Risk factors for development of new compression fractures in adjacent vertebrae include location at the thoracolumbar junction, shorter distance from treated vertebrae, and greater degree of height restoration.[134] These findings may have an impact on how percutaneous vertebroplasty should be approached. Maximal filling of the compressed vertebral body may not be necessary, with one study showing that only 2 mL of cement is sufficient for restoring vertebral body strength.[135] Vertebral body height increase after cement injection during vertebroplasty has also been documented.[136] Loss of height of multiple vertebrae leads to kyphosis. Therefore, restoration of height may help retard progressive kyphosis.[20]

Voormolen and colleagues[137] found that new vertebral compression fractures after vertebroplasty occurred in 24% of patients, with half of the new compression fractures occurring adjacent to the treated levels. The presence of two preexisting vertebral compression fractures was a risk factor for the development of a new vertebral compression fracture. New-onset fractures developing after vertebroplasty tended to occur in the inferior endplate of the vertebra immediately cephalad to the treated level.[138] Sandwich fractures, defined as fracture of an untreated vertebra between two vertebrae that had been previously augmented, have been found to occur with a 37.9% fracture rate in one study.[105] Uebelhart and colleagues[139] found that prophylatically performing vertebroplasty in a nonfractured vertebra located between two previously injected ones did not prevent its collapse.

Refractures of cemented vertebrae after vertebroplasty occurred in 63% of 98 osteoporotic patients in one recent study. Significant anterior vertebral height restoration increases the risk of subsequent fracture in cemented vertebrae.[140] New vertebral compression fractures have been found to be common in patients with a low body mass index, suggesting that osteoporosis is a mechanism of fracture. Increased risk of vertebral compression fractures has also been found to be associated with proximity to the treated vertebrae and greater kyphosis correction.[141] Maehara and colleagues[142] found that performing contrast-enhanced MR imaging after percutaneous vertebroplasty did not improve detection of new compression fractures of adjacent vertebrae. In a study of 30 patients with vertebral compression fractures caused by osteoporosis, it was found that a combination of high levels of bone resorption markers and normal levels of bone formation markers may be associated with increased risk of new recurrent fractures after percutaneous vertebroplasty.[143]

In 76 consecutive patients who underwent percutaneous vertebroplasty for osteoporotic compression fracture, it was found that, although cement distribution patterns did not significantly affect initial clinical response, a higher incidence of new compression fractures was seen in patients with treated vertebrae exhibiting a cleft pattern.[144] A retrospective study of 57 patients showed that a targeted exercise program after percutaneous vertebroplasty significantly decreased fracture recurrence. Refracture rates were also lower in the rehabilitation group compared with the vertebroplasty-only group.[145] In a review of the available data in the literature pertaining to whether or not vertebroplasty predisposes patients to additional vertebral fractures, Trout and Kallmes[146] concluded that there was no definite answer. They stated that all osteopenic patents with spontaneous vertebral fractures are at high risk of new fractures, with or without vertebroplasty and that the potential risk for new fractures should be discussed before vertebroplasty in all patients.

During percutaneous vertebroplasty, the PMM cement vapor levels measure 5 ppm per 1-hour procedure, compared with the recommended maximum exposure of 100 ppm over the course of an 8-hour workday.[147] Rare complications of PMM vapor cement exposure include coughing, increased airway resistance, sensitizing occupational asthma, and acute bronchospasm.[147,148] Using a ductless fume hood in well-ventilated surroundings has been recommended to reduce the exposure of medical workers who may be sensitive to PMM cement vapor.[148] Systemic reactions due to PMM cement during hip arthroplasty are well known.[149,150] Transient hypotension and acute respiratory distress syndrome have been reported in association with vertebroplasty.[151] Aebli and colleagues[152,153] found that potential cardiovascular complications may occur during multilevel vertebroplasty, and that deteriorating baseline mean arterial blood pressure was a consequence of vertebral body pressurization rather than a consequence of the use of PMM cement, and suggested placing a needle in the contralateral pedicle to decompress the vertebral body during PMM cement injection. However, in a retrospective review of their cases, Kaufmann and colleagues[154] did not find an association between PMM cement injection during percutaneous vertebroplasty and systemic cardiovascular derangement. General and specific techniques for avoiding or preventing complications have been extensively reviewed in the literature.[20,95,155,156]

The prolonged fluoroscopic exposures during vertebroplasty results in increased dosages of ionizing radiation.[157–160] Kruger and Faciszewski[157] evaluated the radiation dose to medical staff during vertebroplasty and highlighted the importance of knowing the basic principles of radiation physics and radiation protection. Mehdizade and colleagues[158] measured radiation doses to the hands, finding that they received greater exposure than expected from traditional apron measurements. Kallmes and colleagues[159] found that using an injection device decreased the radiation dose to the practitioner's hands per unit time of injection but total dose per injection was equivalent between using 1-mL syringes and injection devices because of the longer injection duration when using injection devices. Perisinakis and colleagues[160] studied patients who underwent vertebroplasty or kyphoplasty, produced data about patient radiation exposure and associated risks, and concluded that these risks may be considerable. The highest dose rates recorded during vertebroplasty have been found for the primary operator's hand and chest when no shielding is used. Occupational dose has been found to be reduced by 76% using mobile shielding.[161] Synowitz and Kiwit[162] also found that a 75% reduction rate of radiation exposure to the operator hands can be achieved by lead glove protection. Stress needs to be placed on the importance of adequate training for fluoroscopy and careful attention to the exposure parameters, such as collimation, pulsed fluoroscopy, and last frame hold. Practitioners should also understand the risks of acute (deterministic) and late (stochastic) radiation effects to patients. Such devices as the dose-area product meter are recommended, with periodic maintenance and calibration of fluoroscopy equipment. Medical physicists have a vital role in establishing guidelines and procedures for determining patient dose during vertebroplasty.[163]

CLINICAL OUTCOME

Following vertebroplasty, pain relief and increased mobility are expected within 24 hours.[10,22] Significant pain relief is expected in more than 70% of patients with vertebral malignancies,[6,7,45,164,165] in more than 90% of patients with osteoporotic fractures,[9,11,13,15,22,75,164,166] and in 80% of patients with hemangioma.[10,11,164] Percutaneous vertebroplasty has been found to be effective among patients older than 80 years suffering spinal pain due to vertebral fractures, regardless of etiology.[167] In the majority of cases, benefits of the procedure include reduction in the amount of medication needed for pain relief, improved physical mobility, and better quality of life.[14,23,68,69,167–174] The reduction of analgesic requirement may, however, not be as great in patients who require narcotics preprocedure and in those who have older fractures.[68] McDonald and colleagues[45] showed that patients with multiple myeloma required less narcotics after vertebroplasty. Studies assessing the mid- and long-term effects, with follow-up of up to 48 months, have shown that postvertebroplasty pain relief is sustained.[96,112,126,127,129,167,169,175]

Dublin and colleagues[176] studied 40 vertebral compression fractures in 20 consecutive patients, and found that percutaneous vertebroplasty was not only useful in pain relief, but was also an effective method for improving vertebral body height, kyphosis angle, and wedge angle. These investigators found that vertebral body height improvement was comparable to that achieved by kyphoplasty. In a study evaluating 102 vertebral bodies in 40 patients over a 1-year period,

vertebroplasty provided vertebral height gain over 1 year, particularly in cases with severe compression. Vertebrae with moderate compression were fixed and stabilized at the pretreatment level over 1 year.[177] However, Chang and colleagues[178] found that the increase in height and wedge angle of the treated vertebral bodies was lost 1 year after vertebroplasty because of new fractures developing in 48% of these patients. Compared to those without a intravertebral cleft, patients with intravertebral clefts show a significant reduction in the kyphosis angle and have a significantly lower risk of cement leakage during vertebroplasty.[107] Repeat percutaneous vertebroplasty has been found to be effective at the same vertebral levels in patients without pain relief who underwent previous vertebroplasty. Absent or inadequate filling of cement in the unstable fractured areas of the vertebral body may be responsible for the unrelieved pain after the initial vertebroplasty.[179] Multilevel (more than four levels) vertebroplasty has been shown to be useful for providing pain relief in elderly patients with osteoporotic fractures.[180]

An evidence-based assessment study of percutaneous vertebroplasty has shown that the costs for this procedure are relatively low compared with open surgical interventions for vertebral compression fractures.[181] There have been many calls for well-designed randomized, controlled trials to demonstrate the efficacy of this procedure and to show that it has a significantly better outcome than other treatment options.[182–185] Wagner[186] has argued, however, that, based on existing data on vertebroplasty in medically refractory osteoporotic vertebral compression fractures, a true, long-term, randomized double-blind study does not seem necessary or ethically justifiable. Nevertheless, two multicenter randomized, controlled trials have been planned, one to assess the cost-effectiveness of vertebroplasty compared with conservative treatment in patients with an acute osteoporotic compression fractures,[187] and the other to compare vertebroplasty with a controlled intervention.[188] Preliminary findings of the first randomized, controlled trial comparing vertebroplasty with optimal pain medication treatment has shown that vertebroplasty is significantly better in terms of pain relief and improved mobility, function, and stature in the short term.[189] Practitioners of vertebroplasty and researchers in this and related fields should continue monitoring the progress of patients undergoing this procedure, report all adverse effects, study the biomechanical effects of the procedure, and conduct audit studies and long-term clinical trials.[20]

KYPHOPLASTY

Kyphoplasty was developed to correct or prevent the resultant kyphotic deformity resulting from vertebral compression fractures, and to restore vertebral body height, in addition to reducing or eliminating pain. This procedure entails percutaneously inserting a balloonlike device known as a balloon tamp into the compressed vertebral body via an 8-gauge cannula (**Fig. 17**) and inflating the device. This elevates the vertebral endplates, restores the vertebral body height, and creates a cavity into which cement is injected.[27–37] The device, the KyphX inflatable bone tamp (Kyphon, Sunnyvale, California) (**Fig. 18**), has been approved by the US Food and Drug Administration for use as a bone tamp for reducing fractures and for creating voids in cancellous bone. The selection and exclusion criteria for patients to undergo kyphoplasty are similar to those for vertebroplasty.[190] The kyphoplasty technique is also similar except that in kyphoplasty, after insertion of the cannula into the posterior aspect of the vertebral body, a drill is introduced to make a channel through which the deflated balloon is inserted. The balloon is then inflated with radio-opaque contrast agent, with continuous control of pressure and volume. After creation of a cavity by the balloon tamp, together with partial or full restoration of the vertebral body height and correction of the kyphotic deformity, the balloon is retracted and cement is injected using a blunt cannula (**Fig. 19**).[190]

An advocated advantage of kyphoplasty is restoration of vertebral body height.[27,30,32,191–194] Short-term results (of up to 18 months follow-up)

have shown that kyphoplasty produces good to moderate pain relief in 83% to 100% of patients.[30,32,193,195–198] Like vertebroplasty, the complications of kyphoplasty are most commonly related to incorrect placement of hardware or cement extravasation, including neurologic complications.[199–201] Similar to vertebroplasty, postkyphoplasty patients who develop neurologic deficits may require revision open surgical intervention.[202] The incidence of cement extravasation during kyphoplasty has been reported to be 8.6% to 33%.[27,29,30,33,192,193,197] Reasons for decreased cement extravasation during kyphoplasty include (1) balloon tamping of a cavity that is surrounded by a shell of impacted cancellous bone, (2) ability to determine amount of cement to be injected because of prior knowledge of the volume of fluid used to inflate the balloon, and (3) lower injection pressure during cement injection.[36,203] The development of new fractures subsequent to kyphoplasty has also been reported.[30,193,204,205] Meta-analyses of clinical studies have shown kyphoplasty to be better than medical management in reducing pain intensity and increasing mobility in patients with vertebral compression fractures.[194,206]

Both vertebroplasty and kyphoplasty are similarly effective and safe in the treatment of severely painful osteoporotic vertebral fractures. Kyphoplasty has not been shown to be better than vertebroplasty in terms of pain relief or quality of life.[207,208] In a meta-analysis of 14 vertebroplasty and 7 kyphoplasty studies representing totals of 1046 vertebroplasty and 263 kyphoplasty patients treated, Gill and colleagues[209] showed that both procedures reduce pain in symptomatic

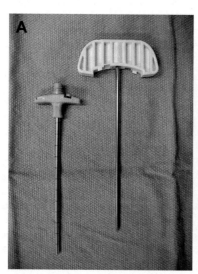
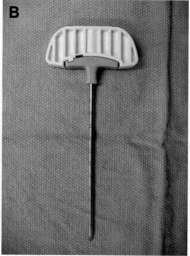

Fig. 17. (*A*) Disassembled and (*B*) assembled components of the needle system used in kyphoplasty.

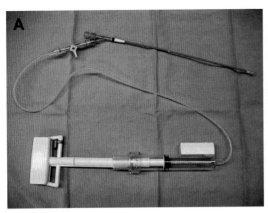
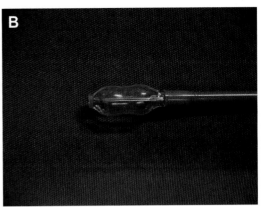

Fig. 18. Components of the KyphX inflatable bone tamp with the balloon deflated (*A*) and inflated (*B*).

osteoporotic compression fractures that have failed conservative treatment, with no difference between the two procedures. In a systematic review and metaregression study, Taylor and colleagues[210] found kyphoplasty and vertebroplasty to be effective in the management of patients with symptomatic compression fractures refractory to conventional medical therapy. There have been calls for a randomized, double-blind trial comparing vertebroplasty and kyphoplasty.[207,209–211]

In a meta-analysis of the literature, Eck and colleagues[212] found that the risk of new fracture for kyphoplasty is 14.1%, similar to the 17.9% for vertebroplasty. Hulme and colleagues,[211] in a systematic literature review, found that pain relief occurred in 87% of patients who had

vertebroplasty and 92% of patients who underwent kyphoplasty. Both had similar amounts of vertebral height restoration, while cement leaks occurred in 41% of treated vertebrae for vertebroplasty and 9% of treated vertebrae for kyphoplasty. In a meta-analysis of the literature, Eck and colleagues[212] found that, although both methods provided significant improvement in visual analog scale pain scores, there was a statistically greater improvement in pain relief with vertebroplasty compared with kyphoplasty. The risk of cement leakage was 19.7% for vertebroplasty versus 7.0% with kyphoplasty. In both of these studies, cement leaks were found to be nonsymptomatic. Cloft and Jensen[213] reviewed the literature and concluded that there was no proven advantage of kyphoplasty over vertebroplasty

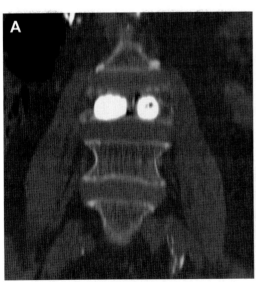
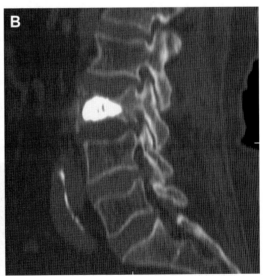

Fig. 19. (*A*) Coronal and (*B*) sagittal CT reconstructions postkyphoplasty demonstrating cement distributed within cavities formed bilaterally within the vertebral body. Despite marked pain relief, no vertebral body height restoration or kyphotic angle correction resulted.

with regard to pain relief, vertebral height restoration, and complication rate. Mathis[208] stated that the claims of superior height restoration by kyphoplasty have not been well substantiated. De Negri and colleagues[214] found, in a prospective non-randomized controlled study, that both vertebroplasty and kyphoplasty offered therapeutic benefit in significantly reducing pain and improving mobility in patients with vertebral fractures, but there was no significant difference between the groups in terms of therapeutic outcome. Kyphoplasty has been estimated to be approximately 2.5 to seven times more expensive than vertebroplasty per vertebra treated, due to additional equipment, general anesthesia, and hospital costs.[213] Based on available data in 2006, Mathis found no substantial scientific or procedural advantage to kyphoplasty that warrants its high cost compared with vertebroplasty.[208]

SKYPHOPLASTY

A third method for percutaneous cement augmentation of the spine is skyphoplasty. It uses a device is also known as the SKy bone expander (Disc Orthopaedic Technology/Disc-O-Tech, Monroe Township, New Jersey). This device shares some similarities with the kyphoplasty device in that it is percutaneously introduced and is used to create a cavity inside the targeted vertebral body. The system is introduced into the vertebra through an 8-gauge cannula, the same size cannula as that used with kyphoplasty. However, the diameter of the skyphoplasty device is slightly larger than that of the kyphoplasty device (**Fig. 20**). This cannula can be introduced with an over-the-guide-wire system or a direct single-step system. Rather than using an inflatable balloon, a stiff plastic tube is deployed through the cannula, placed inside the vertebral body and compressed in an accordion

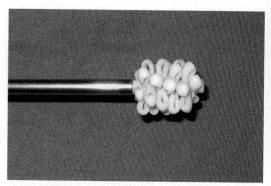

Fig. 21. Popcornlike crenulated configuration of the stiff polymer unit of the SKy bone expander.

fashion into a popcornlike crenulated configuration, thereby creating a cavity (**Fig. 21**). In some instances, elevation of depressed fragments occurs, allowing for some height restoration. The device is then removed and the cavity is filled with cement using a cement application device similar to that employed in kyphoplasty (**Fig. 22**). This device at present come in only two sizes, one with a 14-mm diameter and the other with a 16-mm diameter. Unlike the device used in kyphoplasty, the skyphoplasty device cannot be repositioned once it has been deployed and the device can only be used once. It is, however, capable of creating higher pressures than those created by the kyphoplasty system and has a readily predictable direction and extent of expansion. Compared to the balloon used in kyphoplasty, the plastic configuration used in skyphoplasty is less dependent on the character of bone and expands in a more predictable fashion. The skyphoplasty device is somewhat longer than that used for vertebroplasty or kyphoplasty, which at times may make fluoroscopy awkward. The manufacturer is currently redesigning the system to correct this problem.

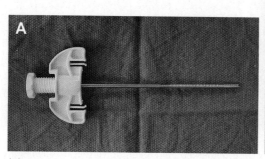

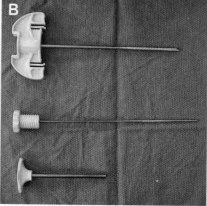

Fig. 20. (A) Assembled and (B) disassembled cannula system used in skyphoplasty.

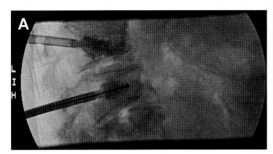
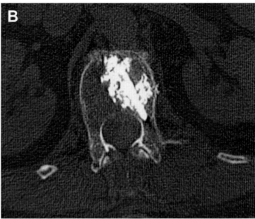

Fig. 22. (*A*) Lateral fluoroscopic image during skyphoplasty demonstrating the deployed stiff polymer (*lower vertebra*) and cement distribution postinjection following removal of the SKy bone expander unit with the bone cannula in place (*upper vertebra*). (*B*) Axial CT image demonstrating typical intravertebral cement distribution postskyphoplasty.

Depending on the size of the vertebral body, a single device may be all that is required to treat a single vertebra. In those instances, a single pedicle access is adequate. The system can also be deployed more rapidly than the Kyphon system, but has the disadvantage of not being reconstrainable for redeployment if repositioning is required or if an additional level needs to be treated.

Skyphoplasty has seen only limited use in the United States, in part because of issues of potential patent infringements by the SKy bone system on Kyphon patents. The system is, however, available in other parts of the world, including Western Europe and Canada. Experience with skyphoplasty is relatively limited and little has appeared in the literature. Tong and colleagues[215] performed skyphoplasty at 12 vertebral levels in 9 patients, and found the SKy bone expander device to be effective and safe in alleviating pain from vertebral compression fractures. Foo and colleagues,[216] in their series of 40 single-level SKy bone expander skyphoplasties in 40 patients, found the procedure to be viable alternative to balloon kyphoplasty. They reported 3 cases of cement extravasation and 1 case in which the SKy bone expander could not be withdrawn from the vertebral body and had to be left in situ. From the published material as well as personal experience and contact with others performing this procedure, it would appear that pain relief using this device is similar to that from vertebroplasty and kyphoplasty. Further experience and studies are ongoing.

SUMMARY

Percutaneous vertebroplasty is a safe, inexpensive, and effective interventional vertebral augmentation technique that provides pain relief and stabilization in carefully selected patients with severe back pain due to vertebral compression. These lesions include osteoporotic fractures, hemangiomas, and pathologic fractures due to malignancy that are not responsive to conservative measures. Adhering to the appropriate indications and recognizing the contraindications to the procedure are important. Complications occur rarely, but can be devastating. They are, however, avoidable with application of a meticulous technique. Percutaneous vertebroplasty has a role in the management pathway of patients presenting with painful vertebral compression fractures. Kyphoplasty uses a balloon tamp to restore vertebral body height, correct kyphotic deformity, and create a cavity into which bone cement is injected. Kyphoplasty is as effective and safe as vertebroplasty in treatment of painful vertebral compression fractures. Skyphoplasty, a modification of kyphoplasty, is a promising new technique.

REFERENCES

1. Galibert P, Deramond H, Rosat P, et al. A method for certain spinal angiomas: percutaneous vertebroplasty with acrylic cement. Neurochirurgie 1987;33:166–8.
2. Deramond H, Darrasson R, Galibert P. Percutaneous vertebroplasty with acrylic cement in the treatment of aggressive spinal angiomas. Rachis 1989; 1:143–53.
3. Kaemmerlen P, Thiesse P, Jonas P, et al. Percutaneous injection of orthopedic cement in metastatic vertebral lesions. N Engl J Med 1989;321:121.
4. Debussche-Depriester C, Deramond H, Fardellone P, et al. Percutaneous vertebroplasty

with acrylic cement in the treatment of osteoporotic vertebral crush fracture syndrome. Neuroradiology 1991;33(Suppl):149–52.

5. Gangi A, Kastler B, Dietemann JL. Percutaneous vertebroplasty guided by a combination of CT and fluoroscopy. AJNR Am J Neuroradiol 1994;15:83–6.

6. Weill A, Chiras J, Simon JM, et al. Spinal metastases: indications for and results of percutaneous injection of acrylic surgical cement. Radiology 1996;199:241–7.

7. Cotten A, Dewatre F, Cortet B, et al. Percutaneous vertebroplasty for osteolytic metastases and myeloma: effects of the percentage of lesion filling and the leakage of methyl methacrylate at clinical follow-up. Radiology 1996;200:525–30.

8. Deramond H, Depriester C, Toussaint P, et al. Percutaneous vertebroplasty. Semin Musculoskelet Radiol 1997;1:285–95.

9. Jensen ME, Evans AJ, Mathis JM, et al. Percutaneous polymethylmethacrylate vertebroplasty in the treatment of osteoporotic vertebral body compression fractures: technical aspects. AJNR Am J Neuroradiol 1997;18:1897–904.

10. Cotten A, Boutry N, Cortet B, et al. Percutaneous vertebroplasty: state of the art. Radiographics 1998;18:311–20.

11. Deramond H, Depriester C, Galibert P, et al. Percutaneous vertebroplasty with polymethylmethacrylate: technique, indications, and results. Radiol Clin North Am 1998;36:533–46.

12. Mathis MJ, Petri M, Naff N. Percutaneous vertebroplasty treatment of steroid-induced osteoporotic compression fractures. Arthritis Rheum 1998;41:171–5.

13. Cyteval C, Sarrabere MP, Roux JO, et al. Acute osteoporotic vertebral collapse: open study on percutaneous injection of acrylic surgical cement in 20 patients. AJR Am J Roentgenol 1999;173:1685–90.

14. Cortet B, Cotten A, Boutry N, et al. Percutaneous vertebroplasty in the treatment of osteoporotic vertebral compression fractures: an open prospective study. J Rheumatol 1999;26:2222–8.

15. Barr JD, Barr MS, Lemley TJ, et al. Percutaneous vertebroplasty for pain relief and spinal stabilization. Spine 2000;25:923–8.

16. Murphy KJ, Deramond H. Percutaneous vertebroplasty in benign and malignant disease. Neuroimaging Clin N Am 2000;10:535–45.

17. Jensen ME, Dion JE. Percutaneous vertebroplasty in the treatment of osteoporotic compression fractures. Neuroimaging Clin N Am 2000;10:547–68.

18. Peh WCG, Gilula LA. Percutaneous vertebroplasty: indications, contraindications, and technique. Br J Radiol 2002;76:69–75.

19. Kallmes DF, Jensen ME. Percutaneous vertebroplasty. Radiology 2003;229:27–36.

20. Peh WCG, Gilula LA. Percutaneous vertebroplasty: an update. Semin Ultrasound CT MR 2005;26:62–4.

21. Heran MK, Legiehn GM, Munk PL. Current concepts and techniques in percutaneous vertebroplasty. Orthop Clin North Am 2006;37:409–34.

22. Afzal S, Dhar S, Vasavada NB, et al. Percutaneous vertebroplasty for osteoporotic fractures. Pain Physician 2007;10:559–63.

23. Banerjee S, Baerlocher MO, Asch MR. Back stab. Percutaneous vertebroplasty for severe back pain. Can Fam Physician 2007;53:1169–75.

24. Syed MI, Shaikh A. Vertebroplasty: a systematic approach. Pain Physician 2007;10:367–80.

25. Melton LJ 3rd. Epidemiology of spinal osteoporosis. Spine 1997;22(Suppl 24):S2–11.

26. Morrison WB, Parker L, Frangos AJ, et al. Vertebroplasty in the United States: guidance method and provider distribution, 2001–2003. Radiology 2007;243:166–70.

27. Lieberman IH, Dudeney S, Reinhardt MK, et al. Initial outcome and efficacy of "kyphoplasty" in the treatment of painful osteoporotic vertebral compression fractures. Spine 2001;26:631–8.

28. Coumans JV, Reinhardt MK, Lieberman IH. Kyphoplasty for vertebral compression fractures: 1-year clinical outcomes from a prospective study. J Neurosurg 2003;99(Suppl 1):44–50.

29. Ledlie JT, Renfro M. Balloon kyphoplasty: one-year outcomes in vertebral body height restoration, chronic pain, and activity levels. J Neurosurg 2003;98(Suppl 1):36–42.

30. Phillips FM, Ho E, Campbell-Hupp M, et al. Early radiographic and clinical results of balloon kyphoplasty for the treatment of osteoporotic vertebral compression fractures. Spine 2003;28:2260–5.

31. Rao RD, Singrakhia MD. Painful osteoporotic vertebral fracture. Pathogenesis, evaluation, and roles of vertebroplasty and kyphoplasty in its management. J Bone Joint Surg Am 2003;85:2010–22.

32. Crandall D, Slaughter D, Hankins PJ, et al. Acute versus chronic compression fractures treated with kyphoplasty: early results. Spine J 2004;4:418–24.

33. Heini PF, Orler R. Kyphoplasty for treatment of osteoporotic vertebral fractures. Eur Spine J 2004;13:184–92.

34. Masala S, Fiori R, Massari F, et al. Kyphoplasty: indications, contraindications and technique. Radiol Med (Torino) 2005;110:97–105.

35. Karlsson MK, Hasserius R, Gerdhem P, et al. Vertebroplasty and kyphoplasty. New treatment strategies for fractures in the osteoporotic spine. Acta Orthop 2005;76:620–7.

36. Shen MS, Kim YH. Vertebroplasty and kyphoplasty. Treatment techniques for managing osteoporotic vertebral compression fractures. Bull NYU Hosp Jt Dis 2006;64:106–13.

37. Ledlie JT, Renfro MB. Kyphoplasty treatment of vertebroplasty fractures: 2-year outcomes show sustained benefits. Spine 2006;31:57–64.

38. Hide IG, Gangi A. Percutaneous vertebroplasty: history, technique and current perspectives. Clin Radiol 2004;59:461–7.

39. Cortet B, Cotten A, Deprex X, et al. Vertebroplasty with surgical decompression for the treatment of aggressive vertebral hemangiomas. Rev Rhum Engl Ed 1994;61:14–20.

40. Cotten A, Deramond H, Cortet B, et al. Preoperative percutaneous injection of methylmethacrylate and N-butyl cyanoacrylate in vertebral hemangiomas. AJNR Am J Neuroradiol 1996;17:137–42.

41. Ide C, Gangi A, Rimmelin A, et al. Vertebral haemangiomas with spinal cord compression: the place of preoperative percutaneous vertebroplasty with methyl methacrylate. Neuroradiology 1996;38: 585–9.

42. Feydy A, Cognard C, Miaux Y, et al. Acrylic vertebroplasty in symptomatic cervical vertebral hemangiomas: report of 2 cases. Neuroradiology 1996;38: 389–91.

43. Zapalowicz K, Radek A, Blaszczyk B, et al. Percutaneous vertebroplasty with methyl methacrylate bone cement in the treatment of spinal angiomas and neoplasms. Ortop Traumatol Rehabil 2003;5: 185–8.

44. Acosta FL, Sanai N, Chi JH, et al. Comprehensive management of symptomatic and aggressive vertebral hemangiomas. Neurosurg Clin N Am 2008; 19:17–29.

45. McDonald RJ, Trout AT, Gray LA, et al. Vertebroplasty in multiple myeloma: outcomes in a large patient series. AJNR Am J Neuroradiol 2008;29:642–8.

46. Pflugmacher R, Schleicher P, Schroder RJ, et al. Maintained pain reduction in five patients with multiple myeloma 12 months after treatment of the involved cervical vertebrae with vertebroplasty. Acta Radiol 2006;47:823–9.

47. Fuwa S, Numaguchi Y, Kobayashi N, et al. Percutaneous pediculoplasty for vertebral hemangioma involving the neural arch: a case report. Cardiovasc Intervent Radiol 2008;31:189–91.

48. Peh WCG, Gelbert MS, Gilula LA, et al. Percutaneous vertebroplasty: treatment of painful vertebral compression fractures with intraosseous vacuum phenomena. AJR Am J Roentgenol 2003;180: 1411–7.

49. Jang JS, Kim DY, Lee SH. Efficacy of percutaneous vertebroplasty in the treatment of intravertebral pseudarthrosis associated with noninfected avascular necrosis of the vertebral body. Spine 2003; 28:1588–92.

50. Cardon T, Hachulla E, Filpo RM, et al. Percutaneous vertebroplasty with acrylic cement in the treatment of a Langerhans cell vertebral histiocytosis. Clin Rheumatol 1994;13:518–21.

51. Rami PM, McGraw JK, Heatwole EV, et al. Percutaneous vertebroplasty in the treatment of vertebral body compression fracture secondary to osteogenesis imperfecta. Skeletal Radiol 2002; 31:162–5.

52. Kremer MA, Fruin A, Larson TC III, et al. Vertebroplasty in focal Paget disease of the spine. Case report. J Neurosurg Spine 2003;99:110–3.

53. Tancioni F, Di Ieva A, Levi D, et al. Spinal decompression and vertebroplasty in Paget's disease of the spine. Surg Neurol 2006;66:189–91.

54. Masala S, Pipitone V, Tomassini M, et al. Percutaneous vertebroplasty in painful Schmorl nodes. Cardiovasc Intervent Radiol 2006;29:97–101.

55. Syed MI, Jan S, Patel NA, et al. Fatal fat embolism after vertebroplasty: identification of the high risk patient. AJNR Am J Neuroradiol 2006;27:343–5.

56. Shimony JS, Gilula LA, Zeller AJ, et al. Percutaneous vertebroplasty for malignant compression fractures with epidural involvement. Radiology 2004; 232:846–53.

57. Appel NB, Gilula LA. Percutaneous vertebroplasty in patients with spinal canal compromise. AJR Am J Roentgenol 2004;182:947–51.

58. Peh WCG, Gilula LA, Peck DD. Percutaneous vertebroplasty for severe osteoporotic vertebral body compression fractures. Radiology 2002;223: 121–6.

59. Cho DY, Lee WY, Sheu PC. Treatment of thoracolumbar burst fractures with polymethyl methacrylate vertebroplasty and short-segment pedicle screw fixation. Neurosurgery 2003;53:1354–60.

60. Chen JF, Wu CT, Lee ST. Percutaneous vertebroplasty for the treatment of burst fracture: case report. J Neurosurg Spine 2004;1:228–31.

61. Yang X, Mi S, Mahadevia AA, et al. Pain reduction in osteoporotic patients with vertebral pain without measurable compression. Neuroradiology 2008; 50:153–9.

62. Wenger M, Markwalder TM. Vertebroplasty combined with pedicular instrumentation. J Clin Neurosci 2008;15:257–62.

63. Maynard AS, Jensen ME, Schweickert PA, et al. Value of bone scan imaging in predicting pain relief from percutaneous vertebroplasty in osteoporotic vertebral fractures. AJNR Am J Neuroradiol 2000; 21:1807–12.

64. Do HM. Magnetic resonance imaging in the evaluation of patients for percutaneous vertebroplasty. Top Magn Reson Imaging 2000;11:235–44.

65. Mathis JM, Barr JD, Belkoff SM, et al. Percutaneous vertebroplasty: a developing standard of care for vertebral compression fractures. AJNR Am J Neuroradiol 2001;22:373–81.

66. Uemura A, Kobayashi N, Numaguchi Y, et al. Pre-procedural MR imaging for percutaneous vertebroplasty: special interest in contrast enhancement. Radiat Med 2007;25:325–8.

67. Kim DH, Vaccaro AR. Osteoporotic compression fractures of the spine: current options and considerations for treatment. Spine J 2006;6:479–87.

68. Kaufmann TJ, Jensen ME, Schweickert PA, et al. Age of fracture and clinical outcomes of percutaneous vertebroplasty. AJNR Am J Neuroradiol 2001; 22:1860–3.

69. Brown DB, Gilula LA, Sehgal M, et al. Treatment of chronic symptomatic vertebral compression fractures with percutaneous vertebroplasty. AJR Am J Roentgenol 2004;182:319–22.

70. Barr JD, Mathis JM, Barr MS, et al. Standard for the performance of percutaneous vertebroplasty. In: American college of radiology standards 2000–2001. Reston (VA): American College of Radiology; 2000. p. 441–8.

71. Della Puppa A, Andreula C, Frass M. Assisted sedation: a safe and easy method for pain-free percutaneous vertebroplasty. Minerva Anestesiol 2008;74: 57–62.

72. Li YY, Hsu RW, Cheng CC, et al. Minimally invasive vertebroplasty managed by a two C-arm fluoroscopic technique. Minim Invasive Ther Allied Technol 2007;16:350–4.

73. Caudana R, Brivio LR, Ventura L, et al. CT-guided percutaneous vertebroplasty: personal experience in the treatment of osteoporotic fractures and dorsolumbar metastases. Radiol Med (Torino) 2008; 113:114–33.

74. Vogl TJ, Proschek D, Schwarz W, et al. CT-guided percutaneous vertebroplasty in the therapy of vertebral compression fractures. Eur Radiol 2006;16: 797–803.

75. Chang WS, Lee SH, Choi WG, et al. Unipedicular vertebroplasty for osteoporotic compression fracture using an individualized needle insertion angle. Clin J Pain 2007;23:767–73.

76. Appel NB, Gilula LA. "Bull's-eye" modification for transpedicular biopsy and vertebroplasty. AJR Am J Roentgenol 2001;177:1387–9.

77. Peh WCG, Gilula LA. Additional value of a modified method of intraosseous venography during percutaneous vertebroplasty. AJR Am J Roentgenol 2003;180:87–91.

78. McGraw JK, Heatwole EV, Strnad BT, et al. Predictive value of intraosseous venography before percutaneous vertebroplasty. J Vasc Interv Radiol 2003;13:149–53.

79. Gaughen JR Jr, Jensen ME, Schweickert PA, et al. Relevance of antecedent venography in percutaneous vertebroplasty for the treatment of osteoporotic compression fractures. AJNR Am J Neuroradiol 2002;23:594–600.

80. Vasconcelos C, Gailloud P, Beauchamp NJ, et al. Is percutaneous vertebroplasty without pretreatment venography safe? Evaluation of 205 consecutive procedures. AJNR Am J Neuroradiol 2002;23: 913–7.

81. Ormsby EL, Dublin AB. Value of the vertebrogram in predicting cement filling patterns with unipedicular percutaneous vertebroplasty. Acta Radiol 2008; 49:344–50.

82. Leibold RA, Gilula LA. Sterilization of barium for vertebroplasty: an effective, reliable, and inexpensive method to sterilize powders for surgical procedures. AJR Am J Roentgenol 2002;179:198–200.

83. Middleton ET, Rajaraman CJ, O'Brien DP, et al. The safety and efficacy of vertebroplasty using Cortoss cement in a newly established vertebroplasty service. Br J Neurosurg 2008;22:252–6.

84. Schallen EH, Gilula LA. Vertebroplasty: reusable flange converter with hub lock for injection of polymethylmethacrylate with screw-plunger syringe. Radiology 2002;222:851–5.

85. Chavali R, Resijek R, Knight SK, et al. Extending polymerization time of polymethylmethacrylate cement in percutaneous vertebroplasty with ice bath cooling. AJNR Am J Neuroradiol 2003;24: 545–6.

86. Kim AK, Jensen ME, Dion JE, et al. Unilateral transpedicular percutaneous vertebroplasty: initial experience. Radiology 2002;222:737–41.

87. Martin JB, Wetzel SG, Seium Y, et al. Percutaneous vertebroplasty in metastatic disease: transpedicular access and treatment of lysed pedicles—initial experience. Radiology 2003;229:593–7.

88. Li AF, Li KC, Chang FY, et al. Preliminary report of transpedicle body augmenter vertebroplasty in painful vertebral tumors. Spine 2006;31: E805–12.

89. Li KC, Li AF, Hsieh CH, et al. Transpedicle body augmenter in painful osteoporotic compression fractures. Eur Spine J 2007;16:589–98.

90. Tong FC, Cloft HJ, Joseph GJ, et al. Transoral approach to cervical vertebroplasty for multiple myeloma. AJR Am J Roentgenol 2000;175:1322–4.

91. Gailloud P, Martin JB, Olivi A, et al. Transoral vertebroplasty for a fractured C2 aneurysmal bone cyst. J Vasc Interv Radiol 2002;13:340–1.

92. Sachs DC, Inamasu J, Mendel EE, et al. Transoral vertebroplasty for renal cell metastasis involving the axis: case report. Spine 2006;31:E925–8.

93. Rodriguez-Catarino M, Blimark C, Willen J, et al. Percutaneous vertebroplasty at C2: case report of a patient with multiple myeloma and a literature review. Eur Spine J 2007;16(Suppl 3):242–9.

94. Mehdizade A, Payer M, Somon T, et al. Percutaneous vertebroplasty through a transdiscal access route after lumbar transpedicular instrumentation. Spine J 2004;4:475–9.

95. Laredo JD, Hamze B. Complications of percutaneous vertebroplasty and their prevention. Skeletal Radiol 2004;33:493–505.

96. Hodler J, Peck D, Gilula LA. Midterm outcome after vertebroplasty: predictive value of technical and patient-related factors. Radiology 2003;227:662–8.

97. Mousavi P, Roth S, Finkelstein J, et al. Volumetric quantification of cement leakage following percutaneous vertebroplasty in metastatic and osteoporotic vertebrae. J Neurosurg Spine 2003;99:56–9.

98. Yeom JS, Kim WJ, Choy WS, et al. Leakage of cement in percutaneous transpedicular vertebroplasty for painful osteoporotic compression fractures. J Bone Joint Surg Br 2003;85:83–9.

99. Vasconcelos C, Gailloud P, Martin JB, et al. Transient arterial hypotension induced by polymethylmethacrylate injection during percutaneous vertebroplasty. J Vasc Interv Radiol 2001;12:1001–2.

100. Harrington KD. Major neurological complications following percutaneous vertebroplasty with polymethylmethacrylate: a case report. J Bone Joint Surg Am 2001;83:1070–3.

101. Ratcliff J, Nguyen T, Heiss J. Root and spinal cord compression from methylmethacrylate vertebroplasty. Spine 2001;26:300–2.

102. Shapiro S, Abel T, Purvines S. Surgical removal of epidural and intradural polymethylmethacrylate extravasation complicating percutaneous vertebroplasty for an osteoporotic lumbar compression fracture. Case report. J Neurosurg Spine 2003;98:90–2.

103. Wu CC, Lin MH, Yang SH, et al. Surgical removal of extravasated epidural and neuroforaminal polymethylmethacrylate after percutaneous vertebroplasty in the thoracic spine. Eur Spine J 2007;16(Suppl 3):326–31.

104. Kelekis AD, Martin JB, Somon T, et al. Radicular pain after vertebroplasty: compression or irritation of the nerve root? Initial experience with the "cooling system". Spine 2003;28:E265–9.

105. Pitton MB, Herber S, Bletz C, et al. CT-guided vertebroplasty in osteoporotic vertebral fractures: incidence of secondary fractures and impact of intradiscal cement leakages during follow-up. Eur Radiol 2008;18:43–50.

106. Jung JY, Lee MH, Ahn JM. Leakage of polymethylmethacrylate in percutaneous vertebroplasty: comparison of osteoporotic vertebral compression fractures with and without an intravertebral vacuum cleft. J Comput Assist Tomogr 2006;30:501–6.

107. Krauss M, Hirschfelder H, Tomandi B, et al. Kyphosis reduction and the rate of cement leaks after vertebroplasty of intravertebral clefts. Eur Radiol 2006;16:1015–21.

108. Lin EP, Ekholm S, Hiwatashi A, et al. Vertebroplasty: cement leakage into the disc increases the risk of fracture of adjacent vertebral body. AJNR Am J Neuroradiol 2004;25:175–80.

109. Bernhard J, Heini PF, Villiger PM. Asymptomatic diffuse pulmonary embolism caused by acrylic cement: an unusual complication of percutaneous vertebroplasty. Ann Rheum Dis 2003;62:85–6.

110. Choe DH, Marom EM, Ahrar K, et al. Pulmonary embolism of polymethyl methacrylate during percutaneous vertebroplasty and kyphoplasty. AJR Am J Roentgenol 2004;183:1097–102.

111. Duran C, Sirvanci M, Aydogan M, et al. Pulmonary cement embolism: a complication of percutaneous vertebroplasty. Acta Radiol 2007;48:854–9.

112. Barbero S, Casorzo I, Durando M, et al. Percutaneous vertebroplasty: the follow-up. Radiol Med (Torino) 2008;113:101–13.

113. Perrin C, Jullien V, Padovani B, et al. Percutaneous vertebroplasty complicated by pulmonary embolus of acrylic cement. Rev Mal Respir 1999;16:215–7.

114. Padovani B, Kasriel O, Brunner P, et al. Pulmonary embolism caused by acrylic cement: a rare complication of percutaneous vertebroplasty. AJNR Am J Neuroradiol 1999;20:375–7.

115. Tozzi P, Abdelmoumene Y, Corno AF, et al. Management of pulmonary embolism during acrylic vertebroplasty. Ann Thorac Surg 2002;74:1706–8.

116. Scroop R, Eskridge J, Britz GW. Paradoxical cerebral arterial embolization of cement during intraoperative vertebroplasty: case report. AJNR Am J Neuroradiol 2002;23:868–70.

117. Reidy D, Ahn H, Mousavi P, et al. A biomechanical analysis of intravertebral pressures during vertebroplasty of cadaveric spines with and without simulated metastases. Spine 2003;28:1534–9.

118. Komemushi A, Tanigawa N, Kariya S, et al. Intraosseous venography with carbon dioxide in percutaneous vertebroplasty: carbon dioxide retention in renal veins. Cardiovasc Intervent Radiol 2008 Mar 21; [Epub ahead of print].

119. Lim SH, Kim H, Kim HK, et al. Multiple cardiac perforations and pulmonary embolism caused by cement leakage after percutaneous vertebroplasty. Eur J Cardiothorac Surg 2008;33:510–2.

120. Chen YJ, Chang GC, Chen WH, et al. Local metastases along the tract of needle: a rare complication of vertebroplasty in treating spinal metastases. Spine 2007;32:E615–8.

121. Chiras J, Depriester C, Weill A, et al. [Percutaneous vertebral surgery. Technics and indications]. J Neuroradiol 1997;24:45–59 [in French].

122. Soyuncu Y, Ozdemir H, Soyuncu S, et al. Posterior spinal epidural abscess: an unusual complication of vertebroplasty. Joint Bone Spine 2006;73:753–5.

123. Vats HS, McKiernan FE. Infected vertebroplasty: case report and review of literature. Spine 2006;31:E859–62.

124. Kwak HJ, Lee JK, Kim YS, et al. Aortic aneurysm complicated with pyogenic spondylitis following vertebroplasty. J Clin Neurosci 2008;15:80–93.

125. Alfonso Olmos M, Silva Gonzalez A, Duart Clemente J, et al. Infected vertebroplasty due to uncommon bacteria solved surgically: a rare and threatening life complication of a common procedure: report of a case and a review of the literature. Spine 2006;31:E770–3.

126. Grados F, Depriester C, Cayrolle G, et al. Long-term observations of vertebral osteoporotic fractures treated by percutaneous vertebroplasty. Rheumatology 2000;39:1410–4.

127. Perez-Higueras A, Alvarez L, Rossi RE, et al. Percutaneous vertebroplasty: long-term clinical and radiological outcome. Neuroradiology 2002;44:950–4.

128. Uppin AA, Hirsch JA, Centenera LV, et al. Occurrence of new vertebral body fracture after percutaneous vertebroplasty in patients with osteoporosis. Radiology 2003;226:119–24.

129. Legroux-Gerot I, Lormaua C, Boutry N, et al. Long-term follow-up of vertebral osteoporotic fractures treated by percutaneous vertebroplasty. Clin Rheumatol 2004;23:310–7.

130. Berlemann U, Ferguson SJ, Nolte LP, et al. Adjacent vertebral failure after vertebroplasty: a biomechanical investigation. J Bone Joint Surg Br 2002;84:748–52.

131. Baroud G, Nemes J, Heini P, et al. Load shift of the intervertebral disc after a vertebroplasty: a finite-element study. Eur Spine J 2003;12:421–6.

132. Polikeit A, Nolte LP, Ferguson SJ. The effect of cement augmentation on the load transfer in an osteoporotic functional spinal unit, finite element analysis. Spine 2003;28:991–6.

133. Baroud G, Heini P, Nemes J, et al. Biomechanical explanation of adjacent fractures following vertebroplasty. [letter]. Radiology 2003;229:606–8.

134. Kim SH, Kang HS, Choi JA, et al. Risk factors of new compression fractures in adjacent vertebrae after percutaneous vertebroplasty. Acta Radiol 2004;45:440–5.

135. Belkoff SM, Mathis JM, Jasper LE, et al. The biomechanics of vertebroplasty: the effect of cement volume on mechanical behaviour. Spine 2001;26:1537–41.

136. Hiwatashi A, Moritani T, Numaguchi Y, et al. Increase in vertebral body height after vertebroplasty. AJNR Am J Neuroradiol 2003;24:185–9.

137. Voormolen MH, Lohle PN, Juttmann JR, et al. The risk of new osteoporotic vertebral compression fractures in the year after percutaneous vertebroplasty. J Vasc Interv Radiol 2006;17:71–6.

138. Trout AT, Kallmes DF, Layton KF, et al. Vertebral endplate fractures: an indicator of the abnormal forces generated in the spine after vertebroplasty. J Bone Miner Res 2006;21:1797–802.

139. Uebelhart B, Casez P, Rizzoli R, et al. Prophylactic injection of methylmetacrylate in vertebrae located between two previously cemented levels does not prevent a subsequent compression fracture in a patient with bone fragility. Joint Bone Spine 2008;75:322–4.

140. Lin WC, Lee YC, Lee CH, et al. Refractures in cemented vertebrae after percutaneous vertebroplasty: a retrospective analysis. Eur Spine J 2008;17:592–9.

141. Lin WC, Cheng TT, Lee YC, et al. New vertebral osteoporotic compression fractures after percutaneous vertebroplasty: retrospective analysis of risk factors. J Vasc Interv Radiol 2008;19:225–31.

142. Maehara M, Tanigawa H, Ikeda K, et al. Gadolinium-enhanced magnetic resonance imaging after percutaneous vertebroplasty does not improve the short-term prediction of new compression fractures. Acta Radiol 2006;47:817–22.

143. Komemushi A, Tanigawa N, Kariya S, et al. Biochemical markers of bone turnover in percutaneous vertebroplasty for osteoporotic compression fracture. Cardiovasc Intervent Radiol 2008;31:332–5.

144. Tanigawa N, Komemushi A, Kariya S, et al. Relationship between cement distribution pattern and new compression fracture after percutaneous vertebroplasty. AJR Am J Roentgenol 2007;189:W348–52.

145. Huntoon EA, Schmidt CK, Sinaki M. Significantly fewer refractures after vertebroplasty in patients who engage in back-extensor–strengthening exercises. Mayo Clin Proc 2008;83:54–7.

146. Trout AT, Kallmes DF. Does vertebroplasty cause incident vertebral fractures? A review of available data. AJNR Am J Neuroradiol 2006;27:1397–403.

147. Cloft HJ, Easton DM, Jensen ME, et al. Exposure of medical personnel to methylmethacrylate vapor during percutaneous vertebroplasty. AJNR Am J Neuroradiol 1999;20:352–3.

148. Kirby BS, Doyle A, Gilula LA. Acute bronchospasm due to exposure to polymethylmethacrylate vapors during percutaneous vertebroplasty. AJR Am J Roentgenol 2003;180:543–4.

149. Philipps H, Cole PV, Lettin AW. Cardiovascular effects of implanted bone cement. Br Med J 1971;3:460–1.

150. Peebles DJ, Ellis RH, Stride SDK, et al. Cardiovascular effects of methylmethacrylate cement. Br Med J 1972;1:349–51.

151. Yoo KY, Jeong SW, Yoon W, et al. Acute respiratory distress syndrome associated with pulmonary cement embolism following percutaneous vertebroplasty with polymethylmethacrylate. Spine 2004;29:E294–7.

152. Aebli N, Krebs J, Schwenke D, et al. Pressurization of vertebral bodies during vertebroplasty causes

cardiovascular complications: an experimental study in sheep. Spine 2003;28:1519–20.

153. Aebli N, Krebs J, Schwenke D, et al. Cardiovascular changes during multiple vertebroplasty with and without vent-hole: an experimental study in sheep. Spine 2003;28:1504–11.

154. Kaufmann TJ, Jensen ME, Ford G, et al. Cardiovascular effects of polymethylmethacrylate use in percutaneous vertebroplasty. AJNR Am J Neuroradiol 2002;23:601–4.

155. Moreland DB, Landi MK, Grand W. Vertebroplasty: techniques to avoid complications. Spine J 2001;1:66–71.

156. Mathis JM. Percutaneous vertebroplasty: complication avoidance and technique optimization. AJNR Am J Neuroradiol 2003;24:1697–706.

157. Kruger R, Faciszewski T. Radiation dose reduction to medical staff during vertebroplasty: a review of techniques and methods to mitigate occupational dose. Spine 2003;28:1608–13.

158. Mehdizade A, Lovblad KO, Wilhelm KE, et al. Radiation dose in vertebroplasty. Neuroradiology 2004;46:243–5.

159. Kallmes DF, Erwin O, Roy SS, et al. Radiation dose to the operator during vertebroplasty: prospective comparison of the use of 1-cc syringes versus an injection device. AJNR Am J Neuroradiol 2003;24:1257–60.

160. Perisinakis K, Damilakis J, Theocharopoulos N, et al. Patient exposure and associated radiation risks from fluoroscopic guided vertebroplasty or kyphoplasty. Radiology 2004;232:701–7.

161. Fitousi NT, Efstathopoupos EP, Delis HB, et al. Patient and staff dosimetry in vertebroplasty. Spine 2006;31:E884–9.

162. Synowitz M, Kiwit J. Surgeon's radiation exposure during percutaneous vertebroplasty. J Neurosurg Spine 2006;4:106–9.

163. Seibert JA. Vertebroplasty and kyphoplasty: do fluoroscopy operators know about radiation dose, and should they want to know? Radiology 2004;232:633–4.

164. Gangi A, Dietemann JL, Guth AS, et al. Computed tomography (CT) and fluoroscopy-guided vertebroplasty: results and complications in 187 patients. Seminars in Interventional Radiology 1999;16:137–42.

165. Cortet B, Cotton A, Boutry N, et al. Percutaneous vertebroplasty in patients with osteolytic metastases or multiple myeloma. Rev Rhum Engl Ed 1997;64:177–83.

166. Martin JB, Jean B, Sugiu K, et al. Vertebroplasty: clinical experience and follow-up results. Bone 1999;25(Suppl):11S–5S.

167. Cahana A, Seium Y, Diby M, et al. Percutaneous vertebroplasty in octogenerians: results and follow-up. Pain Pract 2006;5:316–23.

168. Amar AP, Larsen DW, Esnaashari N, et al. Percutaneous transpedicular polymethylmethacrylate vertebroplasty for the treatment of spinal compression fractures. Neurosurgery 2001;49:1105–14.

169. Zoarski GH, Snow P, Olan WJ, et al. Percutaneous vertebroplasty for osteoporotic compression fractures: quantitative prospective evaluation of long-term outcomes. J Vasc Interv Radiol 2002;13:139–48.

170. Evans AJ, Jensen ME, Kip KE, et al. Vertebral compression fractures: pain reduction and improvement in functional mobility after percutaneous polymethylmethacrylate vertebroplasty- retrospective report of 245 cases. Radiology 2003;226:366–72.

171. Kumar K, Verma AK, Wilson J, et al. Vertebroplasty in osteoporotic spine fractures: a quality of life assessment. Can J Neurol Sci 2005;32:487–95.

172. Kose KC, Cebesoy O, Akan B, et al. Functional results of vertebral augmentation techniques in pathological vertebral fractures of myelomatous patients. J Natl Med Assoc 2006;98:1654–8.

173. Prather H, Van Dillen L, Metzler JP, et al. Prospective measurement of function and pain in patients with non-neoplastic compression fractures treated with vertebroplasty. J Bone Joint Surg Am 2006;88:334–41.

174. Anselmetti GC, Corrao G, Monica PD, et al. Pain relief following percutaneous vertebroplasty: results of a series of 283 consecutive patients treated in a single institution. Cardiovasc Intervent Radiol 2007;30:441–7.

175. Voormolen MH, Lohle PN, Lampmann LE, et al. Prospective clinical follow-up after percutaneous vertebroplasty in patients with painful osteoporotic compression fractures. J Vasc Interv Radiol 2006;17:1313–20.

176. Dublin AB, Hartman J, Latchaw RE, et al. The vertebral body fracture in osteoporosis: restoration of height using percutaneous vertebroplasty. AJNR Am J Neuroradiol 2005;26:489–92.

177. Pitton MB, Morgen N, Herber S, et al. Height gain of vertebral bodies and stabilization of vertebral geometry over one year after vertebroplasty of osteoporotic vertebral fractures. Eur Radiol 2008;18:608–15.

178. Chang CY, Teng MM, Wei CJ, et al. Percutaneous vertebroplasty for patients with osteoporosis: a one-year follow-up. Acta Radiol 2006;47:568–73.

179. Ho SC, Teng GJ, Deng G, et al. Repeat vertebroplasty for unrelieved pain at previously treated vertebral levels with osteoporotic vertebral compression fractures. Spine 2008;15:640–7.

180. Yu SW, Yang SC, Kao YH, et al. Clinical evaluation of vertebroplasty for multiple-level osteoporotic

spinal compression fracture in the elderly. Arch Orthop Trauma Surg 2008;12:97–101.

181. Levine SA, Perin LA, Hayes D, et al. An evidence-based evaluation of percutaneous vertebroplasty. Manag Care 2000;9:56–63.

182. Jarvik JG, Deyo RA. Cementing the evidence: time for a randomized trial of vertebroplasty. AJNR Am J Neuroradiol 2000;21:1373–4.

183. Hirsch JA, Do HM, Kallmes D, et al. Simplicity of randomized, controlled trials of percutaneous vertebroplasty. Pain Physician 2003;6:342–3.

184. Hochmuth K, Proschek D, Schwarz W, et al. Percutaneous vertebroplasty in the therapy of osteoporotic vertebral compression fractures: a critical review. Eur Radiol 2006;16:998–1004.

185. Buchbinder R, Osborne RH. Vertebroplasty: a promising but as yet unproven intervention for painful osteoporotic spinal fractures. Med J Aust 2006;185:351–2.

186. Wagner AL. Vertebroplasty and the randomized study: where science and ethics collides. AJNR Am J Neuroradiol 2005;26:1610–1.

187. Klazen CAH, Verhaar HJJ, Lampmann LEH, et al. VERTOS II: percutaneous vertebroplasty versus conservative therapy in patients with painful osteoporotic vertebral compression fractures; rationale, objectives and design of a multicenter randomized controlled trial. Trials 2007;8:33.

188. Gray LA, Jarvik JG, Heagerty PJ, et al. Investigational Vertebroplasty Efficacy and Safety Trial (INVEST): a randomized controlled trial of percutaneous vertebroplasty. BMC Musculoskelet Disord 2007;8:126.

189. Voormolen MHJ, Mali WPTM, Lohle PNM, et al. Percutaneous vertebroplasty compared with optimal pain medical treatment: short-term clinical outcome of patients with subacute or chronic painful osteoporotic vertebral compression fractures. The VERTOS study. AJNR Am J Neuroradiol 2007;28: 555–60.

190. Wong WH, Olan WJ, Belkoff SM. Balloon kyphoplasty. In: Mathis JM, Deramond H, Belkoff SM, editors. Percutaneous vertebroplasty. New York: Springer; 2002. p. 109–24.

191. Tomita S, Kin A, Yazu M, et al. Biomechanical evaluation of kyphoplasty and vertebroplasty with calcium phosphate cement in a simulated osteoporotic compression fracture. J Orthop Sci 2003;8: 192–7.

192. Rhyne A 3rd, Banit D, Laxer E, et al. Kyphoplasty: report of eighty-two thoracolumbar osteoporotic vertebral fractures. J Orthop Trauma 2004;18: 294–9.

193. Gaitanis IN, Hadjipavlou AG, Katonis PG, et al. Balloon kyphoplasty for the treatment of pathological vertebral compression fractures. Eur Spine J 2005;14:250–60.

194. Bouza C, Lopez T, Magro A, et al. Efficacy and safety of balloon vertebroplasty in the treatment of vertebral compression fractures: a systematic review. Eur Spine J 2006;15:1050–67.

195. Wilhelm K, Stoffel M, Ringel F, et al. Preliminary experience with balloon kyphoplasty for the treatment of painful osteoporotic compression fractures. Rofo 2003;175:1690–6.

196. Fourney DR, Schomer DF, Nader R, et al. Percutaneous vertebroplasty and kyphoplasty for painful vertebral body fractures in cancer patients. J Neurosurg 2003;98(Suppl 1):21–30.

197. Berlemann U, Franz T, Orler R, et al. Kyphoplasty for treatment of osteoporotic fractures: a prospective non-randomized study. Eur Spine J 2004;13: 496–501.

198. Lane JM, Hong R, Koob J, et al. Kyphoplasty enhances function and structural alignment in multiple myeloma. Clin Orthop Relat Res 2004;426: 49–53.

199. Garfin SR, Reilley MA. Minimally invasive treatment of osteoporotic vertebral body compression fractures. Spine J 2002;2:76–80.

200. Nussbaum DA, Gailloud P, Murphy K. A review of complications associated with vertebroplasty and kyphoplasty as reported to the Food and Drug Administration medical device related Web site. J Vasc Interv Radiol 2004;15:1185–92.

201. Majd ME, Farley S, Holt RT. Preliminary outcomes and efficacies of the first 300 consecutive kyphoplasties for the treatment of painful osteoporotic vertebral compression fractures. Spine 2005;5: 244–55.

202. Patel AA, Vaccaro AR, Martyak GG, et al. Neurologic deficit following percutaneous vertebral stabilization. Spine 2007;32:1728–34.

203. Theodorou DJ, Theodorou SJ, Duncan TD, et al. Percutaneous balloon kyphoplasty for the correction of spinal deformity in painful vertebral body compression fractures. Clin Imaging 2002;26: 1–5.

204. Fribourg D, Tang C, Sra P, et al. Incidence of subsequent vertebral fracture after kyphoplasty. Spine 2004;29:2270–6.

205. Harrop JS, Prpa B, Reinhardt MK, et al. Primary and secondary osteoporosis' incidence of subsequent vertebral compression fractures after kyphoplasty. Spine 2004;29:2120–5.

206. Taylor RS, Fritzell P, Taylor RJ. Balloon kyphoplasty in the management of vertebral compression fractures: an updated systematic review and meta-analysis. Eur Spine J 2007;16:1085–100.

207. Deramond H, Saliou G, Aveillan M, et al. Respective contributions of vertebroplasty and kyphoplasty to the management of osteoporotic vertebral fractures. Joint Bone Spine 2006;73: 610–3.

208. Mathis JM. Percutaneous vertebroplasty or kypho-plasty: Which one do I choose? Skeletal Radiol 2006;35:629–31.

209. Gill JB, Kuper M, Chin PC, et al. Comparing pain reduction following kyphoplasty and vertebroplasty for osteoporotic vertebral compression fractures. Pain Physician 2007;10:583–90.

210. Taylor RS, Taylor RJ, Fritzell P. Balloon kypho-plastsy and vertebroplasty for vertebral compres-sion fractures: a comparative systematic review of efficacy and safety. Spine 2006;31:2747–55.

211. Hulme PA, Krebs J, Ferguson SJ, et al. Vertebro-plasty and kyphoplasty: a systematic review of 69 clinical studies. Spine 2006;31:1983–2001.

212. Eck JC, Nachtigall D, Humphreys SC, et al. Compari-son of vertebroplasty and balloon kyphoplastsy for treatment of vertebral compression fractures: a meta-analysis of the literature. Spine J 2008;8:488–97.

213. Cloft HJ, Jensen ME. Kyphoplasty: an assessment of a new technology. AJNR Am J Neuroradiol 2007; 28:200–3.

214. De Negri P, Tirri T, Paternoster G, et al. Treatment of painful osteoporotic or traumatic vertebral com-pression fractures by percutaneous vertebral augmentation procedures: a nonrandomized com-parison between vertebroplasty and kyphoplasty. Clin J Pain 2007;23:425–30.

215. Tong SC, Eskey CJ, Pomerantz SR, et al. "SKypho-plasty": a single institution's initial experience. J Vasc Interv Radiol 2006;17:1025–30.

216. Foo LS, Yeo W, Fook S, et al. Results, experience and technical points learnt with use of the Sky Bone Expander kyphoplasty system for osteopo-rotic vertebral compression fractures: a prospective study of 40 patients with a minimum of 12 months of follow-up. Eur Spine J 2007;16:1944–50.

Index

Radiol Clin N Am 46 (2008) 637–641
doi:10.1016/S0033-8389(08)00120-6

Moving?

Make sure your subscription moves with you!

To notify us of your new address, find your **Clinics Account Number** (located on your mailing label above your name), and contact customer service at:

E-mail: elspcs@elsevier.com

800-654-2452 (subscribers in the U.S. & Canada)
1-407-563-6020 (subscribers outside of the U.S. & Canada)

Fax number: 407-363-9661

Elsevier Periodicals Customer Service
6277 Sea Harbor Drive
Orlando, FL 32887-4800

*To ensure uninterrupted delivery of your subscription, please notify us at least 4 weeks in advance of move.